MANAGEMENT OF EPILEPSY – RESEARCH, RESULTS AND TREATMENT

Edited by **Mintaze Kerem Günel**

Management of Epilepsy – Research, Results and Treatment
Edited by Mintaze Kerem Günel

Published by InTech

Janeza Trdine 9, 51000 Rijeka, Croatia

Publishing Process Manager Dragana Manestar

Technical Editor Teodora Smiljanic

Cover Designer InTech Design Team

Additional hard copies can be obtained from orders@intechopen.com

Management of Epilepsy – Research, Results and Treatment,
Edited by Mintaze Kerem Günel
p. cm.
ISBN 978-953-307-680-5

For EU product safety concerns:
IN TECH d.o.o., Prolaz Marije Krucifikse Kozulić 3, 51000 Rijeka, Croatia,
info@intechopen.com or visit our website at intechopen.com.

Meet the editor

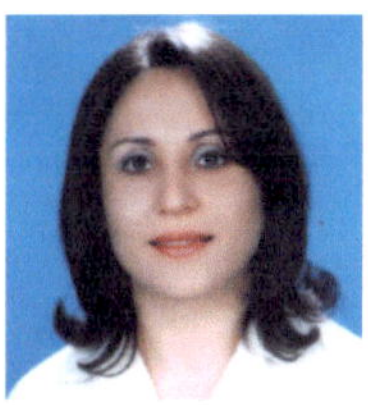

Dr. Mintaze Kerem Günel graduated from Hacettepe University, School of Physical Therapy and Rehabilitation in 1989. He had his doctorate degree with thesis called "Effectiveness of Johnstone Pressure Splints in Children with Spastic Cerebral Palsy". Since 1993, he has been clinically studying Cerebral Palsy Unit. He works with a unit participating to long term study in premature children followed by multidisciplinary team in Hacettepe University, Children Hospital. Since 1993. he is a member of EACD (European Academy of Childhood Disability) and a national coordinator of Turkey as well. Since 1993 he has attended meetings of EACD with oral or poster presentation studies in different countries of Europe. EACD 2012 is held in Istanbul, Turkey, for which Dr. Kerem Günel is secretary in meeting. He currently works as a professor and a vice-president of Department of Physiotherapy and Rehabilitation at Faculty of Health Sciences, Hacettepe University.

Contents

Preface

Epilepsy is one of the most common neurological disorders, with a prevalence of 4-10/1000. The book contains practical methods to approaching the classification and diagnosis of epilepsy and provides information on management. It is a comprehensive book which guides the reader through all the aspects of epilepsy, both practical and academic, covering all issues of diagnosis and management of epilepsy in children in a clear, concise, and practical fashion. The book is organized so that it can either be read from cover to cover for a comprehensive tutorial or be kept desk side as a reference to epilepsy. Each chapter introduces a number of related epilepsy diagnosis, treatment and co-morbidities of each one, followed by examples. The book unites chapters which explore extended clinical knowledge about epilepsy, from clinical features to treatment and practice.

Dr. Mintaze Kerem Günel
Faculty of Health Sciences,
Department of Physiotherapy and Rehabilittaion at Hacettepe University,
Turkey

Part 1

Epileptic Seizures

1

Epileptic Seizures Detection Based on Empirical Mode Decomposition of EEG Signals

Lorena Orosco, Agustina Garcés Correa and Eric Laciar Leber
Faculty of Engineering - National University of San Juan
Argentina

1. Introduction

Epilepsy is a chronic neurological disorder that affects more than 50 million people world wide, characterized by recurrent seizures (World Health Organization [WHO], 2006). An epileptic seizure is a transient occurrence of signs and/or symptoms due to abnormal excessive or synchronous neuronal activity in the brain (Fisher *et al.*, 2005 & Berg *et al.*, 2010). This electrical hyperactivity can have its source in different parts of the brain and produces physical symptoms such as short periods of inattention and loose of memory, a sensory hallucination, or a whole-body convulsion. The frequency of these events can vary from one in a year to several in a day. The majority of the patients suffer from unpredictable, persistent and frequent seizures which limit the independence of an individual, increase the risk of serious injury and mobility, and result in both social isolation and economic hardship (Friedman & Gilliam, 2010). In addition, the patients with epilepsy have an increased mortality risk of approximately 2 to 3 times that of the general population (Ficker, 2000).

The first line of treatment for epilepsy is with multiple anti-epileptic drugs and it is effective in about 70% of the cases. From the 30% remaining affected individuals only less than 10% could benefit from surgical therapy leaving a 20% of the total of people with epilepsy who will continue suffering sudden, incontrollable seizures and for whom other forms of treatment are being investigated (Theodore & Ficker, 2004; WHO, 2006).

For any of the reasons exposed before the seizure detection is an important component in the diagnosis of epilepsy and for the seizures control. In the clinical practice this detection basically involves visual scanning of Electroencephalogram (EEG) long recordings by the physicians in order to detect and classify the seizure activity present in the EEG signal. Usually these are multichannel records of 24 to 72 hours length which implies a very time consuming task and it is also kwon that the conclusions are very subjective so disagreement between physicians are not rare.

The seek here is to detect automatically in long term EEG records those segments of the signal that present epileptic seizures for the shake of reducing the high amount of information to be analyzed by the neurologists. Thus them could focus their attention in these part of the information so a more precisely and quick diagnosis can be made. Seizure detection is also a useful tool for treatments such us timely drug delivery, electrical stimulation and seizure alert systems.

Automated seizure detection, quantification and recognition have been of interest of the biomedical community researchers since the 1970s. In some initial works a number of parameters of EEG waves such us amplitude, sharpness and duration were measured and evaluated (Sanei & Chambers, 2007). This first approach is sensitive to artefacts so in the following years numerous and diverse techniques have been employed and refined to improved epileptic seizures detection.

Artificial Neural Networks (ANN) have been used both to detect abnormal patterns in the EEG (Schuyler *et al.*, 2007 & Bao *et al.*, 2009) and as seizure parameters classifier (Tzallas *et al.*, 2007). Wavelet Transform is also widely used for epilepsy detection (Adeli *et al.*, 2007). Others studies combine Approximate Entropy and Lempel-Ziv Complexity (Abásolo *et al.*, 2007 & Zandi *et al.*, 2009), and Time Frequency Distributions (Tzallas *et al.*, 2007).

In the studies referenced in the previous paragraphs, it had been proposed different seizure detectors that had been tested in particular EEG databases each. In some cases the epileptic EEG records were of a few seconds long. Other techniques were implemented in rats' EEGs with induced seizures were also used. The most recently works used long term epileptic EEGs for a small number of patients or grouped by the type of epilepsy they suffer. In this sense due to seizure detection algorithms were not evaluated on the same database to date so no standardization exists about the good performance of an epileptic seizure detector (Varsavsky *et al.*, 2011).

The aim of this chapter is to examine the recent Empirical Mode Decomposition (EMD) technique for the extraction of features of epileptic EEG records to be used in two seizure detectors. The algorithms will be tested in 21 multichannel EEG recordings of patients suffering different focal epilepsies. Along the sections of this chapter it will be described the used EEG records, the EMD algorithm as well as the features extracted to be used in the developed seizures detectors, the obtained results and finally the conclusions and discussion will be exposed.

2. The EEG database

The EEG database contains invasive EEG recordings of 21 patients suffering from medically intractable focal epilepsy. The data were recorded during invasive pre-surgical epilepsy monitoring at the Epilepsy Center of the University Hospital of Freiburg, Germany (Freiburg, 2008). In order to obtain a high signal-to-noise ratio, fewer artifacts, and to record directly from focal areas, intracranial grid-, strip-, and depth-electrodes were used. The EEG data were acquired using a Neurofile NT digital video EEG system with 128 channels, 256 Hz sampling rate, and a 16 bits A/D converter. Notch or band pass filters have not been applied in the acquisition stage.

The available EEG records include only 6 channels (3 focal electrodes and 3 extrafocal electrodes). The records are divided into segments of 1 hour long. In this study, only the 3 focal channels were used. A total of 87 seizures from 21 patients (8M, 13F, age: 29.9 ± 11.9 years) were analyzed. The details of the database are summarized in Table 1.

3. Empirical Mode Decomposition

In the last years, a technique called Empirical Mode Decomposition (EMD) has been proposed for the analysis of non-linear and non-stationary series (Huang *et al.*, 1998). The EMD adaptively decomposes a signal into oscillating components or Intrinsic Mode Functions (IMFs). The EMD is in fact a type of filter bank decomposition method whose sub bands are built as needed to separate the different natural components of the signal. In the field of biomedical signal processing EMD has been used for the analysis of respiratory mechanomyographic signals (Torres *et al.*, 2007), for denoising in ECG records (Beng *et al.*, 2006). Particularly, this technique was implemented to extract features from EEG signals for mental task classification (Diez *et al.*, 2009), it was used to obtain adaptive bands on EEG signals (Diez *et al.*, 2011) and also for epileptic seizure detection in EEG signals in 5 patients with temporal lobe focal epilepsy (Tafreshi *et al.*, 2008). In this sense the authors of this chapter have previously developed algorithms based on EMD for seizure detection and they have been tested in 9 long EEG records of patients with temporal focal epilepsy (Orosco *et al.*, 2009) and in 21 patients with different epilepsies (Orosco *et al.*, 2010).

#Patient	Sex	Age	Origin	Number of seizures
1	F	15	Frontal	4
2	M	38	Temporal	3
3	M	14	Frontal	5
4	F	26	Temporal	5
5	F	16	Frontal	5
6	F	31	Temporo/Occipital	3
7	F	42	Temporal	3
8	F	32	Frontal	2
9	M	44	Temporo/Occipital	5
10	M	47	Temporal	5
11	F	10	Parietal	4
12	F	42	Temporal	4
13	F	22	Temporo/Occipital	2
14	F	41	Fronto/Occipital	4
15	M	31	Temporal	4
16	F	50	Temporal	5
17	M	28	Temporal	5
18	F	25	Frontal	5
19	F	28	Frontal	4
20	M	33	Temporo/Parietal	5
21	M	13	Temporal	5

Table 1. Freiburg EEG Database.

3.1 The EMD algorithm

The EMD is a general nonlinear non-stationary signal decomposition method. The aim of the EMD is to decompose the signal into a sum of Intrinsic Mode Functions (IMFs). An IMF is defined as a function that satisfies two conditions (Huang *et al.*, 1998):

1. In the entire signal, the number of extrema and the number of zero crossings must be equal or differ at most by one.

2. At any point, the mean value of the envelope defined by the local maxima and the envelope defined by the local minima must be zero (or close to zero).

The major advantage of the EMD is that the IMFs are derived directly from the signal itself and does not require any a priori known basis. Hence the analysis is adaptive, in contrast to Fourier or Wavelet Transform, where the signal is decomposed in a linear combination of predefined basis functions.

Given a signal x(t) such us it is showed in figure 1, the algorithm of the EMD can be summarized in the following 6 steps (Huang *et al.*, 1998):

1. Find local maxima and minima of $d_0(t)=x(t)$.
2. Interpolate between the maxima and minima in order to obtain the upper and lower envelopes $e_u(t)$ and $e_l(t)$, respectively.
3. Compute the mean of the envelopes $m(t)=(e_u(t)+ e_l(t))/2$.
4. Extract the detail $d_1(t)= d_0(t)-m(t)$
5. Iterate steps 1-4 on the residual until the detail signal $d_k(t)$ can be considered an IMF (accomplish the two conditions): $c_1(t)= d_k(t)$
6. Iterate steps 1-5 on the residual $r_n(t)=x(t)- c_n(t)$ in order to obtain all the IMFs $c_1(t)$,.., $c_N(t)$ of the signal.

The procedure terminates when the residual $c_N(t)$ is either a constant, a monotonic slope, or a function with only one extrema.

The result of the EMD process produces N IMFs ($c_1(t)$, …, $c_N(t)$) and a residue signal ($r_N(t)$):

$$x(t) = \sum_{n=1}^{N} c_n(t) + r_N(t) \tag{1}$$

Figure 2 shows the complete process of EMD for the example signal x(t). It can be observed that the lower order IMFs capture fast oscillation modes of the signal, while the higher order IMFs capture the slow oscillation modes.

The EMD is a technique essentially defined by an algorithm and there is not an analytical formulation to obtain the IMFs. Furthermore, several algorithmic variations have been proposed in order to obtain the IMFs decomposition. In this work it had been used the algorithm proposed by Flandrin (2007) & Rilling *et al.* (2009), in which, in order to accomplish the second IMF condition, it is utilized a criterion that compares the amplitude of the mean of the upper and lower envelopes with the amplitude of the corresponding IMF. This criterion is based on two thresholds (θ_1 and θ_2) and a tolerance parameter (α). It were also used the default values proposed by Rilling *et al.* (2009): $\alpha=0.05$, $\theta_1=0.05$ and $\theta_2=0.5$.

3.2 EMD applied to EEG analysis

For the purposes of this work the EMD of the EEG signals was achieved computing IMF1 to IMF5 for every segments of each channel. After several initial tests it was concluded that IMF4 and IMF5 do not contributed to seizure detection, so they were discarded. Thus IMF1, IMF2 and IMF3 of each segment of EEG signals were used in further analysis.

Figure 3 shows an example of a 300 s EEG segment without seizure for one channel and their first 3 IMFs obtained with the described EMD method. Figure 4 illustrates a 300 s EEG segment with an epileptic seizure of the same patient and their corresponding first 3 IMFs. In figure 3 it can be observed how the energy of the IMF remains approximately between the same levels along the showed time period while for the EEG segment of figure 4 the mode functions highlight the increased energy during the seizure.

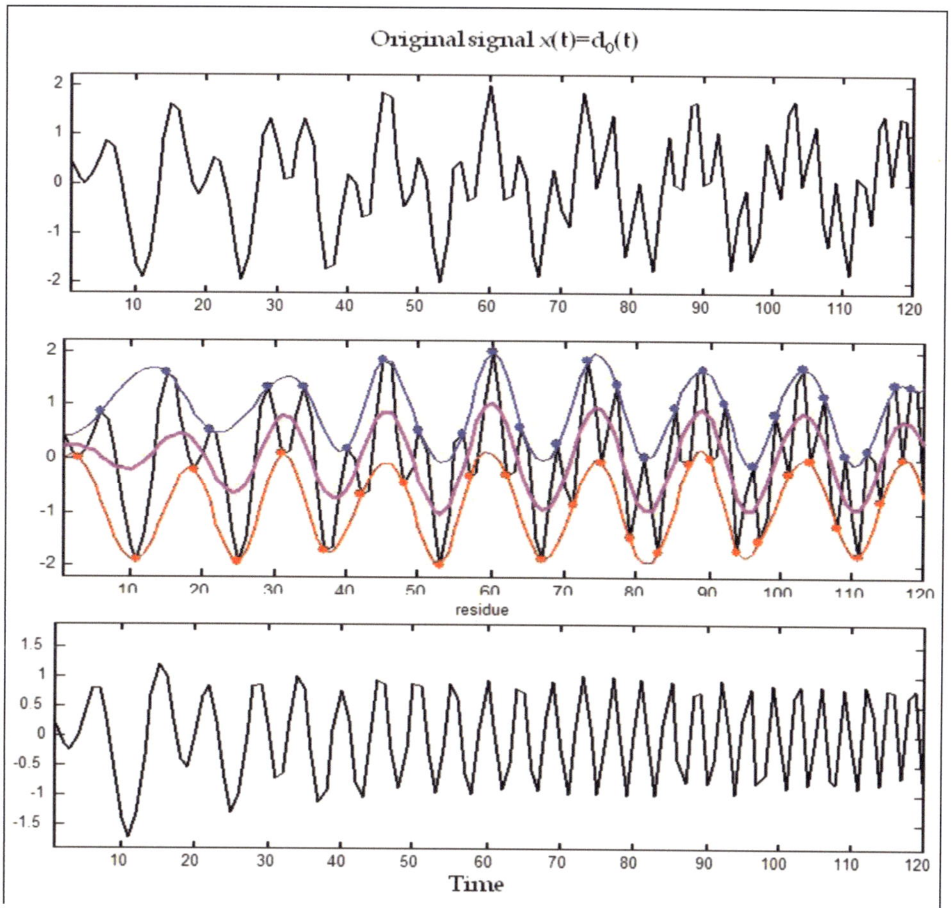

Fig. 1. Step 1, 2, 3 and 4 of the EMD algorithm. In the top pannel the original signal, in the middle pannel the upper (blue) and the lower (red) envelopes are showed as well as the mean of them (magenta). In the bottom pannel the obtained residue. The figure is a modified reproduction of figures available in http://perso.ens-lyon.fr/patrick.flandrin/emd.html

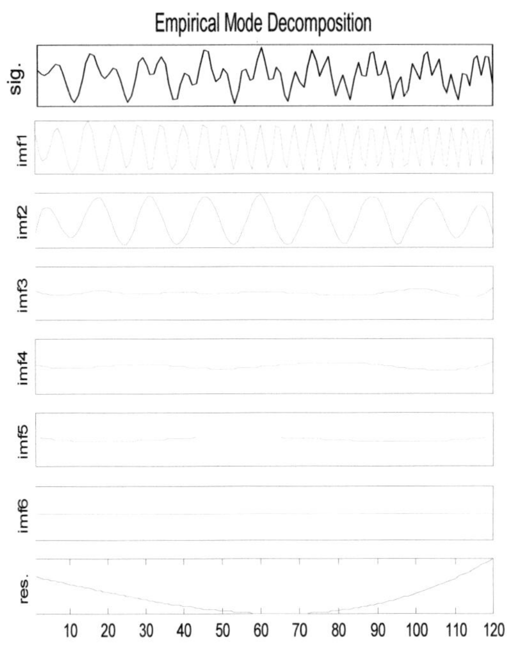

Fig. 2. Original signal x(t) and the result of its EMD computation. The figure is a modified reproduction of figures available in http://perso.ens-lyon.fr/patrick.flandrin/emd.html

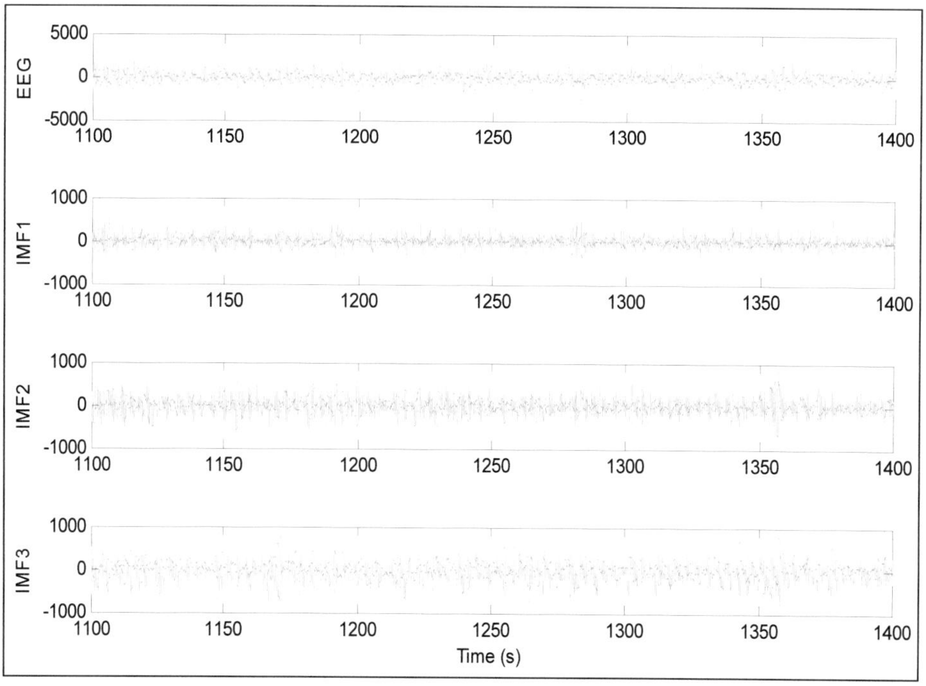

Fig. 3. EEG segment without seizure for one channel and IMF1 to IMF3 of the signal.

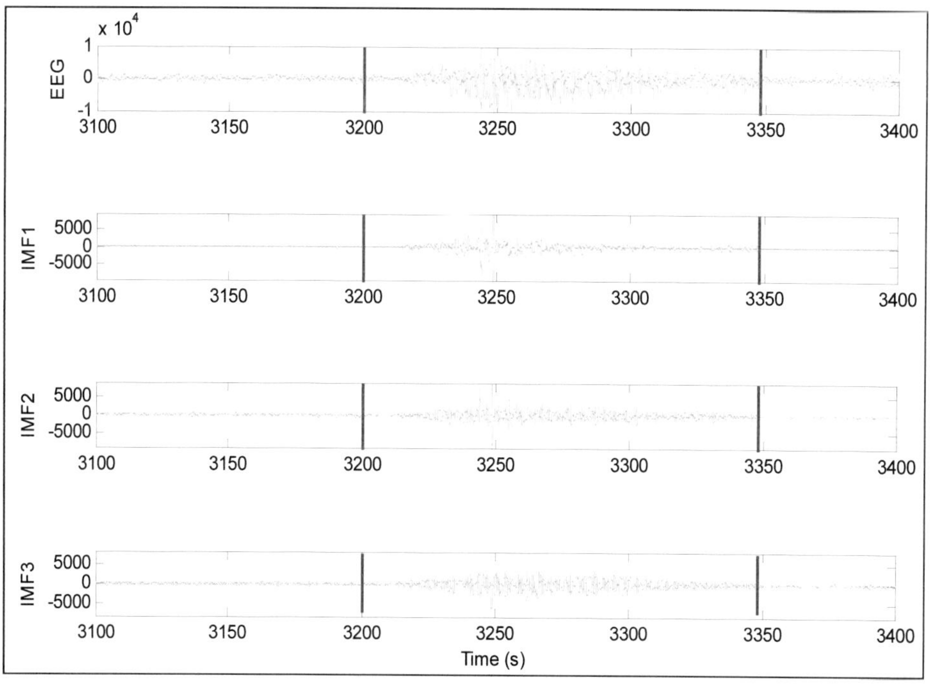

Fig. 4. EEG segment with a seizure for one channel and IMF1 to IMF3 of the signal. Red lines indicate the seizure time endpoints established by the neurologists.

4. Features and detectors

In this chapter two different epileptic seizure detectors based on the EMD of EEG signals will be described. In the first detector, the algorithm computes the energy of each IMF and performs the detection based on an energy threshold and a minimum seizure duration decision. The second detector consists on the extraction of several time and frequency features of IMFs, subsequently a feature selection based on a Mann-Whitney test and Lambda of Wilks criterion is performed and in a last stage linear discriminant analysis (LDA) of the selected parameters is used to classify epileptic seizure and normal EEG segments. In figure 5 the block diagrams of both detectors are showed.

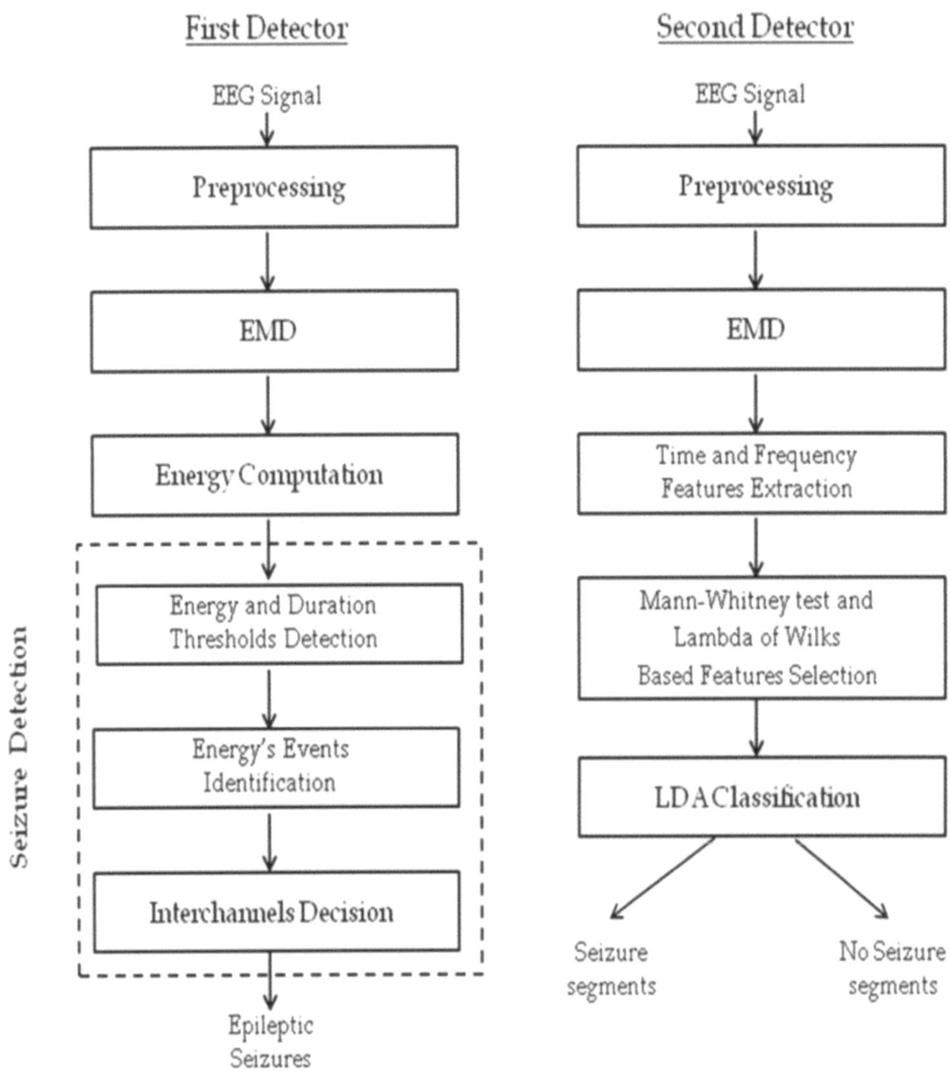

Fig. 5. Block diagrams of two epileptic seizure detectors.

4.1 Preprocessing and EMD

All EEG records were initially filtered with a second order, bidirectional, Butterworth, 50 Hz notch filter in order to remove the power line interference. Then, the EEG signals were band-pass filtered with a second order, bidirectional, Butterworth filter with a bandwidth of 0.5 - 60 Hz.

Next, all EEG records were resampled to 128 Hz in order to reduce computation time of EMD decomposition. This operation does not have any influence on the results since the bandwidth of the signal of interest does not exceed the 60 Hz.

Finally, the EMD of EEG signals was achieved as described in section 3.2.

4.2 First detector

The detector presented in this section and schematized in the left side of figure 5 can be separate in 4 main blocks. The first and second stages consist on the preprocessing of EEG signal and the EMD computation as described in 4.1. The third stage implies the energy computation and the last one, and the most complex, is the seizure detection strategy itself.

4.2.1 Energy computation

The first proposed algorithm takes the IMF1, IMF2 and IMF3 of the EEG signals of each channel and computes the energy serie (EN*i*) of each IMFi as shown in (2).

$$ENi(n) = \frac{1}{L}\sqrt{\sum_{m=n-L/2}^{n+L/2-1} (IMFi(m))^2} \quad i = 1, 2, 3 \tag{2}$$

In equation (2) i denotes the *i-th* IMF, n is its sample number and L is the length in samples for the energy computing window. In this work a 15 s moving, overlapped window (L=1920 samples) is used. Thus, once this computation ends three energy series (EN1, EN2 and EN3) for all EEG segments of each channel are obtained (see Figures 6 and 7).

4.2.2 Seizure detection method

In first place it will be describe what is called as an ***event***. An *event* is define here like the energy series portions that overcomes a certain threshold for more than 30 s. The threshold is computed as (3)

$$Thr\_ENi = \text{mean}\ (ENi) + 1.5\text{*std}\ (ENi) \tag{3}$$

where mean(*ENi*) and std(*ENi*) are the mean and the standard deviation values of the *i-th* energy serie considering the whole EEG channel.

Thus the first stage in this seizure detector is determined all the *events* present in each energy series of each channel.

The second decision step is identifying those *events* present in at least two of the three ENs of each channel. This criterion is used in order to discard possible artifacts that could be present in only one ENi.

Finally, in a third stage an interchannel decision is done by choosing the *events* (selected in the previous stage for each channel) that are present in at least two of the three studied channels.

Hence all events that satisfy the three decision stages are detected as epileptic seizures.

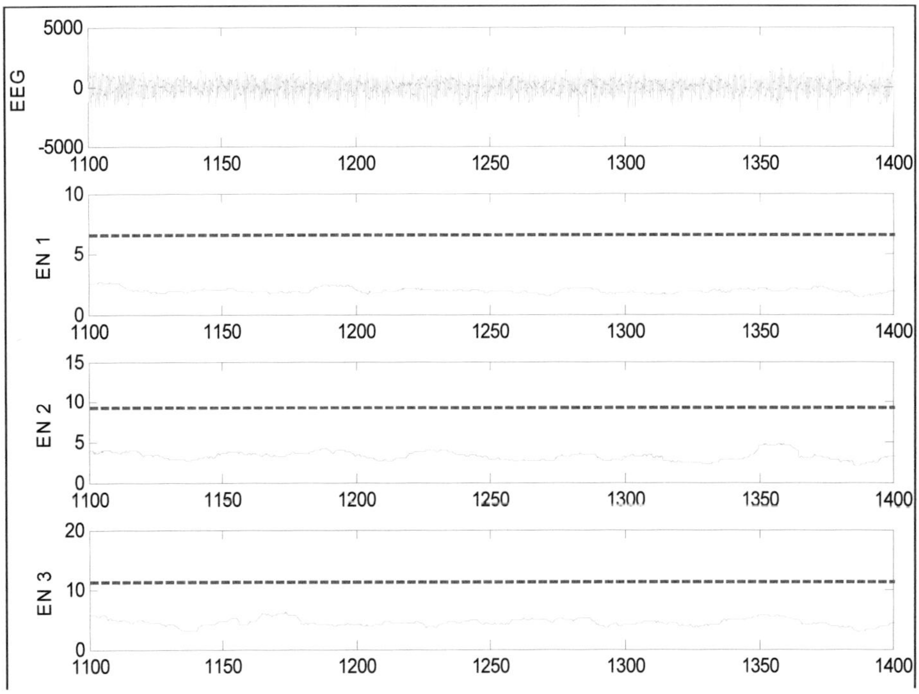

Fig. 6. A no seizure EEG segment of one channel and EN1 to EN3 series of the signal EMD

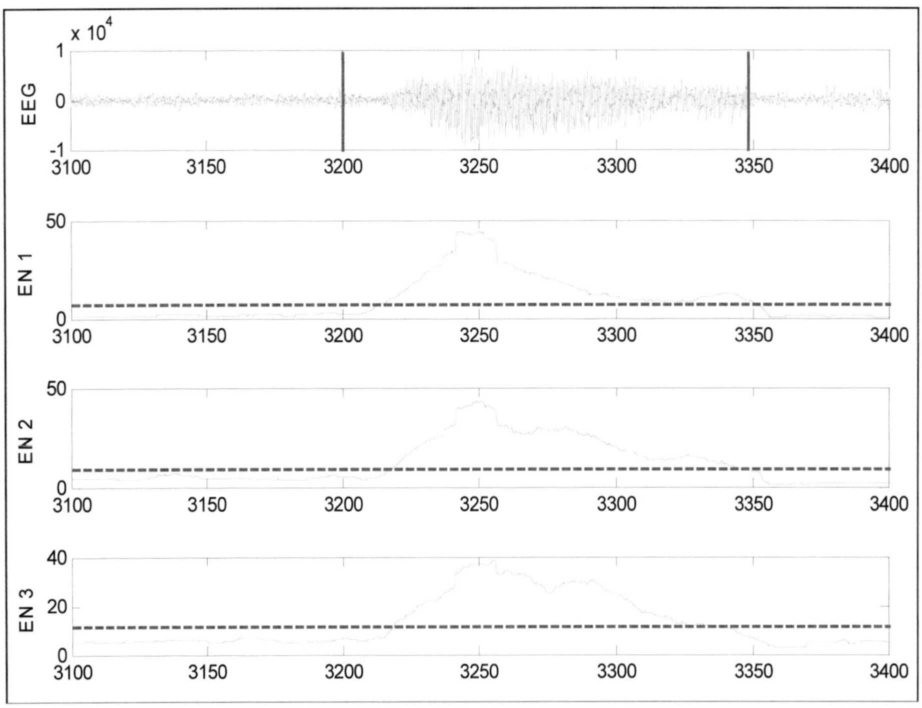

Fig. 7. A seizure EEG segment of one channel and EN1 to EN3 series of the signal EMD

Figure 6 illustrates the energy series (ENi) of the IMFs showed in figure 3. It is observed that the energy for each of the three IMFs does not overcome its corresponding threshold (computed by equation (3)), which is indicated with the red dashed line. So no event is detected in this EEG channel as well it is not detected in neither of the other channels (that are not showed here) so no seizure is present for this segment, corresponding with the database information.
In figure 7 the energy series (ENi) of the IMFs showed in figure 4 are illustrated. In this case the energy rise above the threshold in the 3 IMFs and lasts more than 30 s satisfying thus the event condition for each case so for this channel the second decision step is also accomplished. If this occurs for at least one of the remaining channels then a seizure is detected. In this example the events are detected in the three channels and also match with the seizure time endpoints established by the neurologists.

4.3 Second detector

In the right side of figure 5 a block diagram of the second detector is illustrated. In this case the preprocessing stage and the EMD computation (describe in Section 4.1) are the same as the first detector.
Next several time and frequency features of the IMFs are computed and then selected using a Mann-Whitney test and Lambda of Wilks criterion. Finally, a linear discriminant analysis (LDA) is performed to discriminate epileptic seizures and normal EEG segments.

4.3.1 Feature extraction

In order to characterize the EEG signals several features were computed upon these 3 IMFs series (IMF1 to 3) calculated for each channel. For each IMF, a set of parameters in time and frequency domains were computed.
In this stage in order to improve the statistical stationary of EEG records each IMF was divided in segments of 15 s. Hence the whole IMFs selected of the all EEG records analyzed computes a total of 45517 segments, 44828 of them without epileptic seizures and 689 segments denoted as having only one epileptic seizure each.
In *time* domain, the following parameters were calculated on each IMF: coefficient of variation (VC), Median Absolute Deviation (MAD), Standard Deviation (STD), Mean Value (MV), Variance (VAR) and Root Mean Square Value (RMS). They are summarized in table 2.
For *frequency* domain, the power spectral density (PSD) of IMF1, IMF2 and IMF3 was estimated by the periodogram method with a Hanning window.
Then, classical parameters of descriptive statistics were computed on the PSD. Therefore, the following frequency features were obtained on the spectrum of each IMF: Central, Mean and Peak Frequencies (CF, MF and PF), Standard Deviation Frequency (STDF), First and Third Quartile Frequencies (Q_1F, Q_3F), Interquartile Range (IR), 95% cumulated energy Frequency (MAXF), Asymmetry Coefficient (AC) and Kurtosis Coefficient (KC) (Marple, 1987). These frequency parameters are listed in table 3.

Time Domain Features					
VC	MAD	STD	MV	VAR	RMS

Table 2. Time Domain Features

Frequency Domain Features									
CF	MF	PF	STDF	Q_1F	Q_3F	IR	MAXF	AC	KC

Table 3. Frequency Domain Features

Resuming, 10 frequency domain parameters and 6 time domain features were computed. Thus, for IMF1 we have 16 parameters for each 15 second segment obtaining in this way a series with the time evolution of each feature. The same procedure is repeated for IMF2 and IMF3. Hence this implies a computation of 48 features series for each EEG channel and a total of 144 series considering the three EEG channels.

4.3.2 Feature selection

In order to reduce the dimensionality problem, the median of the individual values of each features series for the three channels were initially computed. For example, we take CF of IMF1 of channel 1, CF of IMF1 of channel 2 and CF of IMF1 of channel 3 and calculate the median of this parameter resulting in one series for this feature in IMF1. The procedure is repeated for all the parameters and IMFs. Thus, the number of the total features series is reduced to 48.

Even though the vector of features was reduced, its dimension is still too large. As a second approach, a stepwise method based on the statistical parameter Lambda of Wilks (WL) is performed. In an *n*-dimensional space constructed with *n* variables and with the matrixes B_{nxn} and W_{nxn} representing the square sum and cross products between groups and within-groups, respectively; the WL can be defined as the ratio between their determinants (Tinsley & Brown, 2000) as it can be see in (4):

$$WL = \frac{|W|}{|W+B|} \tag{4}$$

In other words, the WL measures the ratio between within-group variability and total variability, and it is a direct measure of the importance of the variables. Therefore, the most important features for the analysis should be selected, i.e. the variables (features) that contribute with more information. Besides, the correlated variables are discarded in this process (Tinsley & Brown, 2000).

With the aim of contrasting significant differences between groups, the value of WL is transformed into the general multivariate statistical F. If F value for a variable is higher than 3.84 (F to get in) this is included in the analysis and once accepted the variable is rejected if its F value is smaller than 2.71 (F to get out).

Once the WL criterion was applied the features selected were 11, their mean and standard deviation values are summarized in Table 4.

4.3.4 Classification

To detect the EEG segments with epileptic seizure a linear discriminant analysis (LDA) was implemented using the classification functions ***h***. These functions are a linear combination of the discriminant variables (X_m) which allows maximize the differences between groups and minimize the differences within-group and are calculated as (5) (Gil Flores *et al.*, 2001):

$$h_k(q) = b_{k0} + b_{k1}X_1(q) + \ldots + b_{km}X_m(q) \tag{5}$$

where k represents the classification groups, i.e., for seizure and no seizure classes (k =2), m is the quantity of features (in this work, m =11) and q is the case to classify. The computing of b coefficients is showed in equations (6) and (7) (Gil Flores *et al.*, 2001).

$$b_{ki} = (n-g)\sum_{j=1}^{q} a_{ij}\,\overline{X}_j \qquad \begin{matrix} g\text{=quantity of groups} \\ n\text{=sample size} \end{matrix} \tag{6}$$

$$b_{k0} = -0.5\sum_{j=1}^{q} b_{kj}\,\overline{X}_j \tag{7}$$

IMF	Feature	No Seizure segments	Seizure segments
	PF	16.14 ± 5.18	14.72 ± 4.66
	STDF	7.88 ± 1.26	7.39 ± 1.28
	IR	9.61 ± 2.66	9.05±2.53
1	AC	0.76 ± 0.44	0.77±0.38
	KC	4.3 ± 1.66	4.42 ± 1.19
	VC	409.85 ± 828.41	59.98 ± 28.99
	MAD	56.93 ± 31.18	537.45 ± 694.97
	STD	208.89 ± 204.06	352.04 ± 337.71
2	STDF	3.60 ± 0.66	3.33 ± 0.68
	Q_1F	4.10 ± 0.81	4.14 ± 0.93
3	STD	1180.95 ± 16434.06	500.14 ± 543.51

Table 4. Selected features

For LDA the 50% of data was used as training group and the rest as validation group. Then, a second test was done inverting the training and validation groups. The results are exposed in Section 6.2 using the mean value of SEN and SPE obtained in the validation phase for the two classification tests.

Let g_1 be the seizure group and g_2 the no seizure group, once the classification functions were computing for each group the classification is done satisfying the following criteria:

If $h_2(q) > h_1(q)$ then case q belongs to g_2 otherwise if $h_2(q) < h_1(q)$ case q belongs to g_1.

5. Results

In this section it will be expose the performance of both proposed seizures detectors. In order to evaluate the achievement of the algorithms the following diagnostic categories were considered on the detection stage: true negative (TN), false positive (FP), true positive (TP), false negative (FN). The obtained values for these indexes are contrasted with the segments indicated in the database as having seizure or no seizure by the neurologists. Then the statistical diagnostic indexes of sensitivity (SEN) and specificity (SPE) were also computing (Altman, 1993). These indexes are defined as follows and stated in equations (8) and (9).

Sensitivity (*SEN*): Is the proportion of epileptic seizures segments correctly detected by the algorithm.

$$SEN(\%) = \frac{TP}{TP + FN} \times 100 \tag{8}$$

Specificity (*SPE*): Is the proportion of segments without seizures correctly identified by the algorithm.

$$SPE(\%) = \frac{TN}{TN + FP} \times 100 \tag{9}$$

5.1 Results of first detector

As a first approach for this algorithm its performance was evaluated in two ways. In first place the detector was tested on the data sorted by epilepsy types and then the EEG signals were evaluated all without a specific arrange.
Then in table 5 are resumed the statistical diagnostic indexes of SEN and SPE computed for the different types of epilepsies individually and for the epilepsies all together.

Epilepsy Type	SEN	SPE
Temporal	56.4%	75.9%
Frontal	12.0%	81.8%
Temporo-Occipital	40.0%	73.3%
Others	53.8%	93.3%
All types togheter	**41.4%**	**79.3%**

Table 5. Statistical diagnostic indexes of SEN and SPE for first detector.

5.2 Results of second detector

In order to improve the results obtained with first detector, the second detection scheme detailed in section 4.3 were tested in the same EEG records. Table 6 shows the mean value of SEN and SPE obtained in the validation phase for the two classification tests described in section 4.3.4.

Epilepsy Type	SEN	SPE
Temporal	65.2%	77%
Frontal	51.7%	78.7%
Temporo-Occipital	56.9%	72.4%
Others	57.5%	87.7%
All types togheter	**69.4%**	**69.2%**

Table 6. Statistical diagnostic indexes of SEN and SPE for second detector.

6. Discussion and conclusions

Epileptic seizure detection in EEG records is a useful and important tool due to their various applications such us epilepsy research treatments like timely drug delivery, electrical stimulation and seizure alert systems besides diagnostic applications. In this sense it is a real need the development of automatic algorithms that could be able to detect seizures independently of its brain source. It is also important to establish some kind of standardization of the detectors using to test them the same database so a robust comparison of their performance could be carried out.

In this chapter two epileptic seizure detection methods based on the Empirical Mode Decomposition (EMD) of EEG signals has been proposed. On one hand, the use of EMD for seizures detection it is a recent approach. In addition, as a contribution to the setted out problem, long term epileptic EEG intracranial records with different focal epilepsies are used to evaluate the performance of both seizures detectors.

The used EMD algorithm in this work is the one proposed by Flandrin (2007) & Rilling *et al.* (2009). This technique seems to be more suitable for epileptic EEG records than others of the signal processing area due to the EEG signal presents nonlinear and non-stationary properties during a seizure. Nevertheless, it was recently reported for this version of the algorithm the problem of what is called mode mixing so to solve this a new approach known as Ensemble EMD (EEMD) has been proposed (Wu & Huang, 2009). There are also some extensions of standard EMD to multivariate signals defined by Rehman & Mandic (2010) as Multivariate EMD. Even though the EMD showed a relatively good performance in seizure detection it was observed that the computation time of EMD for each segment is quite time-computing extensive which could represent a disadvantage for analyzing long EEG records. It can be noted that the proposed EMD technique has still much aspects to explore and innovate so its performance could be further improve.

In order to have a complete evaluation of the detectors' performance they both were first tested making a discrimination of the EEG signals by epilepsy type and then the data were used all without a specific arrange. For the first detector the values of SPE obtained were high, arising up to 90% for the epilepsies grouped like "Others" while the SEN results were non-satisfactory, been 56.8% the highest value for temporal lobe epilepsy records. Whereas the performance of this detector for the complete set of data showed a global SEN and SPE values of 41.4% and 79.3%, respectively.

The results shown in Table 6 indicate that the second detector have remarkably improved the SEN values compared with those obtained for the first detector for all classes of epilepsies. With respect to the ESP values, the results of the second detector were better for temporal lobe epilepsy signals and decrease slightly for the remaining classes of epilepsies. So the global performance of the second detector (SEN = 69.4% and SPE = 69.2%) can be considered satisfactory better than the first one because both values are in the same order.

Other authors had also recently used the Freiburg´s database for seizure detection so a comparison of their works with ours could be made. Henriksen *et al.* (2010) in their research uses features of Wavelet Transform (WT) of 16 patients (instead of the 21) of the database and classified them by a support vector machine in order to implement an automatic seizure detection algorithm. They obtained a global SEN of 86% and a false detection rate of 0.39/h, but the SPE value is not reported. In a recent work Vardhan & Majumdar (2011) introduce a differential operator to accentuate the seizure part of depth electrode recordings (ECoG) relative to the non-seizure one. The technique was only applied to 5 patients of Freiburg´s database. For 4 patients, they reported 18 of 20 true detections and 2 false detections. The results for the remaining patient were not reported. Finally, Chua *et al.* (2011) applied the Gotman algorithm (Gotman, 1999) to 15 patients of the database and it was adjusted for epilepsy type with the aim of improve the off-line automated seizure detection methods that will decrease the workload of EEG monitoring units. The obtained values were 78% of SEN and a true positive rate of 51%.

Summarizing, even though some of the detectors described in the previous paragraph obtained higher values of SEN than the ones developed in this chapter it has to be said that all the referenced cases use selected records of the database while the authors of this chapter had tested their algorithms using all 21 EEG recordings available in Freiburg database.

It may also be highlighted that the values of SEN and SPE of first and second detectors could be improved in order to obtain a more reliable application. In this sense, more tests and some adjustments on the algorithms must be made done to be suitable for medical diagnosis. It could be concluded that the developed methods based on EMD are promissory tools for epileptic seizure detection in EEG records.

7. Future works

As future extension of this research in first place the EMD computation time must be reduced may be taking time windows of few seconds to calculate it instead of 1 h EEG segments. It is also needed to improve the values of SEN and SPE so more effort on the features and classifiers must be done.

8. Acknowledgment

This work has been supported by grants from Agencia Nacional de Promoción Científica y Tecnológica (ANPCYT - PICT 2006-01689) and Universidad Nacional de San Juan, both institutions from Argentina. The first author is supported by ANPCYT, whereas the second and third authors are supported by CONICET of Argentina.

9. References

Abásolo, D.; James, C. & Hornero, R. (2007). Non-linear Analysis of Intracranial Electroencephalogram Recordings with Approximate Entropy and Lempel-Ziv Complexity for Epileptic Seizure Detection, *Proceedings of the 29th Annual International IEEE EMBS Conference,* pp. 1953-1956, ISBN: 978-1-4244-0787-3, Cité Internationale, Lyon, France August, 2007

Adeli, H.; Ghosh-Dastidar, S. & Dadmehr, N. (2007). A Wavelet-Chaos Methodology for Analysis of EEGs and EEG Subbands to Detect Seizure and Epilepsy, *IEEE Transaction On Biomedical Engineering,* vol. 54, no. 2, (February 2007), pp 205-211. ISSN: 0018-9294

Altman,D. G. (1993). Some common problems in medical research, In: *Practical statistics for medical research,* Chapman & Hall (Ed.), pp. 396-439, London, UK

Bao, F.; Gao, J.; & Hu, J. (2009). Automated Epilepsy Diagnosis Using Interictal Scalp EEG. , *Proceedings of the 31st Annual International IEEE EMBS Conference,* pp. 6603-07, ISBN: 978-1-4244-3296-7, Minneapolis, Minnesota, USA, September, 2009

Berg, A.; Berkovic S.; Brodie M.; *et al.* (2010). Revised terminology and concepts for organization of seizures and epilepsies: Report of the ILAE Commission on Classification and Terminology, 2005–2009. *Epilepsia*, Vol.51, No.4, (April 2010), pp. 676–685

Chua, E.; Patel, K.; Fitzsimons, M. & Bleakley, C. (2011). Improved patient specific seizure detection during pre-surgical evaluation, *Journal of Clinical Neurophysiology*, Vol.122, No.4, (April 2011), pp. 672–679

Diez, P.; Mut, V.; Laciar, E.; Torres, A. & E. Avila. (2009). Application of the Empirical Mode Decomposition to the Extraction of Features from EEG Signals for Mental Task Classification, *Proceedings of the 31st Annual International IEEE EMBS Conference*, pp. 2579-2582, ISBN: 978-1-4244-3296-7, Minneapolis, Minnesota, USA, September, 2009

Diez, P.; Laciar, E. ; Torres, A. ; Mut, V. & Avila E. (2011). Adaptive bands on EEG signals extracted with Empirical Mode Decomposition, *V Latin-American Congress On Biomedical Engineering (CLAIB2011)*, La Habana, Cuba, May 16-21, 2011, In press.

Ficker, D. (2000). Sudden unexplained death and injury in epilepsy. *Epilepsia*, Vol.41, Suppl.2, pp. S7-S12

Fisher, R.; Van Emde Boas, W. & Blume, W.; *et al.* (2005). Epileptic Seizures and Epilepsy: Definitions Proposed by the International League Against Epilepsy (ILAE) and the International Bureau for Epilepsy (IBE). *Epilepsia*, Vol.46, No.4, (April 2005), pp. 470–472

Flandrin P. (2007). EMD Matlab 7.1 codes with examples, Available from : http://perso.ens-lyon.fr/patrick.flandrin/emd.html

Freiburg EEG Data Base. (2008). Available from: https://epilepsy.uni-freiburg.de/freiburg-seizure-prediction-project/eeg-database

Friedman, D. & Gilliam, F. (2010). Seizure-related injuries are underreported in pharmacoresistant localization-related epilepsy. *Epilepsia*, Vol. 51, Issue 1, (January 2010), pp. 43–47

Gil Flores, J.; Garcia Jimenez, E. & Rodriguez Gómez, G. (2001). *Discriminant Analysis* (in Spanish), La Muralla S.A., Madrid, España. ISBN:84-7133-704-5

Gotman, J. (1999). Automatic detection of seizures and spikes, *Journal of Clinical Neurophysiology*, Vol.16, No.2, (March 1999), pp. 130–140

Henriksen, J.; Remvig, L. & Madsenc, R. *et al.* (2010). Automatic seizure detection: going from sEEG to iEEG, *Proceedings of the 32nd Annual International IEEE EMBS Conference*, pp. 2431-2434, ISBN: 978-1-4244-4124-2, Buenos Aires, Argentina, August/September, 2010

Huang, N.; Shen, Z. & Long, S. *et al.* (1998). The empirical mode decomposition and the Hilbert spectrum for nonlinear and non stationary time series analysis, *Proceedings of the Royal Society of London. Series A: Mathematical, Physical and Engineering Sciences*, vol. 454, no. 1971, (March 1998), pp. 903-995, doi:10.1098/rspa.1998.0193 Key: citeulike:2681232

Marple L.S. (1987). *Digital spectral analysis with applications*, Prentice-Hall. Signal Processing Series. Alan V. Oppenheim, Series Editor. New Jersey

Orosco, L.; Laciar, E. & Garcés Correa, A. *et al.* (2009). An Epileptic Seizures Detection Algorithm based on the Empirical Mode Decomposition of EEG *Proceedings of the 31st Annual International IEEE EMBS Conference*, pp. 2651- 2654, ISBN: 978-1-4244-3296-7, Minneapolis, Minnesota, USA, September, 2009

Orosco, L.; Garcés Correa, A. & Laciar, E. (2010). Multiparametric Detection of Epileptic Seizures using Empirical Mode Decomposition of EEG Records, *Proceedings of the 31nd Annual International IEEE EMBS Conference,* pp. 951-54, ISBN: 978-1-4244-4124-2, Buenos Aires, Argentina, August/September, 2010

Rehman, N. & Mandic, D. (2010). Multivariate empirical mode decomposition, *Proceedings of the Royal Society of London. Series A: Mathematical, Physical and Engineering Sciences,* Vol. 466, No. 2117, (May 2010), pp. 1291-1302

Rilling, G.; Flandrin, P. & Gonçalvès, P. (2003). On Empirical Mode Decomposition and its Algorithms, *Proceedings of the IEEE-Eurasip Workshop on Nonlinear Signal and Image Processing,* Vol.3, pp. 8-11

Sanei, S. & . Chambers, J. (2007). *EEG Signal Processing,* Wiley, England.

Schuyler, R.; White, A.; Staley, K. & Cios, K. (2007). Epileptic Seizure Detection. Identification of Ictal and Pre-Ictal States Using RBF Networks with Wavelet-Decomposed EEG Data, *IEEE Engineering in Medicine and Biology Magazine,* (March/April, 2007), pp. 74-81.

Tafreshi, A.K. Nasrabadi, A.M. Omidvarnia, A.H. (2008). Epileptic Seizure Detection Using Empirical Mode Decomposition, *Proceedings of the IEEE International Symposium on Signal Processing and Information Technology,* pp. 238-242, ISBN: 978-1-4244-3554-8, Sarajevo, December 2008

Theodore, W. & . Fisher, R. (2004). Brain Stimulation for Epilepsy. *The Lancet Neurology,* Vol. 3, Issue 2, (February 2004), pp. 111-118

Tinsley H.E.A, Brown S.D. (2000). *Handbook of applied multivariate statistics and mathematical modeling,* 1st Edition, Elsevier Academic Press. ISBN:0-12-691360-9

Torres, A.; Jané, R.; & Fiz, J. *et al.* (2007). Analysis of Respiratory Mechanomyographic Signals by means of the Empirical Mode Decomposition, *Journal of Physics: Conference Series,* vol. 90, 2007, pp. 1-8. doi:10.1088/1742-6596/90/1/012078 Available from: http://www.iop.org/EJ/toc/1742-6596/90/1

Tzallas, A.; Tsipouras, M. & Fotiadis, D. (2007). The Use of Time- Frequency Distributions for Epileptic Seizure Detection in EEG Recordings, *Proceedings of the 29th Annual International IEEE EMBS Conference,* pp. 3-6, ISBN: 978-1-4244-0787-3, Cité Internationale, Lyon, France August, 2007

Vardhan, P. & Majumdar, K. (2011). Automatic Seizure Detection in ECoG by DB4 Wavelets and Windowed Variance: A Comparison, *Proceedings of the International Conference on Communications and Signal Processing,* pp. 227-230, Calicut, India, February, 2011

Weng, B.; Blanco-Velasco, M. & Barner, K. E. (2006). ECG Denoising Based on the Empirical Mode Decomposition, *Proceedings of the 28th Annual International IEEE EMBS Conference,* pp. 903 - 906, ISBN: 978-0-7695-3398-8, New York City, New York, USA, August, 2006

World Health Organization. (2006). Programmes and projects. Available from: http://www.who.int/mediacentre/factsheets/fs999/en/index.html

Wu, Z. & Huang, N. (2009). Ensemble empirical Mode Decomposition: A noise-assisted data analysis method, *Advances in Adaptive Data Analysis,* Vol.1, No.1, pp. 1–41, World Scientific Publishing Company

Zandi, A.; Dumont, G.; Javidan, M. & Tafreshi, R. (2009). An Entropy-Based Approach to Predict Seizures in Temporal Lobe Epilepsy Using Scalp EEG, *Proceedings of the 31st Annual International IEEE EMBS Conference,* pp. 228-231, ISBN: 978-1-4244-3296-7, Minneapolis, Minnesota, USA, September, 2009

2

Solitary Epileptic Seizures in the Clinical Practice

Branislav Kollár and Katarína Klobučníková
1st Department of Neurology, Faculty of Medicine, Comenius University, Bratislava Slovak Republic

1. Introduction

An epileptic seizure may be conceptualized as a paroxysmal pathological process in the brain of a heterogeneous etiology with heteromorphic clinical and electrophysiological manifestation.The cases of epileptic seizures are classified according to The International Classification of Epileptic Seizures (ICES) published for the first time by The International League Against Epilepsy (ILAE) in 1970 and revised in 1981 (Commission on Classification and Terminology of the International League Against Epilepsy, 1981). This classification is a clinical one related to semiology of the seizures not to their etiology. Therefore it is necessary to exclude an acutely occurring cause responsible for occurrence of the seizure. In such cases we talk about the so-called acute symptomatic seizures. The underlying cause may be structural (e.g. head trauma), metabolic, toxic (e.g. alcohol), or an acute CNS infection, etc.. The most frequent acute symptomatic seizures are the febrile seizures. In fact, the acute symptomatic seizures occur more frequently than epilepsy ("unprovoked" seizures). The risk of occurrence during one's life is very high - approximately 5% in males and 2.5% in females. If the acutely occurring cause has been withdrawn or cured without a residuum in the form of a brain lesion, the seizures do not recur (Dasheiff, 1987; Fromm, 1987). The antiepileptic medication is necessary for suppressing the seizures in the acute stage but usually there is no need for treatment continuation after the complete cure of the underlying disease. If the acutely occurring cause was not responsible for epileptic seizure we talk about a so-called unprovoked seizure. If the unprovoked epileptic seizure occurs in relation to a preceding neurological insult, the disorders is regarded as secondary to this insult; we call it the late symptomatic epileptic seizure or late symptomatic epilepsy in case of seizure recurrence. A general principle of treatment for the symptomatic (secondary) epileptic seizures has been a primary effort for resolution of the underlying disease that is the etiological factor responsible for the seizures. Given that it is impossible, the antiepileptic treatment in accordance with the treatment guidelines for individual seizure types (together with adherence to right living, behavioural precautions and concomitant solutions of the social and psychological issues) is indicated (Hovorka et al. 2004a; Hovorka et al. 2004b; Ošlejšková, 2007). Approximately 5% of the population experiences one unprovoked epileptic seizure in the lifetime (Forsgren et al., 1996; Hauser et al. 1993). The febrile seizure before the age of 5 occurs in approximately 5% of population (Hauser et al. 1996). Only about 25% of people experiencing the first unprovoked seizure see the doctor and nearly always the seizure is a generalized tonic-clonic one. Most of the people have no risk factors for the onset of epilepsy, normal neurological examination as well as normal initial EEG (Pedley et al., 1995). The occurrence of the first unprovoked epileptic seizure requires always a thorough evaluation. The risk of misdiagnosis is high as non-epileptic seizures make 20-33% of newly-diagnosed cases.

EEG is an important non-invasive examination method that informs about electrical activity of the brain. It plays an important role in differential diagnostics of seizures. The greatest diagnostic benefit of EEG belongs to diagnosis of epilepsy. Finding of interictal epileptiform graphoelements supports the diagnosis of epilepsy with specificity of 96% (Vojtěch, 2008). In patients who experienced the first unprovoked epileptic seizure 30-40% catchment of specific epileptiform EEG abnormalities after the first EEG examination was most often reported in the literature (King et. al., 1998; Shinnar et al., 1994). Higher catchment was reported in EEG realized within 24 hours from experienced seizure than after 24 hours (51% versus 34%) (King et. al., 1998). Abnormal EEG occurs more frequently in patients with partial seizures than in patients with generalized seizures and in patients with late symptomatic etiology of epilepsy than in patients with idiopathic epilepsy (Shinnar et al., 1994).

Imaging examinations represent one of the basic methods in diagnostics of patients with epileptic seizures. Their development has significantly contributed to accurate diagnostics and classification of epileptic syndromes. It is necessary to realize that these methods can help reveal etiology of seizures and determine etiopathogenetic diagnosis. The fact that each patient after first epileptic seizure must undertake these examination is common and generally accepted. MRI is an advantageous imaging method for CNS. At present this method is the first choice method. MRI can reveal structural lesions and brain anomalies which CT examination, that is less sensitive, cannot (heterotopias, demyelinizations, anomalies of gyrifications, vascular malformations, etc.) (Bořuta et al., 2007). MRI is markedly more advantageous in patients with temporal epilepsy where it is able to express even very tiny structural changes and mesial temporal sclerosis (Carrilho et al., 1994). In addition, in MRI examination patients are not exposed, in contrast to CT, to radiation load. CT advantages involve better availability, relatively low price, possibility to examine non-cooperating patients because the examination takes only several seconds and it is less sensitive to movable artifacts. Moreover, CT has less contraindications comparing to MRI. MRI cannot be realized in patients with metal implants and clips, pacemaker, uncontrollable claustrophobia. Result can be adulterated if the patient does not cooperate.

In the past we also evaluated the findings of various modification of EEG examination and imaging methods in our patients who experienced solitary unprovoked epileptic seizure (Kollar et. al., 2009). We found that catchment of epileptiform manifestations in native EEG in patients who experienced solitary unprovoked epileptic seizure (14.29%) is lower than reported in literature (*King et al., 1998*; Shinnar et al., 1994; *Vojtěch, 2008*). It might be explained by accepted fact of transient incidence of abnormalities in EEG records. That is the reason that transient incidence of epileptiform EEG abnormalities in patients with epilepsy is considered the factor participating on different results of particular studies. High percentage of non-specific (non-epileptiform) abnormal EEG records in our cohort of patients who experienced solitary epileptic seizure was in agreement with literature data (Kollár et al., 2009). The results of our study - see Table 1.

It is very important to realize the limits of EEG examination. Firstly - normal EEG finding does not rule out clinical diagnosis of epilepsy and presence of epileptiform EEG abnormality does not confirm that the patient has epilepsy. Recurrent occurrence of abnormal interictal EEG findings in the group of non-epileptic seizures is also known (Kuba et al., 2001). That´s why EEG must be recognized as the method that plays a very important role in diagnostics of epilepsy or paroxysmal disorders, however, as the adjuvant examination method its role is limited. In clinically clear epileptic manifestations EEG can confirm, or in specific cases support, clinically clear diagnosis of epilepsy. In clinically absent typical epileptic manifestations high cautiousness is needed in evaluation of the diagnosis (incorrect evaluation or over-evaluation of EEG finding).

	Normal	NFA	NGA	EFA	EGA
EEG (n=84)	41 (48.81 %)	23 (27.38 %)	8 (9.52 %)	8 (9.52 %)	4 (4.77 %)
EEG after SD (n_1=59)	35 (59.33 %)	9 (15.25 %)	6 (10.17 %)	6 (10.17 %)	3 (5.08 %)
LTM-EEG after SD (n_2=46)	35 (76.09 %)	6 (13.04 %)	2 (4.35 %)	2 (4.35 %)	1 (2.17 %)

Table 1. Interictal EEG findings, EEG findings after SD and LTM-EEG after SD in patients who experienced solitary unprovoked epileptic seizure (Kollar et al., 2009). (Abbreviations see in part 5).

Statistical comparing of diagnostic benefits of CT and MRI examinations of the brain in our group of patients confirmed, as in the other works, that MRI examination of the brain in patients who experienced solitary unprovoked epileptic seizure is definitely the first choice method. The results of our evaluation - see Table 2,3.

	UNPROVOKED SOLITARY EPILEPTIC SEIZURES	
	Number of patients	Number/ whole (%)
CT brain	21	
Normal	5	23.81 %
Pathology	16	76.19 %
MRI brain	6	
Normal	2	0.33 %
Pathology	4	0.67 %
Realized CT and MRI	57	
CT normal MRI normal	28	49.12 %
CT normal MRI pathol.	12	21.05 %
CT pathol. MRI pathol./ closer specification CT by MRI examination	17/12	29.83 %
CT pathol. MRI normal	0	0 %

Table 2. Findings of CT and MRI examinations of the brain in patients after solitary unprovoked epileptic seizure (Kollar et al., 2009).

	Benefit
CT of brain (n=57)	5 (8.77 %)
MRI of brain (n=57)	29 (50.88 %)

Table 3. Patients after solitary unprovoked epileptic seizure in which both imaging methods were realized (Kollar et. al., 2009).

Statistical evaluation of benefits of MRI examination comparing to CT examination by binomic test of proportions: $p<0.0001$ – high significant difference between proportions (Kollar et. al., 2009).

In the past we noticed, by the EEG finding evaluation in our group of outpatients with epilepsy, that only in a small amount of cases the EEG findings corresponded completely with the clinical image of epileptic seizure (Kollar et al., 2010). In relation to the imaging methods and their diagnostic agreement with clinical syptomatology of epileptic seizure and EEG findings, it is interesting that in the study of King et al. (1998), who evaluated the imaging of MRI abnormalities after the first epileptic seizure in 300 members of a group, consisting of both children and adults, they determined that, with patients having clinically diagnosed partial seizure, an epileptogenic lesion on the MRI was identified in 17% of cases. In 50 patients with clinical diagnosis of generalized seizure a structural lesion was identified in only one case and in the case of 49 patients with generalized epileptiform activity on EEG no structural lesion on MRI was identified. These facts covey to us the need to try and establish in our own group of patients the clinical typology of epileptic seizure, EEG findings and results of imaging methods. After this we determined the part of patients with complete diagnostic concordance between clinical image of epileptic seizure and results of auxiliary diagnostic methods (Kollar et al., 2010). The summary of all watched data in the group of patients after solitary epileptic seizure - see Table 4. The evaluation of clinical typology of epileptic seizures and results or realized examination - see Table 5.

The group of patients	n	The clinical type of epileptic seizure (ILAE,1981) 1 A	1 B	1 C	2 A	2 B	2 C	2 D	2 E	3	MT	EEG: EEG N	EEG NNA	EEG NFA	EEG ENA	EEG EFA	EEG after SD N	EEG after SD NNA	EEG after SD NFA	EEG after SD ENA	EEG after SD EFA	EEG after SD 0	LTM-EEG after SD N	LTM-EEG after SD NNA	LTM-EEG after SD NFA	LTM-EEG after SD ENA	LTM-EEG after SD EFA	LTM-EEG after SD 0	CT/MRI N	CT/MRI P	CT/MRI 0
Solit. unprov. EPI	84	5	3	25	/	/	40	8	/	/	/	41	8	23	4	8	34	6	9	3	6	25	35	2	6	1	2	38	45/30	33/33	6/21

Table 4. The summary of all watched data in the group of patients after solitary unprovoked epileptic seizure (Kollar et al., 2010). (Abbreviations see in part 5).

The full diagnostic coincidence between the clinical picture of epileptic seizure, EEG examination (native interictal EEG, or EEG after SD or LTM-EEG after SD) and results of imaging methods (CT or MRI of the brain) we found only in 11 from 84 patients (13,1%)

after solitary epileptic seizure. The receiving diagnosis of unclear seizure status was determined in 57 out of 116 patients (49,14%) dismissed, as mentioned in 10 years' time period, with the diagnosis of solitary epileptic seizure. These percentages, together with a high part of unclear receiving diagnosis (the disturbance of consciousness of unclear etiology) in the patients, who were dismissed from our clinic with diagnosis of solitary epileptic seizure, suggests that the diagnosis of this group of patients is often problematic.

Coincidence	Solitary unprovoked EPI (n=84)
Clinical typology + EEG (EEG after SD, LTM-EEG afterSD)	16 (19,05%)
Clinical typology + CT, MRI	52 (61,90%)
Clinical typology + EEG + CT, MRI	11 (13,10%)

Table 5. The evaluation of clinical symptomatology of epileptic seizures with EEG, CT and MRI findings (Kollar et. al., 2010).

From unclear seizure status, which is accepted on the neurological departments, the more considerable part is made by unepileptic seizure status (Angus-Leppan, 2008; Perrig & Jallon, 2008). The correct diagnosis of seizure disorders require the strict observance of standard diagnostic proceeding (Martiniskova et al., 2009). The necessity are detailed anamnesis, adequate "erudition" of medical doctors working in this part of medicine, the right interpretation of auxiliary diagnostic methods results and in many cases the quality of cooperation between the doctors from other specializations (Bajaček et al., 2010; Hovorka et al., 2007; Kollar et al., 2010). Our results repeat the confirmation that diagnostic of seizure disorders with or without the disturbance of consciousness belong between the more difficult performances in the clinical praxis.

2. Solitary unprovoked epileptic seizure – the risk factors of probable seizure recurrence. To treat or not to treat the patient after the first unprovoked epileptic seizure?

2.1 Introduction

At least 5% of the general population experience one unprovoked epileptic seizure during their life (Forsgren et al., 1996; Hauser et al., 1982; Hauser et al., 1993). This is in contrast with an approximately 3-4% cumulative incidence of epilepsy (at least two unprovoked epileptic seizures) and with an approximately 4% incidence of the acute symptomatic seizures (Hauser et al., 1996). The risk of seizure recurrence after the first epileptic seizure has been shown to be most frequently 30-40% (range 23-71%) (Annegers et al., 1986; Engel & Starkman, 1994; Hauser et al., 1990; Kollar et al., 2006; Mann, 2005). This figure oscillates notably depending on certain risk factors. There are multiple risk factors mentioned in the literature. Berg & Shinnar (1991), referring to already published studies and meta-analyses, stated that multiple factors influence the recurrence risk of epileptic seizures - see Table 6.

Etiology	patients with tumours and inflammatory diseases of CNS have the highest risk of seizure recurrence; patients with focal (structural) lesions of CNS have higher risk of seizure recurrence than patient without focal neurological damage
Type of seizure	patients with partial seizures, particularly associated with Todd's post-ictal paresis, have higher percentage of seizure recurrence
EEG	appearance of the specific epileptiform abnormalities increases the risk
Duration of the follow-up	the risk decreases with time elapsed, the highest risk is in the first six months after the first seizure
Objective neurological examination	"positive finding" is an unfavourable factor (evidence of a structural lesion)
Febrile convulsion	history of febrile convulsions poses a higher risk of seizure recurrence
Family history	family history of epilepsy has been considered to be an unfavourable factor
Antiepileptic treatment	the lower risk of seizure recurrence with treatment initiation after the first seizure
Psychosocial environment	significant for the prognosis of the disease

Table 6. Factors influencing the risk of epileptic seizure recurrence (Berg & Shinnar, 1991).

2.2 Material and methods

We evaluated 116 patients (68 men, 48 women; age range 18-81 years) after a solitary epileptic seizure that had been hospitalized at our neurological department since January 1, 1997 to January 1, 2007. There were 84 patients having experienced an unprovoked seizure and 32 with an acute symptomatic epileptic seizure. The baseline information was obtained using a retrospective analysis of the medical records; eligible patients were contacted by telephone or by sending the questionnaire via the post. We evaluated the likelihood of seizure recurrence in 72 patients. Duration of the follow-up was 2 - 12 years. A certain portion of patients were followed prospectively at our outpatient department, others were monitored by their neurologists. We determined the number of patients in whom the seizure reoccurred, and time period between the first and the second epileptic seizures. We evaluated the following recurrence risk factors: incidence of the febrile convulsions; incidence of epilepsy in patients' relatives; period of the day, when the seizure appeared; objective neurological examination; the clinical type of seizure; EEG findings; aetiology of the seizure and the influence of antiepileptic treatment initiation after the first seizure. The logistic regression was used for the statistical assessment of the data obtained.

2.3 Results

The individual risk factors and their relation to the seizure recurrence after the first unprovoked epileptic seizure are shown in the Table 7.

The summary of the logistic regression:

i. Patients with the partial epileptic seizure had 5 times higher recurrence risk (OR = 5.12, 95 % CI: 0.79 - 32.89).

		Patients with seizure recurrence after the first epileptic seizure	Patients without seizure recurrence	Patients with seizure recurrence/ patients with seizure recurrence + without recurrence	Statistically significant factor in terms of the seizure recurrence?
Etiology	idiopathic + cryptogenic	12	18	12/30 (40%)	No
	late symptomatic	14	28	14/42 (33.3%)	
Period of the day, when the seizure appears	day-wakeful condition	17	32	17/49 (34.7%)	No
	sleep-arousal	9	14	9/23 (34.7%)	
Clinical type of the seizure	generalized	14	29	14/43 (32.5%)	No
	partial	12	17	12/29 (41.4%)	
EEG findings	normal + non-epileptic abnormality	20	36	20/56 (35.7%)	No
	epileptic abnormality	6	10	6/16 (37.5%)	
Objective neurological examination	normal	19	34	19/53 (35.8%)	No
	pathological	7	12	7/19 (36.8%)	
History of the febrile convulsions	Yes	0	2	0/2 (0%)	
	No	26	34	26/60 (43.3%)	
Family history of epilepsy	Yes	3	2	3/5 (60%)	No
	No	23	64	23/67 (34.3%)	
Antiepileptic treatment initiation after the first unprovoked epileptic seizure	Yes	6	31	6/37 (16.2%)	Yes
	No	20	15	20/35 (66.5%)	
Seizure recurrence after the first epileptic seizure within …	3 months	17		17/72(23.6%)	
	6 months	18		18/72 (25%)	
	1 year	24		24/72(33.3%)	
	3 years	25		25	
	5 years	26		26	

Table 7. The individual risk factors and their relation to the seizure recurrence after the first unprovoked epileptic seizure in our group of 72 patients.

ii. Patients with epileptiform EEG findings had 5 times higher recurrence risk (OR = 5.84, 95 % CI: 0.98 -34.62).

iii. The antiepileptic treatment initiation after the first seizure seems to be the only statistically significant protective factor as the patients in our group had 7 times lower recurrence risk compared to the patients without medication (OR= 0.13; 95% CI: 0.03 - 0,6).

After the first unprovoked epileptic seizure we recorded the seizure recurrence in 26/72 patients (36.1%); in 24/26 patients (92.3%) the seizure recurred within 12 months after the first unprovoked seizure.

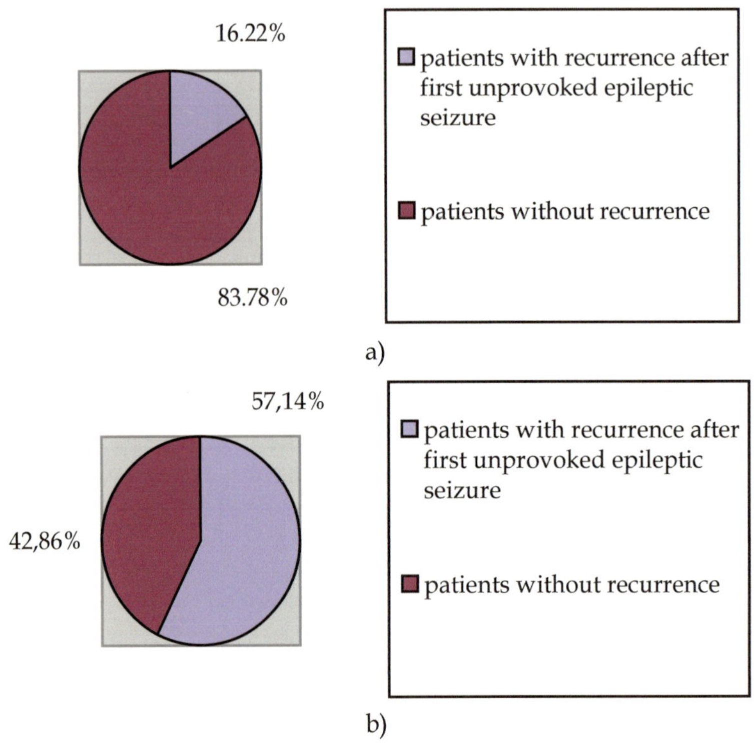

Fig. 1. Comparing the risk for recurrence in the group of patients , in which:
a) an antiepileptic treatment has been prescribed after first unprovoked epileptic seizure (n = 37)
b) an antiepileptic treatment has not been prescribed after first unprovoked epileptic seizure (n=35)

2.4 Discussion

The antiepileptic treatment initiation after the first unprovoked seizure was the only significant factor decreasing the risk of seizure recurrence (7 times lower in our study) (OR = 0.13, 95% CI: 0.03-0.6) in our group of 72 patients. The influence of antiepileptic treatment initiation on the reduction of seizure recurrence has also been reported in earlier studies (Elwes et al., 1985; Kollar et al., 2006). On the contrary, the significance of this factor was not shown in other studies (Bora et al., 1995; Hopkins et al., 1988; Musicco et al., 1997). In our patients there were risk factors of the seizure recurrence showing a clinical, but not statistical, significance - the type of epileptic seizure (5 times higher recurrence risk in patients after the first partial epileptic seizure: OR = 5.12; 95%, CI: 0.79 - 32.89) and EEG findings (5 times higher recurrence risk in patients with epileptiform EEG findings: OR = 5.84; 95% CI: 0.98 - 34.62). In consistence with the conclusions of Berg & Shinnar (1991) we observed a decrease of the recurrence risk of seizure with time that elapsed since the first seizure. The recurrence risk after the first unprovoked seizure was the highest within 12 months (24/26 patients, 92.3%). The differences in results of the studies evaluating the risk factors of seizure recurrence after the first unprovoked epileptic seizure may be attributed to unequal methods and baseline criteria, as well as to diverse durations of the follow-up. The meta-analyses performed help us orient ourselves in this area (Berg & Shinnar, 1991). In case of the first unprovoked epileptic seizure appearance there is a vital need for a thorough evaluation (Kollar et.al., 2009; Martiniskova et al., 2009).

3. Conclusion

The antiepileptic treatment initiation in patients after the solitary unprovoked epileptic seizure was the only statistically significant factor decreasing the risk of seizure recurrence in our group of patients. Based on the recent knowledge and despite of this finding we propose an individual, rather than automatic, antiepileptic treatment initiation, considering all risks, likelihood of seizure recurrence, social and psychological factors, employment and the potential side effects of the treatment.

4. Acknowledgment

This work is partially supported by the Slovak Science Grant Agency (VEGA No 1/0755/09, VEGA No 1/4266/07).

5. Abbreviations

Abbreviations in Table 1.

n = whole number of patients who underwent interictal EEG examination
n_1 = number of patients who underwent EEG after SD
n_2 = number of patients who underwent LTM-EEG after SD
(The numbers of patients are not identical, in same cases of diagnosed epileptic disorder or epileptic focus the whole EEG diagnostic algorithm was not needed.)
NFA = non-epileptiform focal EEG abnormality
NGA = non-epileptiform generalized EEG abnormality
EFA = epileptiform focal EEG abnormality
EGA = epileptiform generalized EEG abnormality

Abbreviations in Table 4.

EEG = native EEG examination
EEG after SD = EEG examination after sleep deprivation with one- hour recording
LTM-EEG after SD = 24-hour eight-channel EEG examination after sleep deprivation
n = number of patients
NFA = non-epileptiform focal EEG abnormality
NGA = non-epileptiform generalized EEG abnormality
EFA = epileptiform focal EEG abnormality
EGA = epileptiform generalized EEG abnormality

N - norm
P - pathology
0 - wasn't realized.
The clinical type of epileptic seizure /ILAE, 1981, being short/:
1 - The partial (focal) seizures:
1A - the simplex partial seizures
1B - the complex partial seizures
1C - the partial seizures with the secondary generalization
2 - The generalized seizures without focal beginning (convulsive or nonconvulsive):
2A - the absence
2B - the myoclonic seizures
2C - the tonic-clonic seizures
2D - the tonic seizures
2E – the atonic seizures
3 - The unclassified epileptic seizures
MT = more types of epileptic seizures

6. References

Angus-Leppan, H. (2008). Diagnosing epilepsy in neurology clinics: A prospective study. *Seizure.* Vol.17 , No. 5, (June 2008), pp. 431-436, ISSN 1059-1311

Annegers, JF.; Shirts, SB.; Hauser, WA. & Kurland, LT (1986). Risk of recurrence after an initial unprovoked seizure. *Epilepsia,* Vol. 27 , No. 1, (February 1986) pp. 43-50, ISSN 1528-1167

Bajaček, M.; Hovorka, J.; Nežádal, T.; Němcová, I. & Herman, E. (2010). Is pseudo-intractability in population of patients with epilepsy still alive in 21 century? Audit of 100 seizure free patients, referred with the diagnosis of pharmacoresistant epilepsy. *Neuroendocrinol Lett,* Vol.31, No.6, (February 2011), pp. 818-822, ISSN 0172-780X

Berg, AT. & Shinnar, S. (1991). The risk of seizure recurrence following a first unprovoked seizure: A quantitative review. *Neurology,* Vol.41, No.7, (July 1991), pp. 965-972, ISSN 0028-3878

Bora, I.; Seckin, B.; Zarifoglu, M.; Turan, F.; Sadikoglu, S. & Ogul, E. (1995). Risk of recurrence after first unprovoked tonic-clonic seizure in adults. *J Neurol,* Vol. 242, No.3, (February 2005), pp. 157- 163, ISSN 0340-5354

Bořuta, P.; Neuschl, V.; Glézlová, A. & Jánska, P. (2007). Úloha magnetickej rezonancie (MR) v diagnostike ochorení centrálneho nervového systému (CNS). [(The role of magnetic resonance imaging in the diagnosing of the central nervous diseases.) (In Slovak with English abstract.)]. *Neurológia,* Vol.2, No.2, (September 2007), pp. 121-126, ISSN 1336-8621

Carrilho, PG.; Yacubian, EM.; Cukiert, A.; Fiore, LA. ; Buchpiguel, CA. ; Jorge, CL.; Scapolan, HB.; Bacheschi, LA. & Marino Junior, R. (1994). MRI and brain spect findings in patients with unilateral temporal lobe epilepsy and normal CT scan. *Arq Neuropsiqiatr,* Vol.52, No.2, (June 1994), pp. 149-152, ISSN 0004-282X

Commission on Classification and Terminology of the International League Against Epilepsy (1981). Proposal for Revised Clinical and Electroencephalographic Classification of Epileptic Seizures. *Epilepsia,* Vol.22, No.4, (August 1981), pp. 489-501, ISSN 0013-9580

Dasheiff, R. (1987). First seizure management-reconsidered: Response III. *Arch Neurol,* Vol.44, No.11, (November 1987), pp. 1190-1191, ISSN 0003-9942

Elwes, RDC.; Chesterman, P. & Reynolds, EH. (1985). Prognosis after a first untreated tonic-clonic seizure. *Lancet,* Vol.326, No.2 (Issue 8458), (October 1985), pp. 752-753, ISSN 0140-6736

Engel, JJR. & Starkman, S. (1994). Overview of seizures. *Emerg Med Clin North Am,* Vol.12, No.4, (April 1994), pp. 895-923, ISSN 0733-8627

Forsgren, L.; Bucht, G.; Eriksson, S. & Bergmark, L. (1996). Incidence and clinical characterization of unprovoked seizures in adults: a prospective population-based study. *Epilepsia,* Vol.37, No. 3, (March 1996), pp. 224-229, ISSN 0013-9580

Fromm, GH. (1987). First seizure management-reconsidered: Response I. *Arch Neurol,* Vol.44, No.11, (November 1987), p. 1189, ISSN 0096-6886

Hauser, WA.; Anderson, WE.; Loewenson, RB. & Mcroberts, SM. (1982). Seizure recurrence after a first unprovoked seizure. *N Engl J Med,* Vol.307, No.9, (August 1982), pp. 522-528, ISSN 0028-4793

Hauser, WA., Rich, SS.; Annegers, JF. & Anderson, VE. (1990). Seizure recurrence after a 1st unprovoked seizure: An extend follow up. *Neurology,* Vol.40, No.8, (August 1990), pp. 1163-1170, ISSN 0028-3878

Hauser, WA.; Annegers, JF. & Kurland, LT. (1993). The incidence of epilepsy and unprovoked seizures in Rochester and Minnesota: 1935-1984. Epilepsia, Vol.34, No.3, (May-June 1993), pp. 453-468, ISSN 0013-9580

Hauser, WA.; Annegers, JF. & Rocca, WA. (1996). Descriptive epidemiology of epilepsy: contributions of population-based studies from Rochester, Minnesota. *Mayo-Clin-Proc.,* Vol.76, No.6, (June 1996), pp. 576-866, ISSN 0025-6196

Hopkins, A; Garman, A. & Clarke, C. (1988). The first seizure in adult life: value of clinical features, electroencephalography, and computerised tomography in predicition of seizure recurrence. *Lancet,* Vol.331, No.8588, (April 1988), pp. 721-726, ISSN 0140-6736

Hovorka, J. ; Herman, E. & Nežádal, T. (2004a). Epilepsie a zásady antiepileptické léčby – část 1. Diagnostika a léčba. [(Epilepsy and basic principles of the treatment- part 1: diagnosis and treatment.) (In Czech with English abstract.)]. *Psychiatr.prax,* Vol.5, No. 3, (September 2004), pp. 123-130, ISSN 1335-9584

Hovorka, J. ; Herman, E. & Nežádal, T. (2004b). Epilepsie a zásady antiepileptické léčby - část 2. Diagnostika a léčba - aspekty psychiatrické. [(Epilepsy and basic principles of the treatment- part 2: diagnosis and treatment.) (In Czech with English abstract.)]. *Psychiatr. prax,* Vol.5, No.4, (December 2004), pp. 181-186, ISSN 1335-9584

Hovorka, J.; Nezadal, T.; Herman, E.; Nemcova, I. & Bajacek, M. (2007). Psychogenic non-epileptic seizures, prospective clinical experience: diagnosis, clinical features, risk factors, psychiatric comorbidity, treatment outcome. *Epileptic Disorders,* Vol.9, Suppl.1, (December 2007), pp. S52-S58, ISSN 1294-9361

Perrig, S. & Jallon, P. (2008). Is the first seizure truly epileptic? *Epilepsia,* Vol.49, Suppl.1, (January 2008), pp. 2-7, ISSN 0013-9580

Kawkabani, A.; Rossetti, AO. & Despland, PA. (2004). Survey of management of first-ever seizures in a hospital based community. Swiss Med Wkly, Vol.134, No.39/40, (October 2004), pp. 586-592, ISSN 1424-3997

King, MA.; Newton, MR.; Jackson, GD.; Fitt, GJ. ; Mitchell, LA.; Silvapulle, MJ. & Berkovic, SF. (1998). Epileptology of the first-seizure presentation: a clinical, electroencephalographic, and magnetic resonance imaging study of 300 consecutive patients. Lancet, Vol.352, No.9133, (September 1998), pp. 1007-1011, ISSN 0140-6736

Kollar, B.; Buranova, D.; Goldenberg, Z.; Klobucnikova, K. & Varsik, P. Solitary epileptic seizure - the risk of recurrence. *Neuroendocrinol Lett*, Vol.27, No.1-2, (April 2006), pp. 16-20, ISSN 0172-780X

Kollár, B. & Klobučniková, K. (2009). Zhodnotenie nálezov „natívneho" interiktálneho EEG EEG, EEG po SD s dobou snímania 1 hodinu a 24-hodinového LTM-EEG po SD u nami hospitalizovaných pacientov po solitárnom nevyprovokovanom epileptickom záchvate, so sporadickými epileptickými záchvatmi a u pacientov s „chronickou" epilepsiou. [(Evaluation of "native" interictal EEG, EEG following a sleep deprivation (SD) with 1-hour recording and 24-hour, long-term monitoring (LTM) following SD findings in hospitalized patients after a solitary unprovoked epileptic seizure and sporadic epileptic seizures and in "chronic" epilepsy patients.) (In Slovak with English abstract.)]. Neurológia, Vol.4, No.2, (September 2009), pp. 106-112, ISSN 1336-8621

Kollar, B.; Martiniskova, Z.; Klobucnikova, K.; Vachalova, I. & Waczulikova, I. (2009). Solitary epileptic seizures in the clinical practice. Part II: Findings of various modifications of EEG examination and imaging methods in patients who experienced solitary unprovoked epileptic seizure. *Neuroendocrinol Lett*, Vol.30, No.4, (September 2009), pp. 487- 490, ISSN 0172-780X

Kollar, B.; Klobucnikova, K.; Fecikova, A. & Borovska, J. (2010). Difficulties in diagnosis of solitary and sporadic epileptic seizures. *Neuroendocrinol Lett*, Vol.31, No.6, (February 2011), pp. 814-817, ISSN 0172-780X

Kuba, R.; Kára, T.; Brázdil, M.; Křížová, J.; Souček, M.; Novák, M. & Rektor, I. (2001). Neurokardiogenní synkopa - interiktální a iktální EEG studie. [(Neurocardiogenic syncope - interictal and ictal EEG study.) (In Czech with English abstract.)]. *Cesk Slov Neurol N*, Vol.64, No.2, (April 2001), pp. 100-108, ISSN 1210-7859

Mann, MW. (2005). Management of first epileptic seizure in adults. *Rev Prat*, Vol.55, No.3, (February 2005), pp. 265- 270, ISSN 0035-2640

Martiniskova, Z.; Kollar, B. ; Vachalova, I.; Klobucnikova, K. ; Waczulikova, I. & Goldenberg, Z. (2009). Solitary epileptic seizures in the clinical practice. Part I: Etiological factors responsible for their occurrence. *Neuroendocrinol Lett*, Vol.30, No.4, (September 2009), pp. 482-486, ISNN 0172-780X

Musicco, M.; Beghi, E.; Solari, A. & Viani, F. (1997). Treatment of first tonic-clonic seizure does not improve the prognosis of epilepsy. First Seizure Trial Group (FIRST Group). *Neurology*, Vol.49, No.4, (October 1997), pp. 991-998, ISSN 0028-3878

Ošlejšková, H. (2007). Zhoršování epileptických záchvatu a epilepsií antiepileptiky - je to možné? [(Worsening of epileptic seizures and epilepsies due to antiepileptic drugs - is it possible?) (In Czech with English abstract.)]. *Cesk Slov Neurol N*, Vol.70, No.2, (April 2007), pp. 137-142, ISSN 1210-7859

Pedley, TA.; Scheuer, ML. & Walczak, TS. (1995). Epilepsy, In: *Merritt´s Textbook of Neurology*, Rowland, LP. (editor), pp. 845-868, Williams and Wilkins, ISBN: 0683074008 Baltimore (9th ed.)

Shinnar, S.; Kang, H.; Berg, AT.; Goldensohn, ES.; Hauser, WA. & Moshe, SL. (1994). EEG abnormalities in children with a first unprovoked seizure. *Epilepsia*, Vol. 35, No.3, (May 1994), pp. 471-476, ISSN 0013-9580

Vojtěch, Z. (2008). Klinická elektroencefalografie v epileptologii. [(Clinical electro-encephalography in epileptology.) (In Czech)]. Neurol. prax, Vol., No.2, (April 2008), pp. 73-78, ISSN 1335-9592

Part 2

Clinical Applications

3

The Clinical Application of Transcranial Magnetic Stimulation in the Study of Epilepsy

Wang Xiao-Ming and Yu Ju-Ming
Institute of Neurological Diseases, North Sichuan Medical College, Sichuan Nanchong
PR China

1. Introduction

Several methods can be used to treat patients with epilepsy: antiepileptic drugs(AED), surgery and neuromodulation. AED is the most common method and also the first choice in the treatment of epilepsy. However, some patients are drug-resistant, or encounter severe adverse effects. In this case, surgery is an alternative to drug therapy for part of these patients. But surgery has several drawbacks: one is its invasive, the other is its high cost, and the third is its requirement for highly equipped medical devices to delineate the epileptiogenic zones. These factors limit its wide use in the clinical field.

Epileptic conditions are characterized by an altered balance between excitatory and inhibitory influences at the cortical level(Tassinari et al.,2003). Antiepileptic drugs work by counteracting such imbalance with different mechanisms(Kwan et al.,2001). It is well known that the excitability of cortical networks can be modulated in humans by trains of regularly repeated magnetic stimuli(Wassermann&Lisanby,2001). Therefore, Repetitive transcranial magnetic stimulation (rTMS), a noninvasive and easily applied technology, could even have therapeutic effect in epileptic patients. Although some conflicting results have been reported, growing evidence shows that low-frequency (<1Hz) rTMS (slow rTMS) can significantly reduce seizure frequency and interictal epileptiform discharges. In this chapter, we aim at providing the reader with the most recent information on the application of TMS in epileptic conditions.

This chapter is composed of 6 sections. First, the different ways and parameters that TMS can be used to investigate cortical pathophysiology are introduced. According to the patterns of stimulation, TMS can be divided into at least 3 categories: single-pulse TMS (sTMS), paired-pulse TMS (pTMS) and repetitive TMS (rTMS). Each TMS may reflect different brain cortical functions or have different physiologic effects. The parameters used as TMS study include motor evoked potential (MEP), motor threshold (MT), cortical silent period (CSP), intracortical inhibition (ICI) and intracortical facilitation (ICF). These parameters can reflect the functional state in motor cortex and motor pathway in different ways.

The second section will discuss the possible antiepileptic mechanisms of rTMS in four aspects: electrophysiology, neurotransmitters, ion channel structure and function, as well as neuronal insults.

The third section will refer to two issues: the effects of different AEDs on TMS parameters; the relationship between the changes of TMS parameters and corresponding AED serum concentrations. The available data suggest that TMS may be a promising tool both in clarifying still-debated mechanisms of action of some AEDs and in optimizing the treatment of patients affected by epileptic seizures.

We will review the therapeutic effect of rTMS on patients with epilepsy in the fourth section. Although conflicting results have been reported, growing evidence supports slow frequency rTMS is effective in reducing seizure frequency and /or decreasing the EEG epileptiform abnormalities. Some problems will be also referred to in this section.

The safety issue of rTMS is another topic for this chapter. Currently available data showed that TMS is a safe technique, both in normal subjects and neurologically impaired patients. No long-lasting effects on cognitive, motor or sensory functions have been reported. As far as seizures are concerned, only 6 seizures have been elicited by rTMS in 6 non-epileptic individuals by the end of 1996. Although high-frequency rTMS may induce accidental seizures in normal subjects and epileptics, slow frequency rTMS has not been shown to induce seizures in patients with epilepsy. The safety issue of TMS will address in a separate paragraph.

The final section will discuss the prospects of rTMS. As a noninvasive, easily applied and safe technology, rTMS may be an effective adjunctive treatment for patients with refractory epilepsy, and may provide a valuable insight into pathophysiological mechanisms underlying epileptic processes and AED-induced changes of the excitability of cortical networks. In addition, rTMS changes induced by different AEDs could be used as a neurophysiological index to optimize the treatment in a given patient. More work is needed to do before wide use of rTMS in the epileptic field.

2. TMS techniques and measures of motor excitability

TMS has mainly three categories: single-pulse TMS (sTMS), paired-pulse TMS (pTMS) and repetitive TMS (rTMS). Single-pulse TMS refers to stimulation with a conventional stimulator, which delivers pulses no faster than 1 Hz. It can be used to obtain motor threshold (MT) and cortical silent period (CSP). Paired-pulse TMS techniques involve a conditioning pulse followed by a test stimulus, which are delivered to the same scalp position through a single coil. It has been used to study intracortical inhibition and facilitation. Repetitive TMS indicates trains of regularly repeated magnetic pulses delivered to a single scalp site(Wassermann,1998). It can also stimulate neurons in unresponsive period, thus preferentially activating tangentially-oriented connecting neurons, which produce excitatory postsynaptic potentials and disrupt the balance between cortical excitability and inhibition.

The parameters used to study experimentally and clinically mainly include motor evoked potential (MEP), motor threshold (MT), cortical silent period (CSP), intracortical inhibition (ICI), and intracortical facilitation (ICF). MEP reflects the excitability of the whole corticospinal system. MEP size increases with contraction of the target muscle, and increases with stimulus intensity in a sigmoid manner. The part of the MEP intensity curve close to MT is determined by the excitability of low-threshold corticospinal neurons, and the high-intensity part of the MEP intensity curve reflects the excitability of high-threshold neurons (Devanne et al.,2002). MEP size may be modulated by inputs to motor cortex from the periphery or other parts of the brain. MEP is a reliable tool to monitor focal cortical excitability.

MT is the minimum stimulus intensity needed to elicit a small motor response in the target muscle, in at least half of 10 consecutive trials. MT can be determined at rest (RMT) or during slight isometric muscle activation (AMT). RMT is determined by the excitability of corticocortical axons and the excitability of synaptic contacts between these axons and corticospinal neurons and between corticospinal neurons and their target motorneurons in the spinal cord. Whereas, AMT is mainly determined by the excitability of corticocortical axons and therefore mainly reflects membrane-related excitability and correlates with ion channels(Hallett ,2007).

CSP refers to a period of silence in the electromyographic pattern of a voluntarily contracted target muscle. Its size reflects the length of intracortical inhibition. The early part of the CSP reflects the inhibitory effect at spinal level, and the late part reflects inhibition at the level of the motor cortex. It is conceived that the late part of the CSP is determined by long-lasting cortical inhibition mediated through the γ-aminobutyric acid type B receptor(Hallett,2007; Ziemann et al.,2006).

Intracortical inhibition (ICI) and intracortical facilitation (ICF) are two parameters provided by pTMS, which reflect neuronal inhibition and excitability, respectively. It is thought that paired-pulse measures reflect mainly synaptic excitability of various inhibitory and excitatory neuronal circuits at the level of the motor cortex. This synaptic excitability is controlled mainly by neurotransmission through the GABA and N-methyl-D-aspartate (NMDA) receptors. Short-interval intracortical inhibition (SICI) and long-interval intracortical inhibition (LICI) underlie separate mechanisms and may reflect inhibition mediated through the $GABA_A$ and $GABA_B$ receptors, respectively(Ziemann et al.,2006; Sanger et al 2001).

3. Possible antiepileptic mechanisms of rTMS

The pathogenic mechanism of epilepsy is very complicated. It may involve several aspects, including the imbalance of cortically excitatory and inhibitory activities, disturbance of neurotransmitter, abnormality of the structure and/or function of ion channels, decrease of endogenous neuropeptides, and metabolic disorder in the brain. Whether rTMS affects epileptic seizure through one or more abovementioned factors is almost unknown. Some pilot researches in this aspect are summarized as follows.

3.1 Electrophysiologic mechanism

Some clinical studies found that RMT and intracortical inhibition in untreated epileptic patients decreased remarkably, and the more the RMT decreased, the more frequently the seizure attacked(Kotova &Vorob'eva,2007). Inghilleri et al reported that CSP in the epileptogenic hemisphere was much shorter than in the contralateral hemisphere(Inghilleri et al.,1998). Cincotta and coworkers found CSP got much longer after receiving 30 minutes, 0.3 Hz rTMS(Cincotta et al.,2003). These studies suggested, for one thing, that imbalance between excitatory and inhibitory neurons existed unquestionably, for another, that rTMS may strengthen the inhibitory effect and therefore regain a new balance, thus leading the seizure decrease or remission. In our recent study, we found that the rats injected intraperitoneally with epileptogenic dose of pilocarpine immediately followed by 40-minute rTMS treatment (0.5 Hz, 95% RMT) had much milder seizure and lower rate of SE development in 90-minute follow-up period, compared with rats without rTMS treatment (not published). This result makes us reasonably infer that the quick antiepileptic effect of rTMS more likely resulted from its direct modulation on the activity of excitatory and inhibitory neurons in the cortex than from its indirect effect by inducing the enhancement of endogenous inhibition. Therefore, Modulating the excitability and inhibition in the cortical neurons may be one of the antiepileptic mechanisms of rTMS.

3.2 Neurotransmitter mechanisms

Neurotransmitters in the brain functionally include excitatory neurotransmitters and inhibitory neurotransmitters, which represent by glutamate andγ-aminobutyric acid, respectively. In normal state, the excitatory neurotransmitters and the inhibitory neurotransmitters maintain a balance. Once the activity of excitatory neurotransmitters becomes hyperactive, or the activity of inhibitory neurotransmitters remarkably decreases, a seizure may occur. N-methyl-D-aspartate (NMDA) receptor-1 is one of the most important glutamate receptors and also the main mediator of calcium ion channel and epileptogenic factor. GAD65 is the key enzyme in the process of GABA synthesis and it has the quality of high specificity and stability. Therefore, NMDAR1 and GAD65 usually act as two marks to evaluate the levels of glutamate and GABA in the brain, respectively.

Zhang et al in the rat pilocarpine seizure model found that the rats pretreated with two-week rTMS (administered at 0.5 Hz, 95%MT) had increased expression of GAD65 and decreased expression of NMDAR1 in the hippocampal CA1, which investigated at 90 minutes after injecting pilocarpine(Zhang et al.,2008). Michael et al in the study of healthy volunteers adopted proton magnetic resonance spectroscopy (MRS) to investigate the effects of high frequency rTMS on brain metabolism. They found that the content of glutamate had a pronounced change not only around the stimulating zone but also the remote areas (ipsilateral and contralateral to the stimulus site) (Michael et al.,2003). Zangen et al in the experimental study also found that the glutamate in the stimulated left prefrontal cortex increased significantly after high frequency rTMS(Zangen&Hyodo,2002). These results suggested that low-frequency and high-frequency rTMS may have different effects on excitatory and inhibitory neurotransmitters or their receptors. The antiepileptic effect of low-frequency rTMS might be related to the upregulation of GAD65 expression and downregulation of NMDAR1 in the hippocampus.

Clinical study on patients with epilepsy revealed a dynamic change for ICI and ICF(Turazzini et al.,2004). The CSP had no longer linear relation with the stimulus intensity when the patients with focal epilepsy were administered at a certain stimulus intensity(Cicineli et al.,2000). Some researchers reported that the changes of GABA receptors are proportional to the changes of ICI, whereas the changes of glutamate receptors are proportional to the changes of ICF(Sanger et al.,2001; Hamer et al.,2005; Issac,2001). In addition, some studies demonstrated that the late part of CSP was determined by LICI, which was mediated through $GABA_B$ receptors.

3.3 Ion channel structure and function mechanisms

It is clear that seizures are linked to membrane potentials, ionic fluxes, and action potential generation. In neurons, action potential generation results primarily from changes in the membrane permeability to four ions: sodium, chloride, calcium, and potassium. These ions enter and exit neurons by way of voltage-dependent channels. Once the ion channel functions abnormally, the ionic concentrations intracellularly and extracellularly will probably change and result in ictal discharges or seizures.

Genetic study has shown that the mutation of the gene coping KCNQ2 and KCNQ3 leads to benign neonatal familial convulsions. But whether or not rTMS is able to affect the gene of ion channels is unknown. Theodore found that rTMS was able to change the flow velocity and distribution of sodium and calcium, and therefore affect membrane permeability (Theodore ,2003). Our most recent study, pretreating rats for two weeks with 0.5 Hz rTMS before making pilocarping-induced model, showed that rTMS can transiently downregulate the expression of sodium channel subunit SCN1A, but upregulate the expression of potassium channel subunit Kcal 1.1 in the hippocampus, and the latter effect maintained at least six weeks (not published). These results suggest that by changing the expression of ion channel genes may be another antiepileptic mechanism of rTMS.

3.4 Protective mechanism

It is well known that the over expression of Bcl-2 can inhibit neuron apoptosis resulted from multiple factors, such as overload of calcium, oxygen free radicals, glutamate and deficiency of neural growth factors(Zhong et al.,1993). This may be one of the self rescue mechanisms. Ke et al found that one-week daily rTMS before making rat pilocarpine seizure model can lead to Bcl-2 upregulation in the hippocampus CA1(Ke et al.,2010). Song et al in a similar study also found that rTMS can inhibit neuronal apoptosis, lessen necrosis resulted from apoptosis in the temporal tissue(Song&Tian,2004). MRS study showed that the hippocampal content of choline-containing compounds (CHO) in the rTMS treated chronic temporal lobe epilepsy (TLE) rats was much lower than that in the rTMS untreated chronic TLE rats. This implied that rTMS delayed or alleviated gliosis in the rTMS treated TLE rats(Song &Tian,2005). Post et al. in their study found that rTMS resulted in a significant increase of secreted amyloid precursor protein (SAPP) in the hippocampal neurons, which is a kind of spanning membrane glucoprotein, similar to cell surface receptor in structure(Postet al.,1999). SAPP has multiple effects, including protecting neurons, promoting cell survival, and stimulating neuronal axon growing. The above-mentioned study suggested that rTMS may have the ability to protect against the insult from TLE. This effect may be its another mechanism in counteracting epilepsy, especially chronic epilepsy.

3.5 Other mechanisms

3.5.1 Metabolism

Some studies showed that both high-frequency rTMS and low-frequency rTMS can change the brain metabolism, not only in the stimulating areas, but also in the remote zones(Michael et al.,2003;Song &Tian,2005; McCann et al.,1998). In a clinical trial, Speer adopted high-frequency rTMS (20 Hz) and low-frequency rTMS (1 Hz) to treat patients with depression, and used positive emission tomography(PET) to measure the brain metabolism. They found that high-frequency rTMS had a better outcome in patients with hypermetabolisms, but low-frequency rTMS had a better outcome in patients with hypometabolisms(Speer et al.,2009). This result suggested that high-frequency rTMS and low-frequency rTMS may affect the brain metabolisms in opposite way: low-frequency rTMS reduces metabolism, high-frequency rTMS enhances metabolism. It is therefore reasonably deduced that the antiepileptic effect of low-frquency rTMS may be related to its ability to reduce the brain metabolism.

3.5.2 Regional cerebral blood flow (rCBF)

Both high-frequency rTMS and low-frequency rTMS can affect the change of regional cerebral blood flow in the stimulated areas. Graff-Guerrero et al described two patients with epilepsia partialis continua(Graff-Guerrero et al.,2004). They investigated these two patients by single photon emission computed tomography (SPECT) before and after rTMS treatment. They found that both have hyperperfusion in the epileptogenic zones before rTMS. But this phenomenon abolished after rTMS treatment. Therefore, modulation of rCBF around the epileptogenic zone may contribute to the control of seizures.

3.5.3 Endogenous antiepileptic mechanism

Anschel et al did an interesting experiment. In this study, they administered a patient with depression with rTMS for 8 consecutive days, then they injected the cerebrospinal flow into the lateral ventricle of rats. They surprisingly found that the flurothyl-kindling effect was significant mitigated(Anschel et al,2003). This result suggested that the CSF of the rTMS treated patient must contain some endogenous antiepileptic substance. Therefore, it reasonably infers that rTMS may have the ability to stimulate the release of some endogenous antiepileptic substances.

4. Effects of AEDs on TMS parameters and their clinical values

4.1 TMS parameters versus AEDs and their possible mechanisms

Extant data show that the effects of different antiepileptic drugs on TMS parameters are variable. It has been found that the MT is increased after acute administration of the voltage-dependent sodium channel blockers carbamazepine (CBZ), lamotrigine (LTG), and phenytoin (PHT)(Boroojerdi et al.,2001), and the maximum MT was observed at the plasma peak time in normal subjects(Ziemann et al.,1996). These findings were also reported in epileptic patients. However, many patients were under chronic AED treatment at the time of TMS testing. This suggests that the increased MT may result from the threshold increasing effect of AEDs in epileptic patients. This view was directly supported by the demonstration that untreated groups of patients with idiopathic generalized epilepsy(IGE)(Reutens et al.,1993) or benign epilepsy with centrotemporal spikes(Nezu et al.,1997) had reduced or normal RMT values compared with healthy controls. However, RMT in the patient groups increased significantly above normal level when remeasured after the commencement of treatment with valproic acid(Reutens et al.,1993; Nezu et al.,1997). In a study on temporal lobe epilepsy patients, RMT significantly increased with the number of AEDs taken by the patients(Hufnagel et al.,1990). In one subgroup of this study, RMT dropped significantly after tapering AED treatment(Hufnagel et al.,1990). On the contrary, some studies found RMT is increased in untreated IGE patients(Gianelli et al.,1994). This elevation of MT may reflect cortical dysfunction after the seizure or is likely a protective mechanism against spread or recurrence of seizures. For these reasons, some researchers applied TMS to evaluate the antiepileptic effects of PHT and CBZ monotherapy. They found a higher MT and a lower MEP in the PHT group than those in CBZ group, which implies PHT may have stronger inhibitory effect on cortical excitability compared with CBZ(Goyal et al.,2004).
In contrast to ion channel blocker intake, a single dose of drugs enhancing γ-aminobutyric acid (GABA)-medicated inhibitory neurotransmission, such as baclofen, diazepam, ethanol, lorazepam, tiagabine, and vigabatrin, does not modify the MT in healthy subjects (Tassinari, 2003), but may change the cortical silent period duration (CSP), intracortical facilitation (ICF), and intracortical inhibition (ICI) (Tassinari,2003). Reis et al found that topiramate, which can enhance the GABA-mediated inhibitory effect and counteract the toxic effect of excitatory amino acid, is able to elevate ICI but does not affect MT and CSP(Reis et al.,2002).

Another study showed that gabapentin had no effect on MT, but reduced the ICF, increased ICI and CSP(Rizzo et al.,2001). This suggests that gabapentin may enhance the GABAergic neurotransmission. In a study on levetiracetam, MT significantly increased, but CSP, ICI, and ICF unchanged(Reis et al.,2004). This implies that levetiracetam may have block effect on sodium channel.

In summary, the relationship between TMS parameters and AEDs is complicated. Ziemann reviewed the literatures and concluded that ion channel blocker AEDs can elevate MT, but have no effect on CSP, ICI and ICF, whereas, enhancing GABAergic AEDs, such as lorazepam, diazepam, vigabatrin, and tiagabine, mainly affect CSP, SICI, ICF, SICF, but have no effect on MT (see table 1)(Ziemann, 2004) MEP can be used as one of the most sensitive indexes in investigating the effects of AEDs.

drug	Mode of action	TMS variables					
		MT	MEP	CSP	SICI	ICF	SICF
CBZ	Na^+	1+	0	1+	0/0	0/1-	0
PHT	Na^+	2+	0/0	0/0			
LTG	Na^+	3+	1-	0	0/0	0/0	0
VPA	Na^+/GABA	0		0	0	0	
LZP	GABA	0/0/0	2-	1+	0/2+	0/1-	1-
DZP	GABA	0/0	1-/0	0/1-	0/1+	1-	1-
TP	GABA	0	1-	0			
VGB	GABA	0	0/0	0/0	0	1-	1-
TGB	GABA	0	0	1+	1-	1+	

carbamazepine: CBZ, phenytoin: PHT, lamotrigine: LTG, valproate: VPA, lorazepam: LZP, diazepam: DZP, thiopental: TP, vigabatrin: VGB, tiagabine: TGB; no clear change: 0, increase: 1+, clear increase: 2+, significant increase: 3+, decrease: 1-, clear decrease: 2-.

Table 1. Effects of antiepileptic drugs on TMS variables

Sohn et al(Sohn et al.,2004) summarized corresponding MEP changes after using sodium channel blocker LTG and GABA receptor agonist thiopental and lorazepam, and transferred these changes into curves. They found that both of the sodium channel blocker and GABA receptor agonist made the curves shift down.

The early part of the CSP is easily affected by spinal inhibitory mechanisms, whereas the late part most probably reflects inhibition specifically at the level of the motor cortex (Hallett,2007; Ziemann et al.,2006). It is thought that this late part of the CSP is determined by long-lasting cortical inhibition (LICI) medicated through the GABA type B receptor. Interestingly, AEDs (CBZ, LZP) with different modes of action may produce similar CSP prolongation, whereas those with the same modes of action (LZP, DZP) may result in different CSP changes, which are shown in table 1(Sohn et al.,2004; Sundaresan et al., 2007). These inconsistent findings suggest further study is needed to clarify the relationship between TMS variables and AEDs.

It is thought that LICI may reflect the long-last inhibition mediated by $GABA_B$ receptors. Therefore, the pronounced enhancement of LICI may be the result of the potentiated neurotransmission mediated through the postsynaptic $GABA_B$ receptors(Werhahn et al.,1999). Short-interval intracortical inhibition (SICI) may reflect the inhibition mediated through $GABA_A$ receptors. Most of the $GABA_A$ receptor agonists, such as LZP, DZP may increase SICI. The duration of SICI correlates with that of the inhibitory postsynaptic potential which is mediated through $GABA_A$ receptors. Combined with inter-stimulus intervals, SICI can be used in ICF evaluation. This suggests that the excitatory interneurons, which mediate ICF, are controlled by inhibitory interneurons, and this influences are dose-dependent(Reis et al.,2004; Ye&Zhang,2000). AEDs of sodium channel blockers exert no clear effect on SICI, as opposed to ICF.

4.2 The relation between TMS variables and the plasma concentrations of AEDs

The relation between RMT and the plasma concentration of AEDs shows a sigmoid(Della Paschoa et al.,2000). A study on 16 healthy subjects taking LTG showed a linear relation between the MT and the LTG plasma concentration (in the range of 430ng to 2500ng/ml)(Tergau et al.,2003). Cantello et al demonstrated that the MT and the plasma concentration, in a study of 15 patients with symptomatic epilepsy taking VPA, had a positive linear relation, whereas a sigmoid relation in 18 healthy subjects (Cantello et al., 2006). Werhahn et al reported that the dose of TGB had a positive linear relation with CSP and ICF. Although TGB can affect SICI, the relation between the dose and SICI is unclear(Werhahn et al.,1999). In a study of CBZ, Turazzini administered 10 patients with symptomatic epilepsy with daily 200mg dose of CBZ, and with an increment of 200mg every other day, then maintained at 800mg daily. They found a linear relation between RMT increases and the serum concentration of CBZ before a stable level after they monitored the changes of serum CBZ and TMS parameters at a certain interval in 2 months(Turazzini et al.,2004). They also found in this study that MEP, CSP, SICI and ICF had no pronounced changes(Turazzini et al.,2004). Lee et al demonstrated a similar effect of CBZ and LTG on MT in the 5-week duration of observation in 20 volunteers, but this was mainly seen at the late stage, and can be explained as follow-up effect(Lee et al.,2005).

4.3 Prospect of TMS in the study of AEDS

TMS variables may be helpful to investigate the unknown mechanisms of some AEDs. Although single- and paired-pulse TMS parameters show sigh variability across subjects, their interside and longitudinal intraindividual variability is lower. Therefore, repeated recordings in the same subjects appear to be a sensitive tool to disclose minor AED-induced changes(Tassinari et al,2003). Furthermore, the threshold intensity varied with the changes of AED dose, or had a positive linear relation with serum levels of AEDs. This suggests that monitoring the change of TMS threshold intensity, just as monitoring the plasma drug concentration and electroencephalography (EEG), could be acted as a tool to guide optimum use of AEDs. In addition, according to the correlation of drug serum concentration and TMS parameters, TMS might be used as an adjunctive means to monitor brain cortical excitability when studying the pharmacodynamics of AEDs. This implies that TMS may be used to evaluate the newly developed antiepileptic drugs.

5. The therapeutic effect of rTMS on patients with epilepsy

5.1 Experimental animal study

A series of animal studies have shown that low-frequency rTMS has antiepileptic effect, and this effect is frequency dependent. Akamatsu et al demonstrated that rTMS of 1000 pulses at

0.5 Hz led to a prolonged latency for seizure development and a lower ratio of status epilepticus after an intraperitoneal injection of pentylenetetrazol in Wistar rats(Akamatsu et al.,2001). Godlevsy and coworkers(Godlevsky et al.,2006) experimented on male WAG/Rij rats with rTMS of 3 impulses at 0.5 Hz and combined recording of electrocorticograms. They found that such stimulation engendered a reduction of spike-wave discharge bursts duration, which was most pronounced in 30 minutes from the moment of cessation of stimulation, but bursts of spike-wave discharges restored up to pre-stimulative level in 90-150 minutes. This result suggested that rTMS possessed an ability to produce short-time suppression of bursts of spike-wave discharges in WAG/Rij rats, a gene model of absence seizure. Rotenberg et al(Rotenberg et al.,2008) tested the anticonvulsive potential of rTMS with different stimulation frequency in the rat kainic acid seizure model. They divided 21 rats into three groups in which individual seizures were treated with rTMS trains at one of three frequencies: 0.25, 0.5 or 0.75 Hz. The rTMS treatments were guided by simultaneous EEG monitoring, that is, rTMS treatment (active rTMS, sham rTMS, or untreat) was administered only when consecutive seizures occurred. They found that KA-induced seizures were abbreviated by 0.75 Hz and 0.5 Hz active EEG-guided rTMS, but neither active 0.25 Hz rTMS nor the control conditions affected seizure duration. This result indicated that rTMS has therapeutic potential, but is frequency dependent. Ke Sha et al(Ke et al.,2010), as well as Huang Min et al(Huang et al.,2009), also investigated the efficacy of a range of rTMS frequencies, but in another model: pilocarping seizure model. They divided rats into different groups according to the rTMS frequency delivered at the treatment, and pretreated each rat with corresponding frequency's rTMS for consecutive two weeks. After finished the pretreatment, each rat was given an intraperitoneal injection of pilocarpine. They demonstrated that pretreatment with TMS at 0.3, 0.5, 0.8, and 1.0 Hz all led to a longer latency of seizure onset, but 0.5 Hz and 0.8 Hz rTMS treatment engendered the longest latency for seizure development and conspicuous anticonvulsive effects.

5.2 Clinical study

Tergau and coworkers(Tergan et al.,1999) first reported the treatment of rTMS on patients with epilepsy in 1999. In their trial, nine patients with medically refractory frontal epilepsy were enrolled. All patients had more than seven focal or secondarily generalized seizures per week in the 6 months before rTMS treatment. After rTMS, which was delivered over the vertex with two trains of 500 pulses at a frequency of 0.33 Hz on 5 consecutive days, weekly seizure frequency dropped significantly from an average of 10.3to 5.8. Seizures did not occur during rTMS. After 6 to 8 weeks, seizure frequency returned to baseline level. Since then, a lot of clinical reports were followed (see Table 2-4). Fregni et al(Fregni et al., 2006) randomly divided 21 patients with refractory epilepsy into active rTMS group and sham rTMS group. rTMs was administered with 5 trains of 1200 pulses and an intensity of 70% rMT at frequency of 1 Hz on 5 consecutive days. They noticed that, compared with sham rTMS group, the seizure frequency and the number of spikes in ictal EEG were significantly reduced, and their cognition was also improved after rTMS. This effect lasted at least 2 months. Santiago-Rodriguez et al(Santiago-Rodriguez et al.,2008) evaluated the number of seizures and interictal epileptiform discharges (IEDs) in 12 patients with focal neocortical epilepsy before, during and after rTMS. rTMS was administered with 900 pulses at 0.5 Hz for 2 consecutive weeks at 120% rMT. They found that the mean seizure frequency decreased from 2.25 per week (basal period) to 0.66 per week (intervention period), a 71%

reduction (p=0.0036). In the 8-week follow-up period the mean seizure frequency was 1.14 per week, which corresponds to a 50% reduction compared with basal period. Moreover, EEG analysis displayed IED frequency was also reduced; it decreased from 11.9 (baseline) to 9.3 (during 2 weeks of rTMS) with a further reduction to 8.2 in the follow-up period. These differences on EEG however were not significant (p=0.190). Joo et al(Joo et al.,2007) investigated the antiepileptic effect of low-frequency rTMS in 35 patients with intractable epilepsy. Patients were divided into a focal stimulation group with a localized epileptic focus, or a non-focal stimulation group with a non-localized or multifocal epileptic focus. Each group was then randomly subdivided into 3000 pulses and 1500 pulses subgroups. rTMS was administered at 0.5 Hz for 5 consecutive days at 100% of rMT. Weekly seizure frequency were determined for 8 weeks before and after rTMS, and the number of interictal spikes before (1st day) and after rTMS (5th days) were also compared. They demonstrated that interictal spikes significantly decreased (-54.9%, p=0.012) and even totally disappeared in 6 patients after rTMS. Although mean weekly seizure frequency was non-significantly decreased after rTMS, longer stimulation subgroups (3000pulses,-23.0%) tended to have fewer seizures than shorter stimulation subgroups (1500pulses,-3.0%), without statistical significance. They also found TMS stimulation site and structural brain lesions did not influence seizure outcome. Wang et al(Wang et al.,2008)randomly divided 30 patients with temporal lobe epilepsy, which was determined with dipole source, into drug group and rTMS group, each group with 15 patients. Drug group were given antiepileptic drug only (AED)(camazepine, 600-800mg daily, three times a day); rTMS group were given rTMS treatment as well as AED (camazepine, 600-800mg daily, three times a day). rTMS was administered using Dantec Maglite-r25 with 500 pulses at 1 Hz for consecutive seven days at intensity of 90% MT. After 7 days of rTMS treatment, both groups continued to take AED. They found that seizure frequency had no significant difference between rTMS group and drug group. However, interictal spikes decreased significantly in rTMS group compared with drug group on the 30 th day after rTMS.

Regrettably, the results of rTMS in the treatment of epilepsy almost exclusively came from interictal epileptic patients. There are very few studies based on ongoing seizures. Nevertheless, Rotenberg and coworkers' study is encouraging(Rotenberg et al.,2009). In their study, seven patients with epilepsia partialis continua (EPC) of mixed etiologies were treated with rTMS over the seizure. rTMS was delivered in high-frequeny (20-100 Hz) bursts or as prolonged low-frequency (1 Hz) trains. The result is that rTMS led to a brief (20-30 min) pause in seizures in three of seven patients and a lasting (no less than one days) pause in two of seven. Seizures were not exacerbated by rTMS in any patient. Only mild side effects including trainsient head and limb pain, and limb stiffening during high-frequency rTMS train occurred.

Above-mentioned studies both clinically and experimentally indicate that rTMS is effective and safe in the treatment of epilepsy. It can not only decrease seizure frequency, but also reduce spikes firing, even terminate ongoing seizures. Some researchers have recommended rTMS to be a method to treat refractory epilepsy. Novertheless, it will be a long way before rTMS really puts to clinical practice. The reason is that current data about effectiveness of rTMS mainly resulted from small size trials, even case report, lack of convincingly large size and randomly controlled trials, and that the parameters (including stimulus frequency, intensity, number of stimuli, train duration, intertrain interval, coil type, and stimulation sites) used in rTMS studies or treatment are different among researchers (see table 5). This may be why some incongruent, even conflicting results occurred.

First author and publish time	Subjects	Epilepsy syndorme	Seizure frequency pre-TMS	Seizure frequency Post-TMS	Epileptiform Discharges Post-TMS
Menkes, 2000	1	ETLE	37/month	Reduction	Reduction
Cantello, 2002	1	Primary generalized	NR	No reduction	Reduction
Rossi, 2004	1	EPC	EPC	Reduction	Reduction
Graff-Guerrero 2004	2	EPC	EPC	Reduction in one of two patients	Reduction
Misawa,2005	1	EPC	EPC	Reduction for two month	NR
Mecarelli, 2006	1	Focal	NR	Reduction	No Reduction
Brighina, 2006	9	Focal=3 Multifocal=6	NR	Reduction only during protocol	NR

ETLE=extra temporal lobe epilepsy; MTLE= mesial temporal lobe epilepsy; TLE=temporal lobe epilepsy; NR=not reported; EPC= Epilepsia partialis continua.

Table 2. Impact of rTMS on epilepsy(Case report study)

First author and publish time	Subjects	Epilepsy syndorme	Seizure frequency pre-TMS	Seizure frequency post-TMS	Epileptiform Discharges Post-TMS
Tergau, 1999	9	TLE=2 ETLE=7	10.3±6.6/w	5.8±6.4/w	NR
Daniele, 2003	4	Frontal=2 Multifocal=2	19/month(focal), 36/month(multifocal)	Reduction(in patients with single focus)	NR
Brasil-Neto, 2004	5	TLE=2 ETLE=3	1.4±0.09/d	Reduction	NR
Fregni 2005	8	TLE=3 Multifocal=4 ETLE=1	3-6.2/w	Reduction for 1 month	Reduction for 1 month
Kinoshita, 2005	7	Focal	16.5±5.2/w	Reduction	NR
Santiago-Rodriguez, 2008	12	Focal	2.25/w	Reduction	No reduction
Rotenberg 2009	7	EPC	EPC	Reduction	NR
Wei Sun 2011	17	Refractory partial	14.09±16.55/w	Reduction	No reduction

d=day;w=week

Table 3. Impact of rTMS on epilepsy(Open-label study)

First author and publish time	Subjects	Epilepsy syndorme	Seizure frequency pre-TMS	Seizure frequency post-TMS	Epileptiform Discharges post-TMS
Theodore 2002	12	Focal	3.4±1.2/w	No reduction	NR
Tergau 2003	17	MTLE/ETLE/ Multifocal/Generalized	NR	Reduction (only0.33 HZ)	NR
Fregni 2006	12	Focal	13.6±10.1/28d	Reduction (at least two month)	Reduction (at least two month)
Joo 2007	35	Focal/Multifocal/Non-localized	9.9±10.1/w (NF group) 7±9.6/w (F group)	Trend for reduction	Reduction
Cantello, 2007	43	Focal	9.1±2.2/w	No reduction	Reduction
Wang 2008	15	TLE	1.9±0.4/w	No reduction	Reduction

Table 4. Impact of rTMS on epilepsy (Double-blinded and sham-controlled study)

6. The safety issue of rTMS

Although extant researches have shown that rTMS is a promising tool in treating epilepsy, its safety and tolerability have been the focus of concerns. rTMS does have the potential for short-term adverse side effects such as headache, tinnitus, insomnia, discomfort at the site of stimulation, but its long-term adverse side effects are unknown. Studies in normal human subjects have shown that rTMS had no long-term adverse effects on blood pressure, heart rate, balance, gait, sensory function, motor function, memory and cognition(Pascual-Leone et al.,1993; Hufnagel et al.,1993), and found no changes in electroencephalogram (EEG), electrocardiogram (ECG), serum hormone(Jahanshahi et al.,1997). Studies of the anatomical effects of rTMS have shown that conventional and diffusion-weighted magnetic resonance imaging are normal following long duration, high-intensity rTMS that exceeded safety guidelines, and MRI is normal following rTMS used for 2 weeks in treating depression (Anand S&Hotson J,2002). Moreover, no pathological changes are seen in resected temporal lobe tissue following approximately 2000 pulses(Gates et al.,1992). In addition, metabolic study showed that proton magnetic responance spectroscope (MRS) revealed no significant alterations of N-acetyl-aspartate, creatine and phosphocreatine, choline-containing compounds, myo-inositol, glucose and lactate, and post mortem histology revealed no changes in microglial and astrocytic activation following rTMS regimen of 1000 stimuli used for 5 consecutive days at 1 Hz(Liebetanz et al.,2003).

Another safety issue of rTMS is its effect on cognition(Anand S&Hotson J,2002). Most safety studies have not reported adverse long-term effects in cognitive function in subjects receiving rTMS. One study found degradation in short term verbal memory immediately following rTMS, but the effect did not persist following the study and was attributed to the short inter-train intervals that were also cause seizures in normal subjects. Performance on standard neuropsychological tests is not adversely affected by rTMS sessions; instead, verbal memory tends to improve and motor reaction time tends to decrease.

First author and publish time	Frequency (Hz)	Intensity	Stimuli	Schedule	Coil form	Position
Tergau, 1999	0.33	100%rMT	500/train	5trains/d* 5d	Round	Vertex
Menkes, 2000	0.5	95%rMT	20/train	5trains/ d*bw*3m	Round	EGF
Cantello, 2002	5	120%MT	NR	Onset of spikes	NR	NR
Theodore, 2002	1	120%MT	900/train	2train/d*7d	Figure-of-eight	EGF
Tergau, 2003	0.33, 1	below MT	1000/train	1train/d*5d	Round	Vertex
Daniele, 2003	0.5	90%MT	100/train	bw*4w,	Figure-of-eight	EGF/ vertex
Rossi, 2004	1	90%rMT	900	Single session	Figure-of-eight	EGF
Brasil-Neto, 2004	0.3	95%MT	20/train	5trains/d*BW*3 m	Round	Vertex
Graff-Guerrero 2004	20	50%, 128%MT	40/train	15days	Figure-of-eight	EGF
Fregni 2005	0.5	65%MSO	600	Single session	Figure-of-eight	EGF/ vertex
Kinoshita 2005	0.9	90%rMT	810/train	2trains/d*5d*/ w*2w	Round	FCz, PCz
Fregni 2006	1	70%MSO	1200/train	1train/d* 5 d	Figure-of-eight	EGF/ vertex
Mecarelli 2006	0.33	100%rMT	500/train	2train/d *5 d	Round	Vertex
Brighina 2006	5	100%rMT	100/train	20d	Figure-of-eight	Near inion
Joo, 2007	0.5	100%MT	3000/train / 1500/train	1train/d* 5 d	Round	Vertex/ temporal
Cantello, 2007	0.3	100%MT/ 65%MSO	500/train	2trains/d*5 d	Round	Vertex
Santiago-Rodriguez, 2008	0.5	120%rMT	900/train	1train/d*2 w	Figure-of-eight	EGF
Wang, 2008	1	90%MT	900/d	7 d	Figure-of-eight	EGF
Rotenberg, 2009	100, 20, 1	100%MT	NR	Difference	Figure-of-eight	EGF

bw=biweek; m=month; MSO=maximum stimulator output intensity; EGF=epileptogenic focus.

Table 5. Brain stimulation parameters

The third safety issue of rTMS is its effect on endocrine system(Anand&Hotson,2002). One study found no change in hormonal levels in humans following rTMS, but a decrease in serum prolactin levels, which is opposite the effect seen after a seizure, and an increase in thyroid-stimulating hormone level, which accompanied an improved mood, were found following rTMS.

The greatest concern with rTMS is the induction of seizures. Even in normal healthy subjects, prolonged, high intensity, rTMS with rate of 10-25 Hz can produce partial seizure with or without secondary generalization. After analyzing thousands of rTMS treated patients, Rosa et al(Rosa et al.,2004) think TMS is safety. They found only 6 patients had an occasional seizure, and the risk factors of seizures elicited by TMS included brain tumor, stroke, inflammation, severe trauma, increased cranial pressure, idiopathic epilepsy, uncontrolled epilepsy, taking some drugs which reduce the threshold of seizures such as tricyclic antidepressants, excessive drinking, and use of stimulant drugs.

The guidelines released by National Healthy Institute of America in 1998 believed that rTMS was relative contradindication to patients with epilepsy, but safe on the condition of strictly controlling stimulating parameters and regular operation(Wassermann,1998). Schrader et al (Schrader et al.,2004) concluded from the analysis of some studies that the peak rate of seizure occurrence related to TMS was 2.8 percent in sTMS, 3.6 percent in pTMS, and the modes of onset were similar to their typical attack; no long-term adverse effects were found and the increased seizure frequency could not exclude the possibilities of intractable epilepsy, decreased use of medication, improper operation and strongly stimulating intensity. Studies of safety evaluation of the combinations of parameters (0.5 Hz, 50 pulses; 8 Hz, 1000 pulses; 20 Hz, 1500 pulses; 25 Hz, 1200 pulses) showed that rTMS delivered in any combination of parameters was safe(Liebetanz et al.,2003; Frye et al.,2008; Post et al.,1999). Bae EH et al(Bae et al.,2007) performed an English-language literature search, and reviewed all studies published from January 1990 to February 2007 in which patients with epilepsy were treated with rTMS. They found that the adverse events attributed to rTMS were generally mild and occurred in 17.1% of subjects; headache was most common, occurring in 9.6%; seizures occurred in 4 patients (1.4%); all but one case were the patients' typical seizures with respect to duration and semiology, and were associated with low-frequency rTMS; a single case had atypical seizure appearing to arise from the region of stimulation during high-frequency rTMS; no rTMS-related episodes of status epilepticus were reported. They concluded that rTMS appeared to be nearly as safe in patients with epilepsy as in nonepileptic individuals.

Based on the consideration of safety, current studies support to use slow-frequency rTMS for the purpose of treatment in epilepsy. As for selecting of parameters, which include stimulus frequency, intensity, intertrain interval, and stimulus site, it should depend on individuals and comply with some norms. Besides, the accurate localization of the stimulus site is also the important part of safety study(Hoffman et al.,2005).

Wassermann (1998) provided a comprehensive report of new guidelines based on the deliberations of an "International Workshop on the Safety of Repetitive Transcranial Magnetic Stimulation, Jun 5-7, 1996." He reiterated three requirements central to research on human subjects, namely, the need for informed consent, the requirements that the potential benefit of the research outweighs the risk as independently assessed by an investigational review board, and the need "for equal distributions of the burdens and the benefits of the research" The research should not be conducted on categories of vulnerable patients or subjects who are likely to bear the burden of the research without the potential for benefit.

Wassermann suggested three types of studies appropriate for rTMS. First are studies where there are reasons to expect direct benefit to patients, such as the treatment of major depression. Second are studies of the pathophysiology of a brain disorder that may add information leading to new therapeutic strategies. These studies would include the participation of normal subjects as controls. Third are studies in normal subjects or patients that are expected to produce original and important observations about brain function that can not be obtained by safer methods.

7. Prospects of rTMS in the study of epilepsy

As a noninvasive, easily applied and safe technology, rTMS may be an effective adjunctive treatment for patients with refractory epilepsy, and may provide a valuable insight into pathophysiological mechanisms underlying epileptic processes and AED-induced changes of the excitability of cortical networks. In addition, rTMS changes induced by different AEDs could be used as a neurophysiological index to optimize the treatment in a given patient. However, the best regimen of rTMS delivering has not been determined. Multiple central collaborative studies are necessary to establish optimum stimulation parameters, such as stimulus frequency, intensity, number of stimuli, train duration, intertrain interval, coil type, and stimulation sites. With study going on, it is probable that rTMS will be an effective therapeutic tool and be widely used in clinical practice. What's more, it is hopeful that the research into mechanisms of epileptogenicity may also break through by using rTMS.

8. References

Akamatsu N, Fueta Y, Endo Y, Matsunaqa K, Uozumi T & Tsuji S.(2001) Decreased susceptibility to pentylenetetrazol-induced seizures after low-frequency transcranial magnetic stimulation in rats. *Neurosci Lett* vol.310,No.(2-3),(2001 Sep),pp.(153-156), ISSN 0304-3940.

Anand S, Hotson J.(2002) Transcranial magnetic stimulation: neurophysiological applications and safety. *Brain cogn* vol.50,No.3,(2002 Dec),pp.(366-386), ISSN 0278-2626.

Anschel DJ, Pascual-Leone A & Holms GL.(2003) Anti-kindling effect of slow repetitive transcranial magnetic stimulation in rats. *Neurosci Lett* vol.351,No.1,(2003 Nov),pp.(9–12), ISSN 0304-3940.

Bae EH,Schrader LM,Machii K, Alonso-Alonso M, Riviello JJ Jr, Pascual-Leone A & Rotenberg A.(2007) Safety and tolerability of repetitive transcranial magnetic stimulation in patients with epilepsy: a review of the literature. *Epilepsy Behav* vol.10,No.4,(2007 Jun),pp.(521-528), ISSN 1525-5050.

Boroojerdi B, Battaglia F, Muellbacher W & Cohen LG.(2001) Mechanisms influencing stimulus-response properties of the human corticospinal system. *Clin Neurophysiol* vol.112,No.5,(2001 May),pp.(931-937), ISSN 1388-2457.

Brasil-Neto JP, de Araujo DP, Teixeira WA, Araujo VP & Boechat-Barros R.(2004) Experimental therapy of epilepsy with transcranial magnetic stimulation: lack of additional benefit with prolonged treatment. *Arq Neuropsiquiatr* vol.62,No.1,(2004 Mar),pp.(21-25), ISSN 0004-282x.

Brighina F, Daniele O, Piazza A, Giqlia G & Fierro B.(2006) Hemispheric cerebellar rTMS to treat drug-resistant epilepsy: case reports. *Neurosci lett* vol.397,No.3,(2006 Apr),pp.(229-233), ISSN 0304-3940.

Cantello R.(2002) Prolonged cortical silent period after transcranial magnetic stimulation in generalized epilepsy. *Neurology* vol.58,No.7,(2002 Apr),pp.(1135-1136), ISSN 0022-3751.

Cantello R, Civardi C, Varrasi C, Vicentini R, Cecchin M, Boccaqni C & Monaco F.(2006) Excitability of the human epileptic cortex after chronic valproate: a reappraisal. *Brain Res* vol.1099,No.1,(2006 Jun-Jul),pp.(160-166), ISSN 0006-8993.

Cantello R, Rossi S, Varrasi C, Ulivelli M, Civardi C, Bartalini S, Vatti G, Cincotta M, Borqheresi A, Zaccara G, Quartarone A, Crupi D, Lagana A, Inghilleri M, Giallonardo AT, Berardelli A, Pacifici L, Ferreri F, Tombini M, Gilio F, Quarato P, Conte A, Manqanotti P, Bonqiovanni LG, Monaco F, Ferrante D&Rossini PM.(2007) Slow repetitive TMS for drug-resistant epilepsy: clinical and EEG findings of a placebo-controlled trial. *Epilepsia* vol.48,No.2,(2007 Feb),pp(366-374), ISSN 0013-9580.

Cicineli P,Mattia D, Spanedda F, Traversa R, Marciani MG, Pasqualetti P, Rossini PM & Bernardi G.(2000) Transcranial magnetic stimulation reveals an interhemispheric asymmetry of cortical inhibition in focal epilepsy. *Neuroreport* vol.11,No.4,(2000 Mar),pp.(701-707), ISSN 0959-4965.

Cincotta M, Borgheresi A, Gambetti C, Balestrieri F, Rossi L, Zaccara G, Ulivelli M, Rossi S,Civardi C & Cantello R.(2003) Suprathreshold 0.3 Hz repetitive TMS prolongs the cortical silent period: potential implications for therapeutic trials in epilepsy. *Clin Neurophysiol* vol.114,No.10,(2003 Feb),pp.(1827–1833), ISSN 1388-2457.

Daniele O, Brighina F, Piazza A, Giqlia G, Scalia S & Fierro B.(2003) Low-frequency transcranial magnetic stimulation in patients with cortical dysplasia-a preliminary study. *J Neurol* vol.250,No.6,(2003 Jun),pp(761-762), ISSN 0022-3077.

Della Paschoa OE, Hoogerkamp A, Edelbroek PM, Voskuyl RA & Danhof M. Pharmacokinetic-pharmacodynamic correlation of lamotrigine, flunarizine, loreclezole, CGP40116 and CGP39551 in the cortical stimulation model.(2000) *Epilepsy Res* vol.40,No.1,(2000 Jun),pp.(41-52), ISSN 0920-1211.

Devanne H, Cohen LG, Kouchtir-Devanne N & Capaday C. (2002) Integrated motor cortical control of task-related muscles during pointing in humans. *J Neurophysiol* vol.87,No.6,(2002 Jun),pp.(3006-3017), ISSN 0022-3077.

Fregni F, Thome-Souza S, Bermpohl F, Marcolin MA, Herzoq A, Pascual-leone A & Valente KD.(2005) Antiepileptic effects of repetitive transcranialmagnetic stimulation in patients with cortical malformations: an EEG and clinical study. *Stereotact Funct Neurosurg* vol.83,No.(2-3),(2005 Jun),pp.(57-62), ISSN 1011-6125.

Fregni F, Otachi PT, Do Valle A, Boqqio PS, Thut G, Riqonatti SP, Pascual-Leone A & Valente KD. (2006)A randomized clinical trial of repetitive transcranial magnetic stimulation in patients with refractory epilepsy. *Ann Neurol* vol.60,No.4,(2006 Oct),pp.(447-455), ISSN 0364-5134.

Frye RE,Rotenberg A,Ousley M & Pascual-Leone A.(2008) Transcranial magnetic stimulation in child neurology: current and future directions. *J Child Neurol* vol.23,No.1,(2008 Jan),pp.(79-96), ISSN 0883-0738.

Gates JR, Dhuna A, & Pascual-Leone A.(1992) Lack of pathologic changes in human temporal lobes after transcranial magnetic stimulation.*Epilepsia* vol.33,No.3, (1992 May-Jun),pp.(504-508), ISSN 0013-9580.

Gianelli M, Cantello R, Civardi C, Naldi P, Bettucci D, Schiavella MP & Mutani R.(1994) Idiopathic generalized epilepsy: magnetic stimulation of motor cortex time-locked and unlocked to 3-Hz spike-and-wave discharges. *Epilepsia* vol.35,No.1,(1994 Jan-Feb),pp.(53-60), ISSN 0013-9580.

Godlevsky LS, Kobolev EV, van Luijtelaar EL, Coenen AM, Stepanenko KI & Smirnow IV.(2006) Influence of transcranial magnetic stimulation on spike-wave discharges in a genetic model of absence epilepsy. *Indian J Exp Biol* vol.44,No.12,(2006 Dec),pp.(949-954), ISSN 0019-5189.

Goyal V, Bhatia M & Behari M.(2004) Increased depressant effect of phenytoin sodium as compared to carbamazepine on motor excitability: a transcranial magnetic evaluation. *Neurol India* vol.52,No.2,(2004 Jun),pp.(224-227), ISSN 0028-3886.

Graff-Guerrero A, Gonzáles-Olvera J, Ruiz-García M, Avila-Ordonez U, Vauqier V & Garcia-Reyna JC.(2004) rTMS reduces focal brain hyperperfusion in two patients with EPC. *Acta Neurol Scand* vol.109,No.4,(2004 Apr),pp.(290-296), ISSN 0001-6314.

Hallett M.(2007) Transcranial magnetic stimulation: a primer. *Neuron* vol.55,No.2,(2007 Jul),pp.(187- 199), ISSN 0896-6273.

Hamer HM, Reis J, Mueller HH, Knake S, Overhof M, Oertel WH & Rosenow F.(2005) Motor cortex excitability in focal epilepsies not including the primary motor area--a TMS study. *Brain* vol 128,No.pt4,(2005 Apr),pp.(811-818), ISSN 0006-8950).

Huang M, Yu JM, Wang XM, & Wang L.(2009) The effects of pretreatment with low-frequency transcranial magnetic stimulation on rats with pilocarpine-induced seizures. *Chinese Journal of physical medicine and rehabilitation.* Vol.31, No,4 ,(2009); pp. (228-231) ISSN 0254-1424.

Hoffman RE,Gueorguieva R,Hawkins KA, Varanko M, Boutros NN, Wu YT, Carroll K & Krystal JH.(2005) Temporoparietal transcranial magnetic stimulation for auditory hallucinations: safety, efficacy and moderators in a fifty patient sample. *Biology Psychiatry* vol.58,No,2,(2005 Jul),pp.(97-104), ISSN 0006-3223.

Hufnagel A, Elgeer CE, Marx W & Ising A.(1990) Magnetic motor-evoked potentials in epilepsy: effects of the disease and of anticonvulsant medication. *Ann Neurol* vol.28,No.5,(1990 Nov),pp.(680-686), ISSN 0364-5134.

Hufnagel A, Claus D, Brunhoelzl C & Sudhop T.(1993)Short-term memory: no evidence of effect of rapid-repetitive transcranial magnetic stimulation in healthy individuals. *J Neurol* vol.240,No,6,(1993 Jun),pp.(373–376), ISSN 0022-3077.

Inghilleri M, Mattia D, Berardelli A & Manfredi M. (1998) Asymmetry of cortical excitability revealed by transcranial stimulation in a patient with focal epilepsy and cortical myoclonus. *Electroencephalogr Clinic Neurophysiol* vol 109,No.1,(1998 Feb),pp.(70-72), ISSN 0013-4694.

Issac M. (2001) The 5-HT2C receptor as a potential therapeutic target for the design of antibesity and antiepileptic target for the design of antiobesity and antiepileptic drugs. *Drugs Future*, 2001;vol 26pp.(389- 393).ISSN0377-8282.

Jahanshahi M, Ridding MC, Limousin P, Profice P, Foqel W, Dressler D, Fuller R, Brown RG, Brow P & Rothwell JC.(1997)Rapid rate transcranial magnetic stimulation-a safe study. *Electroenceph clin Neurophysiol* vol.105,No.6,(1997 Dec),pp.(422-429), ISSN 0013-4694.

Joo EY, Han SJ, Chung SH, Cho JW, Seo DW & Hong SB.(2007) Antiepileptic effects of low-frequency repetitive transcranial magnetic stimulation by different stimulation durations and locations. *Clin Neurophysiol* vol.118,No.3,(2007 Mar) pp.(702-708), ISSN 1388-2457.

Ke Sha, Zhao HN, Wang XM , Zhang JQ, Chen F, Wang YX, Zhao XQ, Huang H & Hu JX.(2010) Pretreatment with low-frequency repetitive transcranial magnetic stimulation may influence neuronal Bcl-2 and Fas protein expression in the CA1 region of the hippocampus. *Neural Regeneration Research* vol. 5,No.12,(2010 May),pp.(895-900), ISSN 1673-5374.

Kinoshita M, Ikeda A, Begum T, Yamamoto J, Hitomi T & Shibasaki H. (2005) Low-frequency repetitive transcranial magnetic stimulation for seizure suppression in patients with extratemporal lobe epilepsy: a pilot study. *Seizure* vol.14,No.6,(2005 Sep),pp.(387-392), ISSN 1059-1311.

Kotova OV, Vorob'eva, OV. (2007) Evoked motor response thresholds during transcranial magnetic stimulation in patients with symptomatic partial epilepsy. *Neurosci Behav Physiol* vol.37,No.9,(2007 Nov),pp(849-852), ISSN 0097-0549.

Kwan P, Sills GJ, Brodie MJ.(2001) The mechanisms of action of commonly used antileptic drugs. *Pharmacol Ther* vol 90,No.1,(2001 Apr), pp.(21-34),ISSN 0163-7258.

Lee HW, Seo HJ, Cohen LG, Baqic A & Theodore WH.(2005) Cortical excitability during prolonged antiepileptic drug treatment and drug withdrawal. *Clin Neurophysiol* vol.116,No.5,(2005 May),pp.(1105-1112), ISSN 1388-2457.

Liebetanz D, Fauser S, Michaelis T, Czeh B, Watanabe T, Paulus W, Frahm J & Fuchs E.(2003) Safety aspects of chronic low-frequency transranial magnetic stimulation based on localized proton magnetic resonance spectroscopy and histology of the rat brain. *J Psychiatr Res* vol.37,No.4,(2003 Jul-Aug),pp.(277-286), ISSN 0022-3956.

McCann UD, Kimbrell TA, Morgan CM, Anderson T, Geraci M, Benson BE, Wassermann EM, Willis MW & Post RM.(1998) Repetitive Transcranial magnetic stimulation for posttraumatic stress disorder. *Arch Gen Psychiat* vol.55,No.3,(1998 Mar), pp.(276-279), ISSN 0003-990x.

Mecarelli O, Greqori B, Gilio F, Conte A, Frasca V, Accornero N&Inghilleri M.(2006) Effects of repetitive transcranial magnetic stimulation in a patient with fixation-off sensitivity. *Exp Brain Res* vol.173,No.1(2006 Aug),pp.(180-184), ISSN 0014-4819.

Menkes DL, Gruenthal M.(2000)Slow-frequency repetitive transcranial magnetic stimulation in a patients with focal cortical dysplasia. *Epilepsia* vol 41,No.2,(2000 Feb),pp.(240-242), ISSN 0013-9580.

Michael N, Gosling M, Reutemann M, Kersting A, Heindel W, Arolt V & Pfleiderer B.(2003) Metabolic changes after repetitive transcranial magnetic stimulation (rTMS) of the left prefrontal cortex: a sham-controlled proton magnetic resonance spectroscopy (IH MRS) study of healthy brain. *Eur J Neurosci* vol.17,No.11,(2003 Jun),pp.(2462-2468), ISSN 0953-816x.

Misawa S, Kuwabara S, Shibuya K, Mamada K & Hattori T.(2005)Low-frequency transcranial magnetic stimulation for epilepsia partialis continua due to cortical dysplasia. *J Neurol Sci* vol.234,No.(1-2),(2005 Jul),pp.(37-39), ISSN 0022-510x.

Nezu A, Kimura S, Ohtsuki N & Tanaka M.(1997) Transcranial magnetic stimulation in benign childhood epilepsy with centro-temporal spikes. *Brain Dev* vol.19,No.2,(1997 Mar),pp.(134-137), ISSN 0387-7604.

Pascual-Leone A, House CM, Reese K, Shotland LI, Grafman J, Sato S, Valls-Sole J, Brasil-Neto JP, Wassermann EM & Cohen LG.(1993) Safety of rapid-rate transcranial magnetic stimulation in normal volunteers. *Electroencephalogr Clin Neurophysiol* vol.89,No.2,(1993 Apr),pp.(120-130), ISSN 0013-4694.

Post A, Mariannne B, Engelmann M & Keck ME.(1999) Repetitive transcranial magnetic stimulation in rats: evidence for aneuro protective effect in vitro and in vivo. *Eur J Neurosci* vol.11,No.9,(1999 Sep) ,pp.(3247-3254), ISSN 0953-816x.

Reis J, Tergau F, Harmer HM, Muller HH, Knake S, Fritsch B, Oertel WH & Rosenow F.(2002) Topiramale selectively decreases motor cortex excitability in human motor cortex. *Epilepsia* vol.40,No.10,(2002 Oct),pp.(1149-1156), ISSN 0013-9580.

Reis J, Wentrup A, Hamer HM, Mueller HH, Knake S, Tergan F, Oertel WH & Rosenow F.(2004) Levetiracetam influences human motor cortex excitability mainly by modulation of ion channel function---a TMS study. *Epilepsy Res* vol.62,No.1,(2004 Nov),pp.(41-51), ISSN 0920-1211.

Reutens DC, Berkovic SF , Macdonell RA&Bladin PF. (1993) Magnetic stimulation of the brain in generalized epilepsy: reversal of cortical hyperexcitability by anticonvulsants. *Ann Neurol* vol.34,No.3,(1993 Sep) ,pp.(351-355), ISSN 0364-5134.

Rizzo V, Quartarone A, Bagnato S, Battaqlia F, Majorana G & Girlanda P.(2001) Modification of cortical excitability induced by gabapentin: a study by transcranial magnetic stimulation. *Neurol Sci* vol.22,No.3,(2001 Jun),pp.(229-232), ISSN 0022-510x.

Rosa MA, Odebrecht M, Rigonatti SP & Marcolin MA.(2004) Transcranial magnetic stimulation：review of accidental seizures. *Rev Bras de Psiquiatr* vol.26,No.2,(2004 Jun),pp.(131-134), ISSN 1516-4446.

Rossi S, Ulivelli M, Bartalini S, Galli R, Passero S, Battistini N & Vatti G.(2004) Reduction of cortical myoclonus-related epileptic activity following slow-frequency rTMS. *Neuroreport* vol.15,No.2,(2004 Feb),pp.(293-296), ISSN 0959-4965.

Rotenberg A, Muller P, Birnbaum D, Harrinqton M, Riviello JJ, Pascual-leone A & Jensen FE.(2008) Seizure suppression by EEG-guided repetitive transcranial magnetic stimulation in the rat. *Clin Neurophysiol* vol.119,No.12,(2008 Dec),pp.(2697-2702), ISSN 1388-2457.

Rotenberg A, Bae EH, Takeoka M, Tormos JM, Schachter SC & Pascual-Leone A.(2009) Repetitive transcranial magnetic stimulation in the treatment of epileosia partialis continua. *Epilepsy Behav* vol.14,No.1,(2009 Jan),pp.(253-257), ISSN 1525-5050.

Sanger TD, Tarsy D, Pascual-Leone A.(2001) Abnormalities of spatial and temporal sensory discrimination in writer's cramp. *Mov Disord* vol.16,No.1,(2001 Jan),pp. (94-99), ISSN 0885-3185.

Santiago-Rodriguez E, Cardenas- Morales L, Harmony T, Fernandez-Bouzas A, Porras-Kattz E & Hernandez A.(2008) Repetitive transcranial magnetic stimulation decreases the number of seizures in patients with focal neocortical epilepsy. *Seizure* vol.17,No.8,(2008 Dec),pp.(677-683), ISSN 1059-1311.

Schrader LM, Stern JM, Koski L, Nuwer MR & Enqel J Jr.(2004)Seizure incidence during single and paired-pulse transcranial magnetic stimulation(TMS) in individuals with epilepsy. *Clin Neurophysiol* vol.115,No.12,(2004 Dec),pp.(2728-2737), ISSN 1388-2457.

Sohn YH, Kaelin-Lang A, Jung HY & Hallett M.(2001) Effect of levetiracetam on human corticospinal excitability. *Neurology* vol.57,No.5,(2001 Sep),pp.(858-863), ISSN 0028-3878.

Song YJ, Tian X.(2004) Effects of low-frequency transcranial magnetic stimulation on apoptosis of temporal lobe and hippocampus in rats with temporal lobe epilepsy. *Chinese Journal of Neuroscience* vol.20,No.1,(2004 Jan),pp.(14-17), ISSN 1008-0872.

Song YJ, Tian X. (2005) Effects of transcranial magnetic stimulation on hippocampus metabolic function in rats with temporal lobe epilepsy. *Chinese Journal of Physical medicine and rehabilitation*, vol.27,No.2,(2005 Feb),pp.(75-78), ISSN 0254-1424.

Speer AM, Benson BE, Kimbrell TK, Wassermann EM, Willis MW, Herscovitch P & Post RM.(2009) Opposite effects of high and low frequency rTMS on mood in depressed patients: relationship to baseline cerebral activity on PET. *J Affect Disord* vol.115,No.3,(2009 June),pp.(386-394), ISSN 0165-0327.

Sun W, Fu W, Mao W, Wang D & Wang Y.(2011) Low-frequency repetitive transcranial magnetic Stimulation for the treatment of refractory partial epilepsy. *Clin EEG Neurosci* vol.42,No.1,(2011 Jan),pp.(40-44), SSIN 1550-0594.

Sundaresan K, Ziemann U, Stanley J & Boutros N.(2007) Cortical inhibition and excitation in abstinent cocaine-dependent patients: a transcranial magnetic stimulation study. *Neuroreport* vol.18,No.3,(2007 Feb),pp.(289-292), ISSN 0959-4965.

Tassinari CA, Cincotta M, Zaccara G & Michelucci R.(2003) Transcranial magnetic stimulation and epilepsy. *Clin Neurophysiol* vol.114, N0.5,(2003 may),pp.(777-798),ISSN 1388-2457.

Tergan F, Naumann U, Paulus W & Steinhoff BJ.(1999) Low-frequency repetitive transcranial magnetic stimulation improves intractable epilepsy. *Lancet* vol.353,No.9171,(1999 Jun),pp.2209, ISSN 0140-6736.

Tergau F, Wischer S, Somal HS, Nitsche MA, Mercer AJ, Paulus W & Steinhoff BJ. (2003) Relationship between lamotrigine oral dose, serum level and its inhibitory effect on CNS: insights from transcranial magnetic stimulation. *Epilepsy Res* vol.56,No.1,(2003 Sep),pp.(67-77), ISSN 0920-1211.

Tergau F, Neumann D, Rosenow F, Nitsche MA, Paulus W & Steinhoff B.(2003) Can epilepsies be improved by repetitive transcranial magnetic stimulation? Interim analysis of a controlled study. *Suppl Clin Neurophysiol* vol.56,(2003),pp.(400-405), ISSN 1567-424x.

Theodore WH, Hunter K, Chen R, Vega-Bermudez F, Boroojerdi B, Reeves-Tyer P, Werhahn K, Kelley KR & Cohen L.(2002). Transcranial magnetic stimulation for the treatment of seizures: a controlled study. *Neurology* vol.59,No.4,pp.(560-562), ISSN 0028-3878.

Theodore WH. (2003) Transcranial magnetic stimulation in epilepsy. *Epilepsy Curr* vol.3,No.6,(2003 Nov), pp.(191-197), ISSN 1535-7511.

Turazzini M, Manganotti P, Del Colle R, Silvestri M & Fiaschi A .(2004)Serum levels of carbamazepine and cortical excitability by magnetic brain stimulation .*Neurol Sci* vol 25,No.2,(2004 Jun),pp.(83-90), ISSN 0022-510x.

Wang XM, Yang DB, Wang SX, Zhao XQ, Zhang LL, Chen ZQ & Sun XR.(2008) Effects of low-frequency repetitive transcranial magnetic stimulation on electroencephalogram and seizure frequency in 15 patients with temporal lobe epilepsy following dipole source localization. *Neural Regeneration Research* vol.3,No.11,(2008),pp.(1257-1260), ISSN 1673-5374.

Wassermann EM.(1998) Risk and safety of repetitive transcranial magnetic stimulation: report and suggested guidelines from the International Workshop on the Safety of Repetitive Transcranial Magnetic Stimulation. *Electroencephaloqr Clin Neurophysiol* vol.108,No.1,(1998 Jan),pp.(1-16), ISSN 0013-4694.

Wassermann EM, Lisanby SH.(2001) Therapeutic application of repetitive transcranial magnetic stimulation: a review. *Clin Neurophysiol* vol.112,No.8,(2001 Agu),pp.(1367-1377),ISSN 1388-2457.

Werhahn KJ, Kunesch E, Noachtar S, Benecke R & Classen J.(1999) Differential effects on motorcortical inhibition induced by blockade of GABA uptake in humans. *J Physiol* vol.517,No.pt2,(1999 Jun),pp.(591-597), ISSN 0022-3751.

Ye J, Zhang WB Qi J, Lian ZC & Han Y.(2000) Pathological observation on temporal lobe and hippocampus in experimental epileptic rats. *Chinese Journal of Neurology and Psychiatry*. Vol.26,No3,(2000),pp.(76-78),ISSN1002-0152.

Zangen A, Hyodo K.(2002) Transcranial magnetic stimulation induces increases in extracellular levels of dopamine and glutamate in the nucleus accumbens. *Neuroreport* vol.13,No.18,(2002 Dec),pp.(2401-2405), ISSN 0959-4965.

Ziemann U, Lonnecker S, Steinhoff BJ & Paulus W.(1996) Effects of antiepileptic drugs on motor cortex excitability in humans: a transcranial magnetic stimulation study. *Ann Neurol* vol.40,No.3,(1996 Sep),pp.(367-378), ISSN 0364-5134.

Ziemann U. (2004) TMS and drugs. *Clin Neurophysiol* vol.115,No.8,(2004 Aug),pp.(1717-1729), ISSN 1388-2457.

Ziemann U, Ilic TV & Jung P.(2006) Long-term potentiation (LTP)-like plasticity and learning in human motor cortex--investigations with transcranial magnetic stimulation (TMS).*Suppl Clin Neurophysiol* vol.59,(2006),pp.(19-25), ISSN 1567-424x.

Zhang JQ, Yu JM, Wang XM, Zhao HN, Huang M, Zhang XD, Zhao XQ, Huang H & Hu JX.(2008) Effects of pretreatment with low-frequency repetitive transcranial magnetic stimulation on expressions of hippocampus GAD65 and NMDAR-1 in rats with pilocarpine-induced seizures. *Chinese Journal of Neuroimmunology and Neurology* vol.15,No.6(2008 Nov),pp.(430-433), ISSN 1006-2963.

Zhong LT, Sarafian T, Kane DJ, Charles AC, Mah SP, Edwards RH & Bredesen DE.(1993) Bcl-2 inhibits death of central neural cells induced by multiple agents. *Proc Natl Acad Sci* vol.90,No.10,(1993 May),pp(4533-4537), ISSN 0027-8424.

Part 3

Epilepsy Research

4

EEG-fMRI Multimodal Integration for Epilepsy Research

Anna M. Bianchi[1], Tiziana Franchin[1,2] and Maria G. Tana[1]
[1]*Department of Bioengineering, IIT Unit, Politecnico di Milano, Milan,*
[2]*Bambino Gesù Children Hospital, IRCCS, Rome,*
Italy

1. Introduction

Epileptologists have now at their disposal a variety of tools for investigating human brain functions. Among the technologies of non-invasive functional imaging that have flowered in the last years, two techniques became particularly popular: the electroencephalogram (EEG) which records electrical voltages from the electrodes placed on the scalp and functional magnetic resonance imaging (fMRI) which records magnetization changes due to variations in blood oxygenation.

Each of these methods have its own advantages and disadvantages and no single method is best suited for all experimental and clinical conditions. EEG is a long-established tool for the non-invasive brain investigation characterized by the high temporal resolution (measured in milliseconds) but very low spatial resolution (measured in square centimetres). In contrast, fMRI provides good spatial resolution (measured in square millimetres) but relatively poor temporal resolution (measured in seconds). Combining EEG and fMRI provides integration of information that results in an enhanced view of the phenomena of interest.

This fusion of information is particularly useful in the context of the study of the epileptic disorders. The EEG was used in the study of epilepsy since it was discovered and it remains nowadays the gold-standard for the diagnosis of epilepsy, the classification of the seizures types and the localization of the generators of the epileptic activity. The EEG measurements recorded on the scalp is visually inspected by the neurophysiologists in order to detect any epileptic pattern such as spikes, spike-wave bursts, seizures, etc. and to diagnose the epilepsy. From a spatial point of view only a topographic localization of the generators of ictal and interictal activity is possible. Because of poor spatial resolution of the EEG technique, in many cases it means just a lateralization of the generators and not their precise localization.

fMRI, first demonstrated in 1990, is a technique that, through the blood oxygen level dependent (BOLD) effect, allows the localization of brain areas in which there is a variation of the level of neuronal activity during an experimental condition compared to a control condition. fMRI is mostly used in the study of sensory, motor and cognitive functions, in which the experimental condition differs from the control condition in a way that is controlled by the experimenter. In the context of epilepsy or spontaneous physiological changes in brain state, one can consider the control condition at the time when the EEG is at baseline and the experimental condition to occur in presence of endogenous electrophysiological phenomena such as an epileptic discharge or a sleep spindle. To define

such an experimental condition, it is necessary to combine fMRI with EEG measurements by recording EEG while the subject is in the MR scanner.
In this way, it is possible to determine the region of the brain in which there is a change in the BOLD signal correlated to modified neuronal activity such as an epileptic discharge recorded on the scalp..
In this chapter, we will present the methods that have been developed for integrated processing of EEG and BOLD signals simultaneously acquired focusing our attention on the application of these methods in the context of epilepsy.
More in details, the chapter is organized into three sections dealing with the following issues: analysis of EEG-fMRI data by General Linear Model (GLM) theory and estimation of the haemodynamic response function correlated to the epileptic discharges; analysis of EEG-fMRI data by separation into Independent Component Analysis; connectivity analysis of the brain networks underlying epileptic activity.

2. Analysis of the haemodynamic response to the epileptic discharges

One of the most popular approaches to combine EEG and fMRI measurements is to include EEG-derived information as regressors of interest in the GLM definition commonly used for fMRI analysis. This type of analysis is usually known as EEG-informed fMRI analysis.
The most widely used approach to perform EEG-informed fMRI analysis consists in analyzing EEG in the time domain and in using information derived from EEG time course into the GLM analysis.
This type of analysis allows for the spatial localization of brain areas involved in spontaneously arising neural activities in which the "stimuli" are not exogenous (i.e. externally generated and controlled) but are "task-free", random and endogenous (i.e. internally generated).
This is the case of pathological disorders such as epilepsy in which EEG-informed regressors can be used to identify and localize the epileptogenic and the irritative areas. In this particular application, the temporal sequence of onset times of epileptic disharges is used to construct regressors forming a design matrix that is than fitted to the fMRI image data.
One of the most critical factors limitating the potential of the above mentioned technique and preventing it from becoming a clinical tool in the context of epilepsy is the few knowledge about the haemodynamic response to the epileptic spikes. The commonly used EEG-informed GLM analysis needs, in fact, the definition of an "a priori" model of neurovascular system impulse response (HRF, Hemodynamic Response Function).
During the GLM analysis of fMRI data, a statistical comparison is made between the real time course of the BOLD signal in each voxel of the acquired volume and an expected time course of the BOLD signal in the same voxel. The latter is obtained convolving a train of impulses synchronized with the epileptic events and an a priori modeled HRF. Such statistical comparison results in a fMRI map representing the resemblance between real data and modeled data. The whole procedure is summarised and depicted in Fig.1.
A wide variety of basis functions has been used to describe the hemodynamic response. The simplest one uses a standard HRF, which is the measured response to a brief stimulus, such as an auditory tone (Glover et al., 1999). Clearly, this model assumes that each event is followed by a stereotyped response, not accounting for differences among patients, among brain regions or among sessions within a single patient, although it is known that these effects can be considerable (Aguirre et al., 1998). There are also no evidences to assume that

the behaviour of the neuro-vascular system in response to an "endogenous" and spontaneous event such as an epileptic discharge, or any other pathological activity, is the same as the one observed in normal subjects, performing sensory or cognitive tasks, in which exogenous and experimentally controlled stimuli are used.

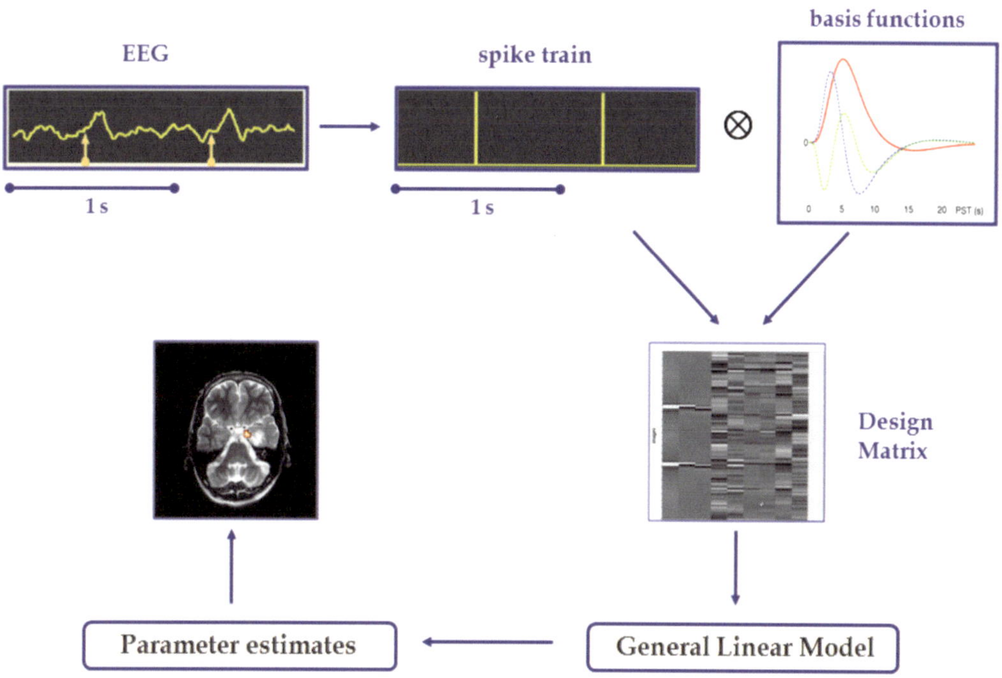

Fig. 1. Statistical analysis of EEG-fMRI data: the epileptic interictal spikes are detected on the EEG signal an impulse train is then created and convolved with a a set of basis functions representing HRF. Convolved impulse trains are used as regressors of interest, and are inserted into the design matrix which is then fitted to the image data. After the estimation of the regression coefficients, inference on relevant contrasts of their estimates was performed by using a t-test or F-test depending if one is testing for one parameter only or several parameters at the same time. The obtained spatial t-maps or F-maps are thresholded for significance level and the resulting maps are the functional images, where the value at each voxel reflects the resemblance between the model and the data and therefore the probability that this region is involved in the generation of the spikes.

In order to overcome these limitations, several approaches were proposed in literature. In this section we will describe the existing techniques that were developed to study the HRF related to epileptic discharges and how these can be applied in the context of the study of epileptic disorders.

2.1 Parametric vs non-parametric estimation of the haemodynamic response function

The techniques to estimate the temporal dynamics and the spatial variability of the HRF can be classified into two main classes: parametric and non-parametric methods.

The parametric methods fix the shape of the HRF by fitting to fMRI data a particular non-linear function of parameters which models typically the delay and the blurring effect of the HRF.

$$HRF(t) = \left(\frac{t}{d_1}\right)^{a_1} \times e^{-\left(\frac{t-d_1}{b_1}\right)} - c \times \left(\frac{t}{d_2}\right)^{a_2} e^{-\left(\frac{t-d_2}{b_2}\right)}$$

where t is the time, b_1, b_2 , d_1, d_2 and c are the parameters whose range of variations are derived from physiological information.

A hybrid method with parametric and non parametric characteristics at the same time was more recently introduced (Gossl et al., 2001). More in detail, this approach is parametric on the temporal scale and, on the other hand, is not parametric on the spatial scale since it uses only general prior to model the spatial extension of the signal.

The parametric methods are not able to fully capture the shape variations of HRF within the brain, since they unavoidably introduce a bias in the HRF estimate.

In order to overcome such limitations another class of HRF estimation techniques were recently introduced. This novel class of methods are known as non-parametric methods.

Non-parametric techniques for HRF estimation make no prior hypothesis about the shape of the impulse response of the neurovascular system.

The first type of non-parametric method that was applied is the simple averaging over time of the BOLD response. However, this classical voxelwise analysis is precluded by the low signal-to-noise ratio of fMRI data. For these reasons further non parametric methods were proposed: averaging over regions (Kershaw et al., 2000), selective averaging (Dale et al., 1997), introduction of non-diagonal models for the temporal covariance of the noise (Burock et al., 2000), or introduction of smoothing FIR filters (Goutte et al., 2000).

In such a context, recently, a Bayesian, non-parametric estimation of the HRF has been proposed (Marrelec et al., 2003), (Ciuciu et al., 2003) in which information based on the underlying physiological knowledge was used within a Bayesian framework only to temporally regularize the problem. In this way estimates of the HRF are derived without introducing bias into the estimation, since only very soft regularizing constraints, which are clearly derived from physiological requirements, are imposed. By using a Bayesian approach, the HRF estimate results from a tradeoff between information brought by the data and by our prior knowledge (Marrelec et al., 2003), (Ciuciu et al., 2003).

One of the points of strength of this approach is the possibility to extend it from a voxelwise formulation of the problem of HRF estimation to a regional level (Makni et al., 2008). The development of an estimation method of cerebral haemodynamic response at a regional level allows a joint procedure of HRF estimation and detection of active brain areas. The possibility to use a joint-detection estimation approach, avoiding the classical procedure based on GLM, allows to overcome the necessity of an "a-priori" model of HRF.

For this reasons and since this Bayesian non-parametric estimation of HRF has been shown to be able to provide a quantification of the haemodynamic response to epileptic discharges (Tana et al., 2007), hereinafter we will concentrate our attention on this particular approach describing it in details in the following paragraph.

2.2 Bayesian non-parametric estimation of the haemodynamic response function

The non-parametric Bayesian HRF estimation approach proposed by (Ciuciu et al., 2003) was first developed in a voxelwise formulation.

The value of the BOLD signal y_{tn} at time $(t_n=nTR)$ $1 \le n \le N$ (TR = time of repetition of MR sequence) measured in the voxel V_i is described by the following convolution model:

$$y_{i,t_n} = \sum_{k=0}^{K} h_{i,k\Delta t} x_{t_n-k\Delta t} + \sum_{q=1}^{Q} p_{t_n,q} l_{q,i} + b_{i,t_n} \quad \text{for } t_n = t_1,\ldots,t_N \tag{1}$$

which in matrix form becomes:

$$y_i = Xh_i + Pl_i + b_i \tag{2}$$

where $\boldsymbol{X}=[x_{tn}, x_{tn-\Delta t}, \ldots, x_{tn-\Delta t}]^t$ is a binary matrix corresponding to the time of occurrence of the events which, in the particular case of epilepsy, can be both interictal and ictal. $\boldsymbol{h}=[h_0, h_{\Delta t}, \ldots, h_{K\Delta t}]^t$ represents the HRF that has to be estimated, $\boldsymbol{Pl}_i$ is the confounding part (deterministic trends) and $\boldsymbol{b}_i$ is a zero-mean Gaussian white noise process $\boldsymbol{b}$ of unknown variance $\boldsymbol{r}_b$.

The likelihood function of this model is given by:

$$L(\underline{y}|\boldsymbol{h}) = (2\pi r_b)^{-\frac{N}{2}} \exp\left(\frac{-\left\| \underline{y} - \underline{X}\boldsymbol{h} - \underline{\boldsymbol{P}}\underline{l} \right\|^2}{2r_b} \right) \tag{3}$$

where:

$$\underline{y} = [y_1^t,\ldots,y_I^t]^t, \underline{X} = [\mathbf{X}_1^t|\ldots|\mathbf{X}_I^t]^t, \underline{P} = diag[\boldsymbol{P}_1,\ldots,\boldsymbol{P}_I], \underline{l} = [l_1^t|\ldots|l_I^t]^t$$

Bayesian formalism is then used to model temporal prior information about the structure of the HRF. Since the underlying process of BOLD response to epileptic events is object of investigation, only basic and soft constraints, that do not contradict current knowledge, can be used (Ciuciu et al., 2003), (Buxton et al., 1997).

More precisely, it is possible to assume that the amplitude of the HRF starts and ends at zero and that its variations are smooth, i.e. that the underlying process evolves rather slowly on the experimental time scale. The first condition is introduced by setting the first and last sample points of the HRF to zero. Quantification of the second condition is achieved by setting a Gaussian prior $p(\mathbf{h},\mathbf{R},\boldsymbol{\theta}) \sim N(0,\boldsymbol{\theta}\mathbf{R})$ with a covariance matrix $\mathbf{R} = (\mathbf{D}_2^t\mathbf{D}_2)$ where $\mathbf{D}_2$ is the finite second-order difference matrix. θ stands for the hyperparameter that adjusted the prior weight.

The trade-off between constraints and the information given by data and that is modeled by the hyperparameter θ, can be set automatically from the data themselves using a Maximum Likelihood Expectation Conditional Maximization algorithm (ECM) (Ciuciu et al., 2003). Also the coefficients of the functions modelling the low frequencies were automatically tuned by using ECM.

The prior and the likelihood function (3) can be fused by using the Bayes rule into the Gaussian a posteriori distribution whose maximum is the Maximum a Posteriori (MAP) estimate of the HRF $\boldsymbol{h}^{MAP}$:

$$p(h \mid \underline{y};\theta,\underline{l}) \sim N(\hat{h}^{MAP},\Sigma)$$

$$\Sigma^{-1} = \frac{1}{r_b}\sum_{i=1}^{I} X_i^t X_i + R_H^{-1} \quad (4)$$

$$\hat{h}^{MAP} = \frac{1}{r_b}\Sigma\sum_{i=1}^{I} X_i^t (y_i - P_i l_i)$$

where $\mathbf{R}_H = \text{diag}[\boldsymbol{\theta}\mathbf{R}]$.

Since the BOLD signal is known, to have some spatial structure, this method of HRF estimation can be also extended, in an appropriate region-based HRF model accounting for the spatial dimension of the data (Ciuciu et al., 2004), (Makni et al., 2004).

2.3 HRF estimation applied to the study of interictal epileptic activity

In the context of the study of fMRI response in epilepsy several attempts have been made to study HRF to epileptic activity and to take into account both the interregional HRF variability and HRF variability between healthy and epileptic patients .

The majority of the studies existing in literature are devoted to the investigation of the BOLD response to interictal epileptic discharges (IED).

One of the first works of this type used a linear estimation approach based on a simple averaging over the time of the BOLD response (Bénar et al., 2002). This method consists mainly in performing the following three steps: detecting activated areas by GLM analysis, obtaining the time courses of the BOLD signal for each region of interest as the spatial average over the voxels of the ROI and, at the end, averaging the extracted BOLD signal over the time using IEDs identified on EEG signal as events. (Bénar et al., 2002) found important variations in amplitude and shape between average HRFs across patients (see Fig. 5 from (Bénar et al. 2002)) that probably could reflect in part different pathophysiological mechanisms. More particularly, findings of (Bénar et al., 2002) showed that average HRF presented a wider positive lobe than the Glover model in three patients and a longer undershoot in two patients and allowed to conclude that the HRF for epileptic spikes can be somewhat different from the standard model and is also different from patient to patient. Although only few patients were analyzed in the work of (Bénar et al., 2002), it opened the door to the necessity to improve the standard GLM analysis with more complex analysis in order to take into account the variability of HRF and the fact that it does not seem to be a standard response to all type of epileptic discharges and, therefore, to all types of pathophysiological mechanisms underlying epileptic activity.

Following the way opened by (Bénar et al., 2002), HRF variability was studied in a wider group of subjects (Bagshaw et al., 2004) and the use of patient-specific haemodynamic response following a *parametric* approach was proposed (Kang et al., 2003).

In particularl, in (Bagshaw et al., 2004), a group of 31 patients with focal epilepsy were analysed and variations of the peak time of HRF were taken into account within a GLM framework. Using multiple HRFs (with the following four different peak times: 3, 5, 7, 9, s) composed of a single gamma function, resulted in an increased percentage of data sets with significant fMRI activations, from 45% when using the standard HRF alone, to 62.5%.

The standard HRF was found to be good at detecting positive BOLD responses, but less appropriate for negative BOLD responses, the majority of which were found to be more accurately modelled by an HRF that peaked later than the standard.
(Kang et al., 2003), (Lu et al., 2006), (Lu et al., 2007) proposed to detect fMRI areas of activation using canonical HRF, to subsequently estimate HRF and to use patient-specific (Kang et al., 2003) and voxel-specific HRF (Lu et al., 2006), (Lu et al., 2007) within a GLM framework.
Using patient-specific and voxel-specific HRF, the found active regions are characterized by similar or larger volume extent and higher adjusted coefficient of multiple determination (Razavi et al. 2003) than the regions resulting from GLM analysis with fixed HRF.were found (Kang et al., 2003), (Lu et al., 2006),; and additional activated areas compatible with EEG and anatomical MRI localization of epileptogenic and lesional regions were also found (Kang et al., 2003), (Lu et al., 2006), (Lu et al., 2007).
All the above mentioned work (Bénar et al., 2002), (Kang et al., 2003), (Lu et al., 2006), (Lu et al., 2007) support the hypothesis that the misspecification of the form of the HRF may have an important impact on the probability of detecting significant BOLD responses in epileptic patients.
It is worth mentioning also a recent work of (Lemieux et al., 2008) where *parametric* estimation of haemodynamic response performed on a group of 30 patients revealed that the shape of the haemodynamic response is very different from the canonical HRF only remotely from the suspected focus of epileptic activity whereas it appeared similar to canonical one in the vicinity of the presumable epileptogenic areas.
Recently the *non-parametric* Bayesian approach described in details in the previous theoretical paragraph was proposed to study HRF to interictal spikes (Tana et al., 2007).
In the study of (Tana et al., 2007) *non-parametric* Bayesian estimation of HRF was applied to a two patients with temporal lobe epilepsy and HRF variability among patients and among regions was studied.
(Tana et al., 2007) observed important variations in the time course of the haemodynamic response both between patients and across the different fMRI areas of a same subject. In Fig. 2 an example is shown of HRF estimation obtained with non-parametric Bayesian method in a subject with a clinical diagnosis of focal epilepsy shown in Fig. 3. It can be noted as the HRFs in region of interest are different from canonical haemodynamic response function defined in (Glover, 1999). In the areas congruent with the scalp EEG alterations the haemodynamic response has an initial pattern similar to the one obtained in classical event-related experiments but it is followed by an increase of fMRI signal activity away from the event. This should be related to deep epileptic activity that is not recorded on the scalp (Bénar et al., 2002). A negative fMRI response was also detected in an area far from the localization of the interictal EEG spikes.
Non-parametric Bayesian estimation appears to confirm that the shape of the HRF of the epileptic spikes may differ from the standard model and it is variable across regions. The fact that the haemodynamic response could be also widespread and found in distant cortical regions from the ones related to the scalp EEG findings could be an artefact or can suggest an underlying biological process that extends beyond the area clinically assumed as focus and, therefore, can suggest the possibility of effects of focal EEG spikes on remote but synaptically connected regions (Lemieux et al, 2008), (Tana et al., 2007). It could be possible to further investigate this issue by means of invasive EEG recordings or by means of methodologies of analysis that do not need the detection of epileptic events on scalp EEG (see section 3).

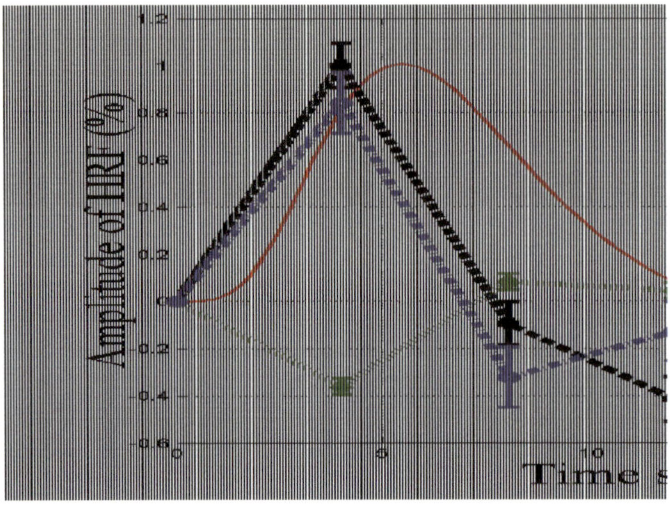

Fig. 2. MAP HRF estimates relatives to the EEG-fMRI areas showed in Figure 3. The graphic shows the standard HRF (red solid line), the HRF of the R polar temporal region (black dashed line - -), the HRF of the R basal frontal region (blue dashdot line . -) and of the L basal frontal region (green dotted line --) (reproduced from (Tana et al., 2007)).

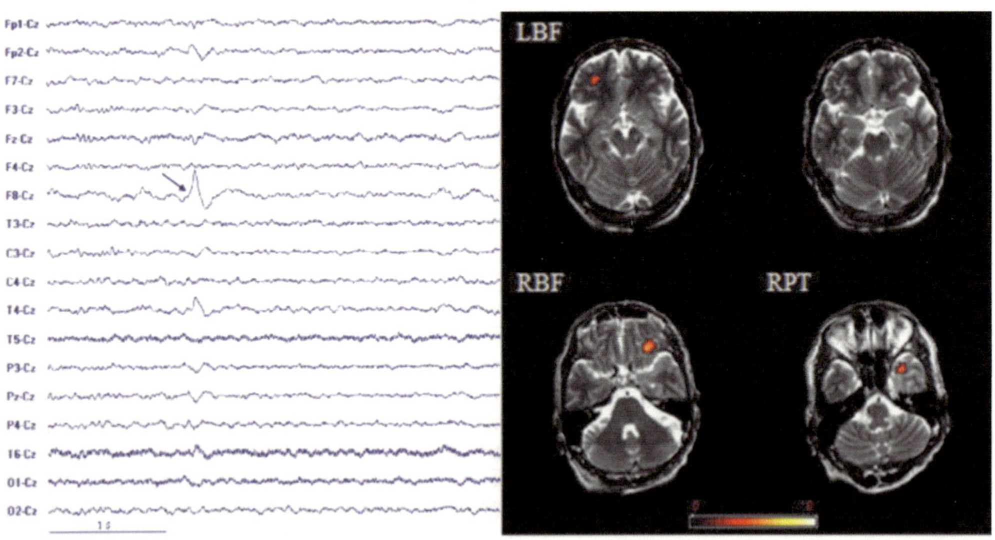

Fig. 3. EEG -fMRI findings in a patient with a diagnosis of temporal lobe epilepsy Left side of the figure illustrates EEG recording with an example of interictal spike. Right side of the figure illustrates F-maps related to spikes superimposed on axial slices of T2-weigthed image. (the images are shown according the neurological convention (right on right)) (adapted from (Tana et al., 2007)).

Summarizing all the results described above, it seems possible to conclude that the issue of estimation of the haemodynamic response to epileptic activity and, particularly the potential effect on the detection efficiency remains still an interesting subject of investigation.

This opens the way for new type of analysis of fMRI data that are free not only from whatever type of "a priori" model of HRF but also from the necessity to detect epileptic events on scalp EEG recordings. The following section of this chapter will be devoted to the description of these techniques and to how they are able to significantly contribute to the investigation of haemodynamic correlates of epilepsy.

3. Independent component analysis of EEG-fMRI data in epilepsy

In contrast to model-based GLM analyses, data-driven techniques applied in fMRI are not constrained by a fixed hypothesis. The most successful one is the Independent Component Analysis (ICA) (McKeown et al., 1998), which separates the data into a large set of independent components showing brain activation patterns with a common time course. Not imposing a-priori models about the shape of the HRF, ICA analysis might find out more information about the BOLD signal.
Let y be the M×N (M=number of scans, N=number of time courses) matrix of the fMRI time series, x the L×N matrix whose rows x_i (i=1,..., L) contain the spatial processes (or sources) that generate y ($L \leq N$). ICA decomposition of fMRI time series is the estimation of the spatial processes by the following linear statistical model:

$$y = Bx + v \tag{5}$$

where v is the noise contribution and $\boldsymbol{B}$ is the unknown mixing matrix . Assuming the hypothesis of the number of sources are minor or equal to the number of observed variables ($L \leq N$), and considering the $\boldsymbol{A}$ matrix to be full rank (Comon, 1994), the problem is reduced to:

$$y = \boldsymbol{A}\, s \tag{6}$$

where s is the matrix of sources and $\boldsymbol{A}$ is the mixing matrix whose columns $\boldsymbol{A}_j$ (j=1,...,L) contain the time courses of the L processes.
All the spatial components, with the possible exception of one, are assumed to be independent and non-Gaussian (Hyvärinen & Oja, 2000): the non-Gaussianity is, hence, the criterion for the blind estimation of the original sources. Several measures are proposed for applying non-Gaussianity in ICA estimation, even if there is no published evidence about different performances in fMRI analysis. The estimation of the significant components (i.e., related to brain activation patterns) is not based on a comparison with a BOLD model or different shapes of HRFs, but on the maximizing of a non-Gaussianity contrast function (Comon, 1994), therefore on the statistical feature of fMRI data.
The critical point is the separation of the significant components related to an investigated process (i.e., spike-related BOLD responses) from no-significant ones (MR artefacts, default state mode).
The first proposal to overcome this limitation was presented for the analysis of interictal fMRI in focal epileptic patients (Rodionov et al., 2007). After IC decomposition, components selection was implemented by an automatic IC classification (De Martino et al., 2007, see Fig. 4) resulting in the following set of labels: (1) the 'BOLD' class, which included components that are thought to consistently reflect task-related, transiently task-related and brain state-related (e.g. default state) neuronal activity; (2) residual motion artefacts; (3) EPI-susceptibility artefacts; (4) physiological noise; (5) noise at high spatial frequency; and (6) noise at temporal high frequency (Rodionov et al., 2007).

The classification was based on a training dataset from healthy volunteers: it was designed for revealing stereotypical components of normal brain activity, misclassified components related to motion, blood vessels, noise, and components related to interictal epileptiform discharges (IEDs). The method was tested on 63 patients with focal epilepsy, who underwent EEG-fMRI recording (Salek-Haddadi et al., 2006). A mean of 16 over 20 ICs were classified as significant BOLD-related sources. Concordance between the ICA and GLM-derived results was assessed based on spatial and temporal criteria on 8 case studies. The remaining ICs were associated to BOLD patterns of spontaneous brain activity, introducing the possibility of an epileptic activity that was not evident on the scalp EEG.

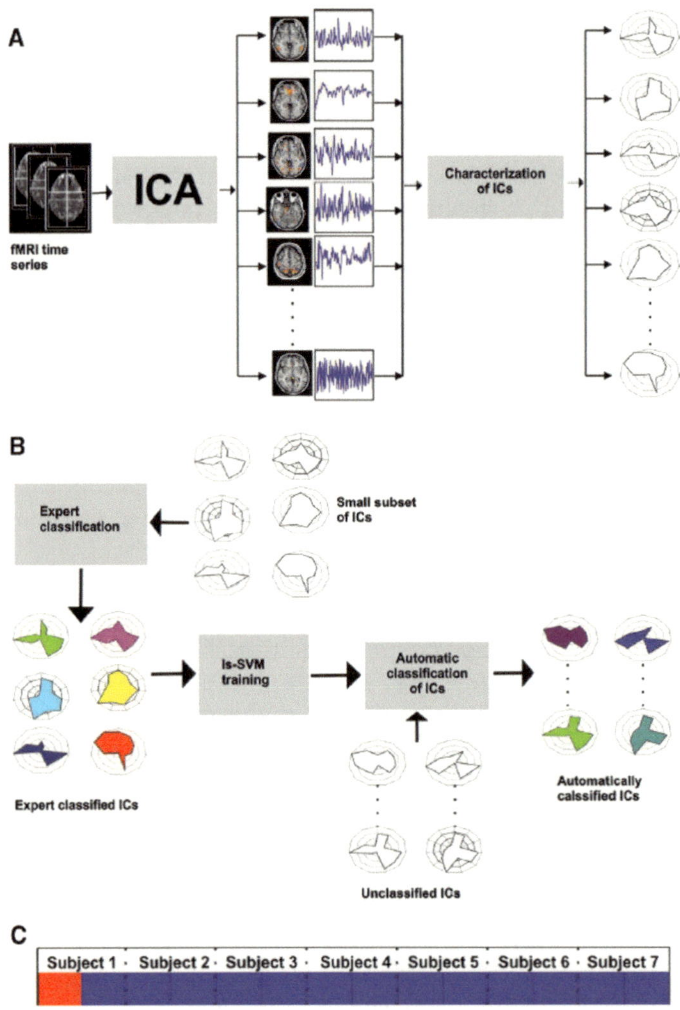

Fig. 4. Separation and classification of fMRI-ICs: (A) ICA of fMRI data and representation of the ICs in a multi-dimensional space of fingerprints. (B) Classification of IC-fingerprints by an ls-SVM-based algorithm, trained on a small subset of data labelled by an expert. (C) Proportion of data which has been used for training (red, 1/14) and testing (blue, 13/14). (De Martino et al., 2007) Reproduced with permission of Elsevier

Using this approach, the potential spike-related components were estimated using the corresponding activation in the GLM analysis and the selection was again depending on the canonical HRF used in the GLM (Moeller et al., 2009). Moreover, the classifier was trained on GLM-activation on a very small number of healthy subjects (De Martino et al., 2007) and the training was implemented on only 7% of the testing dataset, decreasing the statistical significance of the model.

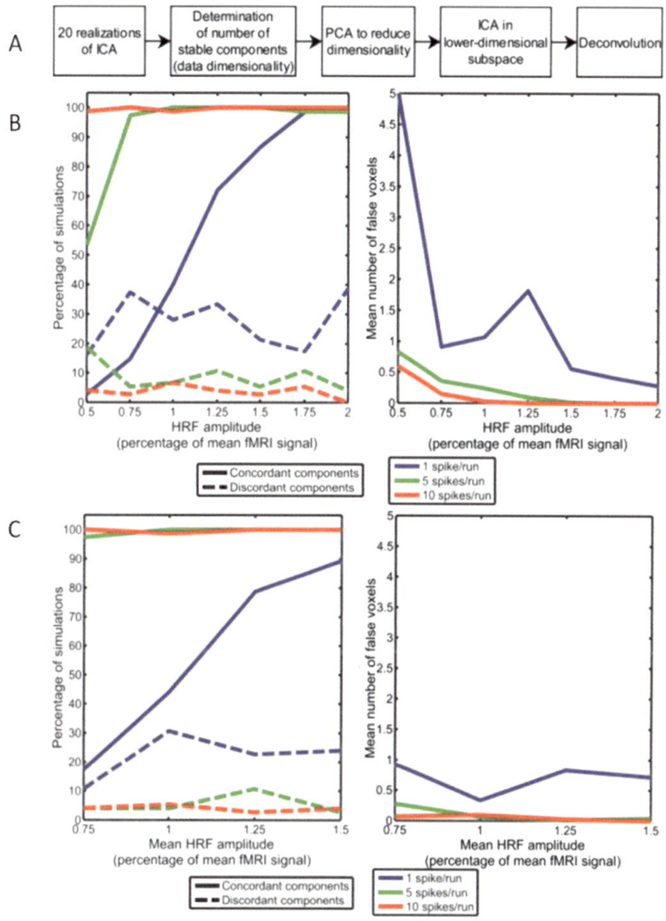

Fig. 5. Data analysis scheme and results of the model-free ICA approach. A) 20 ICA decompositions are applied to the fMRI data for determining the number of reproducible components. A lower-dimensional subspace is obtained by PCA and an additional ICA is then performed for identifying which components well-represented the simulated epileptic activity. The deconvolution is then applied to detect time courses that showed significant changes following the spike timings, without constraining the HRF to a canonical shape. B) (left) Percentage of simulations with constant HRF amplitudes where significant components were found. (right) Mean number of falsely activated voxels in concordant components. C) (left) Percentage of simulations with varying HRF amplitudes where significant components were found, either correctly matching the simulated activation region. (right) Mean number of falsely activated voxels in concordant components. (LeVan & Gotman, 2009) Reproduced with permission of Wiley

(LeVan and Gotman, 2009) introduced a more independent ICA method using deconvolution for identifying component time courses significantly related to simulated focal spikes without constraining the shape of the HRF. Artificial time courses were obtained by generating spikes at random tims and convolving them with a canonical HRF computed from the difference of two gamma functions (Glover, 1999), and varying the location of the activation, the number of simulated spikes per run, and the HRF amplitude. The robustness of traditional analysis methods based on the GLM when the HRF is mis-specified was evaluated adding an additional dataset based on a non-canonical HRF. Fig. 5 shows a schematic representation of the data processing and the obtained results related to the percentage of simulations with constant and variable HRF amplitudes, and the related mean number of falsely activated voxels in concordant components.

Components matching the simulated activation regions were found in 84.4% of simulations, while components at discordant locations were found in 12.2% of simulations; large artefacts occurring simultaneously with spikes are the majority of the false activations. This method mainly depends on the simulation parameters because, when the number of spikes was low, concordant components could only be identified when HRF amplitudes were large.

An application of this method was in detecting dynamic ictal BOLD responses in focal seizures (LeVan et al., 2010), for investigating HRFs with clear peaks - but varying latency – and differentiating the ictal focus from propagated activity. Components related to seizures of 15 patients (suffering of focal ictal discharges or generalised spike and slow waves and sharp and slow wave discharges) were identified by fitting an HRF to the component time courses at the time of the ictal EEG events. HRFs with a clear peak were used to derive maps of significant BOLD responses and their associated peak delay (LeVan et al., 2010). The prominence of the HRF peak was defined considering as baseline the data more than 5 s before or after the peak, and computing the ratio of the peak amplitude to the standard deviation of the baseline. The so-obtained ICA maps were significantly correlated with the GLM maps for each patient (Spearman's test, $p<0.05$), for a further confirm. The ictal BOLD responses identified by ICA consisted of the presumed epileptogenic zone, but in more widespread area (about 20.3% in addition of the average value). The introduction of an ICs classification method based on the peak delay showed that BOLD response clusters corresponded to early HRF peaks were concordant with the suspected epileptogenic focus, while late HRF peaks to ictal propagation (Fig. 6).

A last attempt of ICA analysis in epilepsy was presented by Moeller et al. (Moeller et al., 2011), where patients with idiopathic generalized epilepsy (IGE) and generalized spike wave discharges (GSW) were studied for the particularity of having hemodynamic behaviour not easily identified with a standard HRF (Moeller et al., 2008). Moreover, GSW are often related with more robust results in regular areas, thus allowing a good comparison between GLM and ICA methods.

After fMRI preprocessing and ICA decomposition (Moeller et al., 2011), ICA time courses were modelled as blocks with the same timings and durations as the GSWs, and convolved with a Fourier basis set (Josephs et al., 1997), assuming that BOLD response to the GSWs could be contained within an interval from 10 s before to 20 s after the marked events, and accommodating the HRF variability. From each temporal IC, a deconvolved HRF was produced by fitting the Fourier basis set. Components significantly related to the GSW were then identified by an F-test ($P < 0.05$, corrected for the number of components), with the motion parameters used as confounds as in the following GLM analysis. HRFs fitted to the

GSW components were then investigated to determine the sign of the HRF peaks, as in (LeVan & Gotman, 2009).

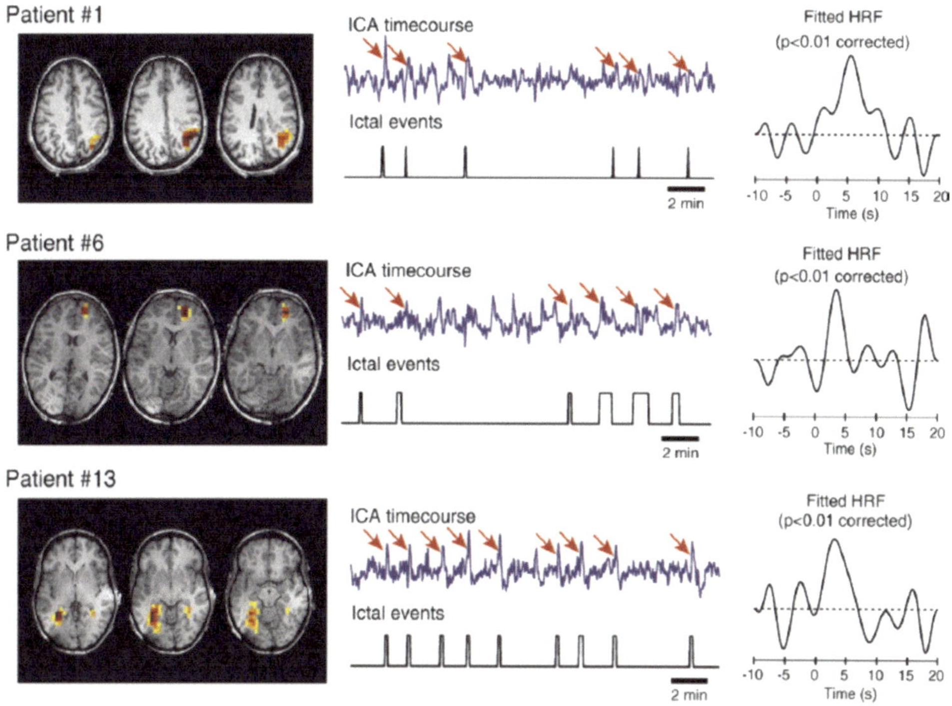

Fig. 6. Spatial topographies, time courses and deconvolved HRFs of seizure-related components extracted by ICA. (LeVan et al., 2010) Reproduced with permission of Elsevier.

In 12 epileptic patients, comparison of GLM maps and ICA maps showed significant correlation and revealed BOLD responses in the thalamus, caudate nucleus, and default mode areas. Few areas of BOLD signal changes that were only detected by ICA in 8 patients (Fig. 7) and showed variable shapes, different from the canonical HRF in most cases, while one component that was only detected by ICA showed an HRF resembling the canonical HRF.

The particular result is that, in patients with a low rate of discharges per minute, GLM maps detected BOLD signal changes within the thalamus and the caudate nucleus, not present in the ICA ones. Even if these results demonstrated that the BOLD response largely resembles the standard HRF and confirmed the adequacy of GLM analysis, it is worth noting that the number of investigated subjects and their variability in epileptic diseases might compromise the final outcome.

4. Brain connectivity and propagation of epileptic activity

One of the challenges of the neurologists in the study of epileptic disorders is the understanding of the propagation of epileptic abnormal activity inside the brain.

The propagation of epileptic seizure and interictal activity is a key concept in epilepsy which indicates the observation of similar patterns or of signals with different patterns but all suspected of reflecting a common underlying phenomenon, on an increasing number of EEG recording channels. (Lemieux et al., 2011).

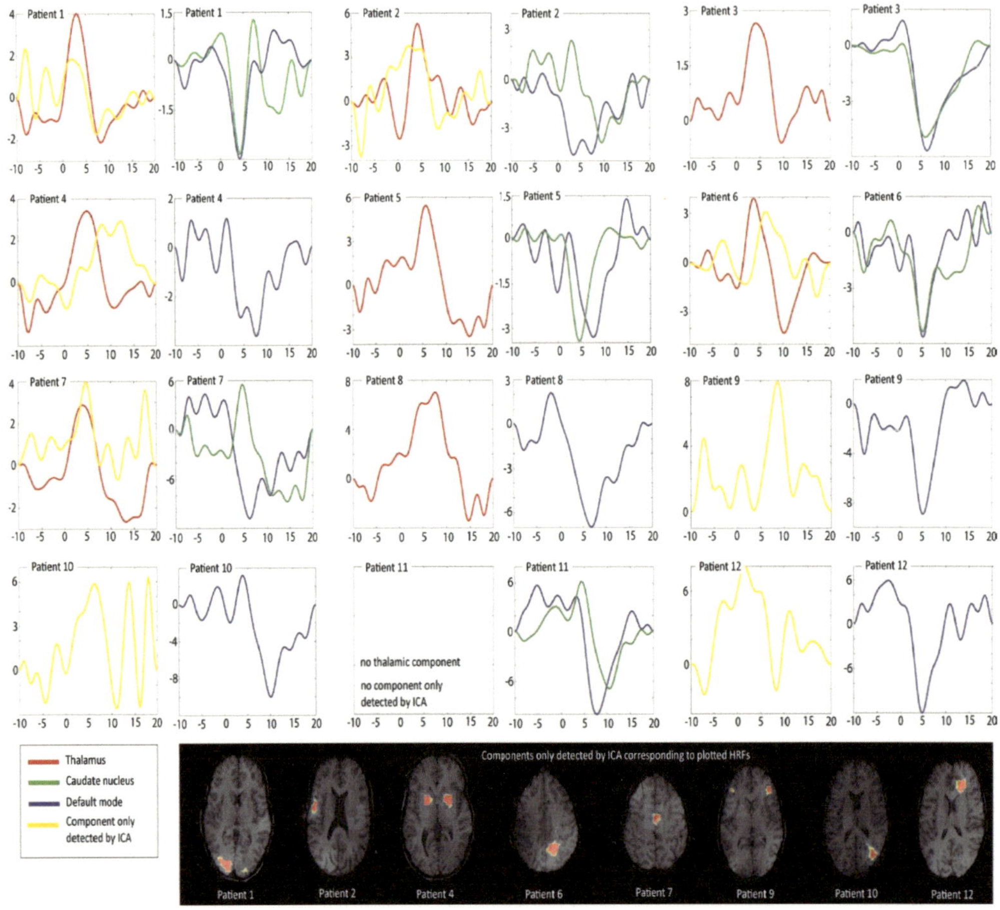

Fig. 7. Comparison between GLM maps and ICA maps revealed a few areas of BOLD signal changes that were only detected by ICA in 8 patients. HRFs for components in the thalamus, caudate nucleus, and default mode areas. Additionally, components that were only detected by ICA are shown with their corresponding HRF. (Moeller et al., 2011) Reproduced with permission of Wiley

The techniques used to extract information about interacting brain areas involved in the phenomenon of propagation, can be classified according to two broad typologies of approaches: functional connectivity and effective connectivity. Functional connectivity is defined as the "temporal correlation between spatially remote neurophysiological events" (Friston et al., 1993) and effective connectivity is defined as "the causal influence that a system exerts over one other" (Friston et al., 1993) and it reveals the strength and the direction of the flow of information between fMRI areas.

Functional connectivity can only partly account for the wide variety of the interaction patterns that can be expressed by the effective connectivity, (Friston et al. 1993). The full understanding of the network interaction structure need of information about the directionality of flows provided only by effective connectivity.

The issue of effective connectivity can be approached by two main typologies of analysis techniques: model-based methods (e.g. Dynamical Causal Modeling or DCM) and data-driven methods (e.g. Granger Causality Analysis or GCA). Both approaches try to estimate directed casual influences between cerebral structures by extracting useful information from the temporal dynamics in the EEG and fMRI signals. Both DCM and GCA approaches have advantages and disadvantages and, in the case of the fMRI signal, it is a current open issue, strongly debated in literature, to establish which is the most suitable method for the investigation of connectivity (David 2009), (Roebroeck et al., 2009).
In this section we will review and describe both methods and their current applications on the investigation of the propagation of epileptic activity.

4.1 Model-based effective connectivity: Dynamical Causal Modeling

The central idea of DCM is to treat the brain as a deterministic non-linear dynamic system that is subject to inputs and produces outputs. DCM relies a dynamic neuronal model of interacting brain regions, whereby neuronal activity in a given brain region causes changes in neuronal activity in other regions according to a graphical model. A further forward model (the so-called balloon model (Friston et al., 2003)) of the relationships between haemodynamic response and neural activity supplements the above mentioned neural model. The use of balloon model allows to include in the analysis the effect of the haemodynamic convolution and to quantify the strength of the interactions within brain networks directly at neural level. The parameters of the model are then inferred using a Bayesian inference scheme, (Stephan et al., 2009).
The point of strength of DCM is that it is able to model the effect of experimental, external, modulatory inputs on network dynamics and but one of its critical features is the effective ability of the proposed neuro-vascular coupling model to capture the real relationships between blood flow changes and oxygen metabolism changes during activation (Marrelec et al. 2006), (Aubert et al., 2002).
Since DCM takes dynamics and modulations into account in the model, its mathematical framework, which is also able to capture nonlinearities and temporal correlations into account, is very complex and, as a consequence, DCM is computationally limited by the number of regions that can be included in the analysis (maximum of eight according to Penny et al. (2004a); three in Mechelli et al. (2003), Penny et al. (2004b), and Ethofer et al. (2006); three and five in Lee et al. (2006)).
In order to overcome this problem, (Penny et al. (2004b) proposed an extension of the DCM framework to perform model comparison within a set of graphs given a priori. How this approach can be generalized to allow for blind model selection from the whole set of structural models (i.e., with no structural model required a priori) remains a central, yet complex, issue (Marrelec et al. 2006).

4.2 Data-driven effective connectivity: Granger Causality Analysis

The most important disadvantage of model-based effective connectivity is that it requires an "a priori" specification of a structural model in the form of a directed graph and that it allows to test hypothesis about connectivity only within a small set of models assumed to be applicable. To overcome this problem GCA was introduced on the basis of the Granger causality concept according to which the activity of a region of interest (ROI)-1 "causes" the activity of a ROI-2 if the knowledge of past values of the ROI-1 time series improves the prediction of the current value of the ROI-2 time-series

GCA does not require any pre-specification or a priori knowledge about the connectivity structure and was successfully applied to fMRI data measuring BOLD response both in bivariate (Roebroeck et al., 2005); (Abler et al. 2006) and multivariate GC models (Deshpande et al., 2008); (Sato et al., 2009); (Deshpande et al. 2009) . (Sato et al., 2010), (Havlicek et al., 2010).

Although the choice between GCA and model-based method like DCM is currently debated in literature (David, 2009), (Roebroeck et al., 2009), at the state of art no theoretical reasons exist to exclude the effectiveness of GCA analysis to infer connectivity on BOLD signal (Roebroeck et al., 2009). GCA approach was indeed successfully applied to fMRI data for studying brain connectivity during cognitive (Roebroeck et al., 2005), (Demirci et al., 2009), (Sato et al., 2010), (Ide et al., 2011), (Shippers et al., 2011), (Seger et al., 2011), sensory (Deshpande et al., 2008), (Stilla et al., 2007), (Stilla et al., 2008), (Havlicek et al., 2010), and motor tasks (Abler et al., 2006), (Sato et al, 2006), (Chen et al., 2009) and for investigating resting-state networks, (Liao et al., 2011), (Jiao et al., 2011) and in pathological conditions like epilepsy (Tana et al., submitted).

One of the methodology more widely used to calculate Granger causality are is based on multivariate autoregressive models which are fitted to the signals (EEG or BOLD) of interest. The multivariate autoregressive (MVAR) recorded from a set of k signals can be expressed as:

$$\mathrm{Y}(t) = \sum_{i=1}^{p} \mathrm{A}(i)\mathrm{Y}(t-i) + \mathrm{E}(t) \tag{7}$$

where $Y(t)=[Y_1(t), Y_2(t),\dots Y_k(t)]$ is a vector wherein Y_k is the time series corresponding the k-channel, $A(i)$ is the matrix of the model parameters, $E(t)$ is the vector containing white noise processes and p is the model order which can be determined using information theory criteria, (Akaike, 1974).

By transforming (7) to the frequency domain, we can obtain the following formulation:

$$\mathrm{Y}(f) = \mathrm{A}^{-1}(f)\mathrm{E}(f) = H(f)\mathrm{E}(f) \tag{8}$$

where $H(f)$ is the transfer matrix of the model whose element H_{ij} represents the connection from the j-th to the i-th channel.

Normalizing the transfer matrix of the model in (8) with respect to the inflows into channel i, we can obtain the Directed Transfer Function (DTF):

$$DTF_{ij}^{2}(f) = \frac{\left|H_{ij}(f)\right|^2}{\sum_{m=1}^{k}\left|H_{im}(f)\right|^2} \tag{9}$$

where $H_{ij}(f)$ is the minor produced by removing i-th row and the j-th column from transfer matrix $H(f)$.

Values of DTF equal to 1 between a pair of channels show maximum direct causal relationships and values of DTF near to 1 indicate that most of the signal in channel i consists of signal from channel j. DTF values of 0 or close to 0 means an absence of causal interrelations between the two channels considered.

DTF gives information only about the causal relationships underlying the networks of the investigated system and it is not able to discriminate direct transmission for a given pair of regions from indirect propagation of information mediated by other regions. To solve this problem , the estimator dDTF can be introduced, (Korzeniewska et al., 2003). It is given by the following equation:

$$dDTF_{ij}(f) = \eta_{ij}(f)\chi_{ij}(f) \tag{10}$$

where $\eta_{ij}(f)$ is the DTF normalized over the full frequency band also known as full frequency direct Directed Transfer Function (ffDTF), (Korzeniewska et al., 2003), and $\chi_{ij}(f)$ is the partial coherence defined as in (Korzeniewska et al., 2003). The partial coherence is a measure of how much the interaction between two brain regions is mediated by other areas.
Multiplying DTF by partial coherence, we can combine the information about the directionality of the interactions within the networks with the information provided by partial coherence function and can clearly identify causal direct connections and distinguish them from causal indirect connections.
Another method to identify causal direct connections is the calculation of the Partial Direct Coherence (PDC) introduced by (Baccalà et al., 2001). PDC is a frequency domain representation of the key concept of Granger causality and is defined as:

$$PDC_{ij}(f) = \frac{\overline{A}ij(f)}{\sqrt{\overline{a}_j^*(f)\overline{a}_j(f)}} \tag{11}$$

where $\overline{A}ij(f)$ is the i, jth element and $\overline{a}_j(f)$ the jth column of the matrix $\overline{\mathrm{A}}(f) = \mathrm{I} - \mathrm{A}(f)$.
$PDC_{ij}(f)$ represents the frequency domain GC from the j-th time series to the i-th time series at frequency f.
Significance of both DTF and PDC values can be assessed employing surrogate data (Deshpande et al., 2008), (Korzeniewzka et al., 2003). To this aim, surrogate data can be generated by transforming the data to the frequency domain, randomizing their phases and transforming back to the time domain, (Theiler et al., 1992). The resulting time series have the same power spectrum but random phases with respect to the original signals.
A null distribution can then be obtained by generating a set of sufficient number (for examples 1000 (Deshpande et al., 2008) of surrogate data and calculating the DTF or PDC from these datasets. The DTF or PDC value obtained for each connection from the original time series have then to be compared with the null distribution for a test of significance (e.g. a two-tailed test (Deshpande et al. 2008).

4.3 Application to epilepsy

Both interictal and ictal activities can be propagated themselves inside the brain and the progressive recruitment of brain areas far from the origin of the epileptiform activity appears as a spread of pathological EEG pattern.
The causes of the progressive spread of the epileptic activity depends on both the connections existing locally and at a wider range scale and also on the capability of the brain region to be recruited by the abnormal neural activity characteristic of an epileptic discharge (Lemieux et al., 2011).

Sometimes, the pattern of propagation can be studied on the basis of general knowledge of anatomical information and correlated with the temporal evolution of clinical symptoms of the ictal episodes. The majority of the times these general clinical considerations are insufficient to understand the real pattern of propagation which can also vary from event to event (Lemieux et al., 2011) and the question of how an initially spatially localized epileptic focus can spread to involve a larger portion of the cortex remains an open issue.

The identification of the pathways for the spread of partial seizures is, therefore, one of the most relevant and interesting field on which the above described brain connectivity technique can be applied.

The majority of studies existing in literature regarding the connectivity in epilepsy are mainly related to the EEG signal as mean to measure and evaluate neural activity.

Regarding functional connectivity, as reported in (Wendling et al., 2010), the first attempts in the field of epilepsy, were done in the middle of the twentieth century (Barlow and Brazier, 1954), just after the introduction of the Fast Fourier Transform algorithm.

In the 70s the propagation of interictal events was studied by calculating cross-correlation in time domain or equivalently the coherence in the frequency domain using first invasive EEG (Brazier et al., 1972) and later scalp EEG recordings (Lopes da Silva et al., 1977).

Coherence function was then used also to study ictal events, and in particular to study the evolution of the partial seizures and their propagation between the two hemispheres (Gotman et al., 1982). The concept of coherence was extended in 90s in time-varying context in order to study the evolution of the degree of synchronization of interictal and ictal activity (Haykin et al., 1996) and (Franaszcuk et al., 1999).

The methods for studying functional connectivity based on cross-correlation function or on its equivalent form in the frequency domain, that is the coherence function, are based on the assumption that the interaction between EEG signals are linear and, in order to capture also non-linear interactions further techniques were developed. Among these, we can mentioned: mutual information (Mars et al., 1983), non linear regression analysis (Wendling et al, 2001), phase synchronization methods (Rosemblum et al., 2004), generalized synchronization methods (Stam et al., 2003). A recent work of (Wendling et al., 2009) have compared the performance of ten of these methods (which can be grouped into three main families: non linear regression, phase synchronization and generalized synchronization) using simulated data in which the degree of coupling can be controlled. The results obtained by applying the various types of methods to simulated data showed that there is not a "universal" method that performs better than the other ones whatever the considered situation (Wendling et al., 2009), (Wendling et al., 2010).

Regarding effective connectivity, GC has been used to study temporal lobe epileptic seizures in the form of DTF applied to electrocortigram (ECoG) recorded with subdural grids and stereotactic EEG (SEEG) recorded with deep electrodes (Franaszczuk et al. 1998).

(Franaszczuk et al. 1998) extends, in particular, the application of the DTF method to compare patterns of flow of seizures with different sites of origin. Analysis of a seizure originating from mesial temporal structures is compared with a seizure originating from lateral temporal neocortex. The DTF method has the potential to determine patterns of flow of activity, including periods when visual analysis of the intracranial ictal EEG may not allow for definitive source localization.

More recently GC was also applied in the form of PDC to scalp EEG signal in order to study temporal lobe epilepsy (Baccalà et al., 2004).

In particular PDC was applied to mesial temporal epileptic seizures and it has been shown that it is able to localize the epileptogenic focus via the simultaneous analysis of multiple EEG channels thanks to the determination of the direction of information flow among signals and thanks to its representation by means of directed graphs, where focal electrodes are associated with high observed rates of pertinence to strongly connected subgraphs.

It is possible to affirm that both DTF and PDC are able to study effective connectivity in epilepsy , to infer epileptic seizure propagation and to identify the focus of epileptic activity (Cadotte et al., 2009).

Differently from EEG, nowadays there are still few application of fMRI effective connectivity studies in the field of epilepsy.

Effective connectivity studies using DCM have been performed in (David et al., 2008) and (Vaudano et al., 2009).

DCM and Baysian model comparison was used in (Vaudano et al., 2009) to investigate the role of thalamus, prefrontal cortex and precuneus in seizure generation. EEG-fMRI data recorded in a group of seven patients with idiopathic generalized epilepsy (IGE) with frequent generalized SW discharges (GSWD) and significant GSWD-correlated haemodynamic signal changes in the thalamus, the prefrontal cortex and the precuneus.

In order to perform Bayesian model selection three dynamic causal models were constructed: GSWD was modelled as autonomous input to the thalamus (model A), ventromedial prefrontal cortex (model B), and precuneus (model C). Bayesian model comparison revealed that, although model C (GSWD as autonomous input to precuneus) is the best in five patients while model A (GSWD as autonomous input to thalamus) prevailed in two cases, at the group level model C dominated.

The findings lead the authors to hypothesize a role for the precuneus as a form of modulator of generalized SW activity, and by extension, of the occurrence of absence seizures, linking spontaneous fluctuations in brain state as reflected by the so-called Default-Mode Network of brain activity to the occurrence of epileptic discharges (Vaudano et al., 2009), (Lemieux et al., 2011).

In a rat model of absence epilepsy (David et al., 2008) performed simultaneous EEG and fMRI measurements, and subsequent intracerebral EEG (iEEG) recordings in regions strongly activated in fMRI (first somatosensory cortex, thalamus and striatum). (David et al., 2008) showed that using DCM, instead of GCA, it is possible to spatially localize the origin of spontaneous spike-and-wave (SW) discharges in the first somatosensory cortex.

More recently, a study of epileptic seizure propagation using GCA was performed in (Tana et al, submitted). In this study, GCA analysis was applied to networks of brain areas showing fMRI activation during epileptic seizures. EEG-fMRI recording was performed on a group of four case studies related to patients with different epileptic pathologies and GCA analysis was applied to networks obtained using different parcellation strategies for the definition of the nodes. In Figure 8, the connectivity pattern of a patient with a diagnosis of occipital lobe epilepsy is shown. The patient shows an area of almost continuous spiking under left occipital lobe revealed by ECoG measurements (not shown in figure) and fMRI activation mainly localized in the left occipital and right parietal lobe. GCA results showed that the source of the connectivity network is the left occipital fusiform gyrus (LOFG) confirming intracranial EEG findings.

The role of LOFG as possible starting point of seizure propagation and, therefore, the ability of GCA to recognize LOFG as epileptogenic focus is also confirmed by the fact that the area identified as GC network source is located within the brain volume removed in successful surgery for epilepsy (Fig. 8b).

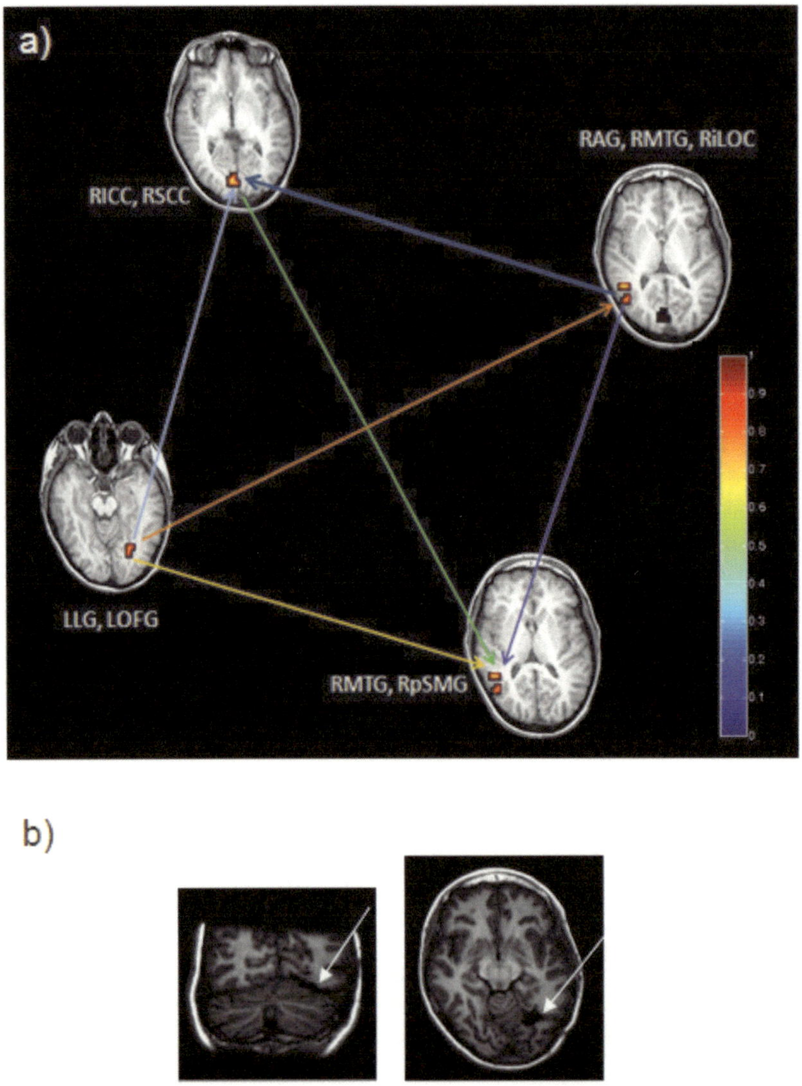

Fig. 8. (a) GC Connectivity graph and fMRI response of a patient with a diagnosis of occipital lobe epilepsy. fMRI findings show both left occipital and right temporal-occipital BOLD activation (radiological convention (left on right)) (The acronyms stand for the following expression: RMTG (right middle temporal gyrus), RpSMG (right supramarginal gyrus, posterior division), LLG (left lingual gyrus), LOFG (left occipital fusiform gyrus), RiLOC (right lateral occipital cortex, inferior division), RAG (right angular gyrus), RICC (right intracalcarine cortex), RSCC (right supracalcarine cortex)); (b) Surgery outcome. White arrow shows the resected area localized in the left occipital lobe. (adapted from (Tana et al., submitted)).

According to GC results, the seizure starting in the left occipital lobe propagates to the contralateral occipital, parietal and temporal regions. The sink of the network (i.e. the area in which the propagation of the seizure terminates) is localized in the contralateral temporo-parietal area.

5. Conclusion

This chapter summarizes various techniques for integrated analysis of EEG and fMRI signals for the investigation of epilepsy. In particular, we describe how the information coming from the EEG can be used for triggering the analysis of the BOLD signal, in order to establish a direct connection between EEG events and haemodynamic activation, and for a precise localization of the brain areas involved in the specific events. This type of analysis is limited by the current little knowledge about the HRF that is necessary to define a model of expected BOLD signal to construct GLM regressors. In order to improve the understanding of the impulse response function of neurovascular system, several techniques have been developed for the estimation of the HRF temporal and spatial characteristics.

To overcome the limitations of classical GLM approach that are also due to the fact that EEG describes only cortical activity and is not always able to detect deep brain events, other methodologies have been proposed in literature, such ICA, calculated on the BOLD signal only.

After the localization of the activated cortical areas during epileptic seizure, it is of extreme interest to study the temporal interactions inside the network formed by activated brain regions and in order to identify the pattern of seizure propagation. Applying connectivity techniques like GCA and DCM to both EEG and, more recently, BOLD signal it is possible to obtain useful information about the localization of the epileptogenic focus, the propagation of the seizure and sometimes to localize also how the seizure terminates.

Even if some problems are still open and several features are under investigation, all the methodologies described in this chapter are promising tools that will allow a deeper investigation of the mechanisms involved in epileptic activity and can found large application in the clinical field as well as in research.

6. References

Abler B, Roebroeck A, Goebel R, Hose A, Schonfeldt-Lecuona C, Hole G, Walter H (2006): Investigating directed influences between activated brain areas in a motor-response task using fMRI, *Magnetic Resonance Imagin,g* Vol.24, pp.181-185.

Akaike, H., (1974). A new look at the statistical model identification, *IEEE Transactions on Automatic Control*, Vol. 19, pp. 716-723.

Aguirre, G.K., Zarahn E. and D'Esposito M. (1998). The variability of human, BOLD hemodynamic responses, *Neuroimage*, Vol. 8, No.4, (November 1998), pp. 360-369, ISSN 1053-8119.

Aubert, A., Costalat, R., (2002). A model of the coupling between brain electrical activity, metabolism, and hemodynamics: application to the interpretation of functional neuroimaging. *NeuroImage*, Vol.17, pp.1162- 1181, ISSN 1053-8119.

Baccalà, L.A., Sameshima, K. (2001). Partial directed coherence: A new concept in neural structure determination. *Biological Cybernetics* Vol.84, pp.463-474.

Baccalà, L.A., Alvarenga, M.Y., Sameshima, K., Jorge, C.L., Castro, L.H. (2004) Graph theoretical characterization and tracking of the effective neural connectivity during episodes of mesial temporal epileptic seizure. J Integr Neurosci 3:379–395.

Bagshaw, A.P., Aghakhani, Y., Bénar, C.-G., Kobayashi, E., Hawco, C., Dubeau, F., Pike, G.B. and Gotman, J. (2004). EEG-fMRI of focal epileptic spikes: analysis with multiple haemodynamic functions and comparison with gadolinium-enhanced MR angiograms. *Human Brain Mapping,* Vol. 22, No. 3, (July 2004), pp.179-192, ISSN 1097-0193.

Barlow, J. S., and Brazier, M. A. (1954). A note on a correlator for electroencephalographic work. *Electroencephalogr. Clin. Neurophysiol.* 6, 321–325.

Bénar, C.G., Gross, D.W., Wang, Y., Petre, V., Pike, P., Dubeau, F. and Gotman, .J (2002). The BOLD response to interictal epileptiform discharges, *Neuroimage,* Vol.17, No.3, (November 2007), pp.1182-1192, ISSN 1053-8119.

Brazier, M. A. (1972). Spread of seizure discharges in epilepsy: anatomical and electrophysiological considerations. *Exp. Neurol.* 36, 263–272.

Burock, M.A. and Dale, A.M. (2000). Estimation and detection of event-related fMRI signals with temporally correlated noise: a statistically efficient and unbiased approach. Hum Brain Mapp, Vol.11, No. 4, pp.249-260, ISSN 1097-0193.

Buxton, R. and Frank, L. (1997). A model for the coupling between cerebral blood flow and oxygen metabolism during neural stimulation. J. Cereb. Blood Flow Metab. Vol.17, No.1, pp.64-72, ISSN 0271-678X.

Cadotte, A.J., Mareci, T.H., DeMarse, T.B., Parekh, M.B., Rajagovindan, R., Ditto, W.L., Talathi, S.S., Dong-Uk Hwang, Carney, P.R., Temporal Lobe Epilepsy: Anatomical and Effective Connectivity," Neural Systems and Rehabilitation Engineering, IEEE Transactions on , Vol.17, No.3, pp.214-223

Chen, H., Liao, W., Gong, Q., Shen, S. (2009). Evaluation of the effective connectivity of supplementary motor areas during motor imagery using Granger causality mapping. *Neuroimage,* Vol.47, No.4, (October 2009), pp.1844-1853, ISSN 1053-8119.

Ciuciu P., Poline J.-B., Marrelec G., Idier J., Pallier C .and Benali H. (2003). Unsupervised robust nonparametric estimation of the hemodynamic response function for any fMRI experiment. *IEEE Transactions on Medical Imaging,* Vol. 22, No.10, (October 2003), pp.1235-1251, ISSN 0278-0062.

Ciuciu, P., Idier, J., Roche, A., Pallier, C. (2004). Outlier detection for robust region-based estimation of the hemodynamic response function in event-related fMRI. Proc. IEEE International Symposium on Biomedical Imaging , (April 2004), pp. 392-395.

Comon, P. (1994). Independent components analysis: A new concept?. *Signal Processing,* Vol. 36, No.3, (April 1994), pp. 287–314, ISSN 0165-1684

Dale, A.,M. and Buckner, R., L. (1997). Selective averaging of rapidly presented individual trials using fMRI. *Human Brain Mapping,* Vol.5, No.5, pp. 29–340, ISSN 1097-0193.

David, O., Guillemain, I., Saillet, S., Reyt, S., Deransart, C., Segebarth, C., and Depaulis, A. (2008a). Identifying neural drivers with functional MRI: an electrophysiological validation. *PLoS Biol.* 6, 2683–2697.

David, O. (2009). fMRI connectivity, meaning and empiricism Comments on: Roebroeck et al. The identification of interacting networks in the brain using fMRI: Model selection, causality and deconvolution. *Neuroimage,* in press.

De Martino, F.; Gentile, F.; Esposito, F.; Balsi, M.; Di Salle, F.; Goebel, R.; Formisano, E. (2007) Classification of fMRI independent components using IC-fingerprints and support vector machine classifiers. *NeuroImage*, Vol.34, No.1, (January 2007), pp. 177–194, ISSN 1053-8119.

Demirci, O., Stevens, M.C., Andreasen, N.C., Michael, A., Liu, J., White, T., Pearlson, G.D., Clark, V.P., Calhoun, V.D. (2009). Investigation of relationships between fMRI brain networks in the spectral domain using ICA and Granger causality reveals distinct differences between schizophrenia patients and healthy controls. *Neuroimage,* Vol. 46, pp.419-431, ISSN 1053-8119.

Deshpande, G., Xiaoping, H., Stilla, R., Sathian, K. (2008): Effective connectivity during haptic perception: A study using Granger causality analysis of functional magnetic resonance imaging data. *Neuroimage,* Vol. 40, pp.1807-1814, ISSN 1053-8119.

Deshpande, G., LaConte, S., James, G.A., Peltier, S., Hu, X. (2009): Multivariate Granger Causality Analysis of fMRI data. *Human Brain Mapping,* Vol. 30, pp. 1361-1373.

Ethofer, T., Anders, S., Erb, M., Herbert, C., Wiethoff, S., Kissler, J., Grodd, W., Wildgruber, D., (2006). Cerebral pathways in processing of affective prosody: a dynamical causal modeling study. *NeuroImage,* Vol. 30, pp.580–587.

Franaszczuk, P. J., and Bergey, G. K. (1998). Application of the directed transfer function method to mesial and lateral onset temporal lobe seizures. *Brain Topography.* 11, 13–21.

Franaszczuk, P. J., and Bergey, G. K. (1999). An autoregressive method for the measurement of synchronization of interictal and ictal EEG signals. *Biological Cybernetics* 81, 3–9.

Friston, K.J., Frith, C.D., Liddle, P.F., Frackowiak, R.S., (1993). Functional connectivity: the principal component analysis of large (PET) data sets. *Journal of Cerebral Blood Flow & Metabolism,* Vol.13, pp.5-14, ISSN 0271-678X.

Friston, K. J., Harrison, L., and Penny, W. D. (2003). Dynamic causal modelling. *Neuroimage* Vol.19, pp. 1273–1302, ISSN 1053-8119.

Glover, G.H. (1999). Deconvolution of impulse response in event-related BOLD fMRI, NeuroImage, Vol. 9, No.4, (April 1999), pp. 416–429, ISSN 10538119

Gossl, C., Fahrmeir, L. and Auer, D.P., (2001). Bayesian modeling of the hemodynamic response function in BOLD fMRI, Neuroimage, Vol.14, No.1 , (July 2001), pp.140–148, ISSN 1053-8119.

Gotman, J. (1987). Interhemispheric interactions in seizures of focal onset: data from human intracranial recordings. Electroenceph. Clin. Neurophysiol. 67, 120–133.

Goutte, C., Arup Nielsen, F., Hansen, L.K. (2000) Modeling the haemodynamic response in fMRI using smooth FIR filters, *IEEE Transactions on Medical Imaging,* Vol. 19, No.12, (December 2000), pp.1188–1201, ISSN 0278-0062

Haykin, S., Racine, R. J., Xu, Y., and Chapman, C. A. (1996). Monitoring neural oscillation and signal transmission between cortical regions using time-frequency analysis of electroencephalographic activity. Proc. IEEE 84, 1295–1301.

Havlicek, M., Jan, J,. Brazdil, M., Calhoun, V.D. (2010). Dynamic Granger causality based on Kalman filter for evaluation of functional network connectivity in fMRI data. *Neuroimage,* Vol.53, pp.65-77.

Hyvärinen, A. &Oja, E. (2000) Independent Component Analysis: Algorithms and Applications. *Neural Networks,* Vol. 13, No.4-5, (June 2000), pp. 411-430, ISSN 0893-6080.

Ide, J.S., Li, C.R. (2011). A cerebellar thalamic cortical circuit for error-related cognitive control. *Neuroimage* Vol. 54, pp. 455-464.

Jiao, Q., Lu, G., Zhang, Z., Zhong, Y., Wang, Z., Guo, Y., Li, K., Ding, M., Liu, Y. (2011). Granger Causal Influence Predicts BOLD Activity Levels in the Default Mode Network. *Human Brain Mapping*, Vol.32, pp.154-161.

Josephs, O.; Tuner, R. & Friston, K.J. (1997) Event-related fMRI. *Human Brain Mapping*, Vol. 5, No.4, (June-July 1997),pp. 243–248, ISSN 1053-8119.

Kang, J.K., Bénar, C.G., Al-Asmi, A., Khani, Y., A., Pike, G.B., Dubeau, F., Gotman, J. (2003). Using patient-specific hemodynamic response functions in combined EEG-fMRI studies in epilepsy. *Neuroimage*, Vol.20, No.2, (October 2003), pp.1162-1170, ISSN 1053-8119.

Kershaw, J., Abe, S., Kashikura, K., Zhang, X. and Kanno, I, (2000). A Bayesian approach to estimating the haemodynamic response function in event-related fMRI. *Neuroimage*, Vol.11, No.5, Supplement 1, (May 2000), pp. S474, ISSN 1053-8119.

Korzeniewska, A., Manczak, M., Kaminski, M., Blinowska, K.J., Kasicki, S. (2003). Determination of information flow direction between brainstructures by a modified directed transfer function method (dDTF), *J. Neurosci. Meth.*, Vol.125, pp.195–207.

Lee, L., Friston, K., Horwitz, B., 2006. Large-scale neural models and dynamic causal modelling. NeuroImage Vol. 30, pp.1243–1254.

Lemieux, L., Laufs, H., Carmichael, D., Paul, J. S., Walker, M. C. and Duncan, J. S. (2008). Noncanonical spike-related BOLD responses in focal epilepsy. Human Brain Mapping. Vol. 29, No.3, (March 2008) , pp. 329–345, ISSN 1065-9471.

Lemieux, L., Daunizeau, J.,Walker, M. (2011). Concepts of connectivity and human epileptic activity, Frontiers in Systems Neuroscience Vol.5, Article 12, (March 2011), pp. ISSN 1662-5137.

LeVan, P. & Gotman, J. (2009) Independent Component Analysis As a Model-Free Approach for the Detection of BOLD Changes Related to Epileptic Spikes: A Simulation Study. Hum Brain Mapping, Vol. 30, No.7, (July 2009), pp. 2021-2031, ISSN 1097-0193

LeVan, P.; Tyvaert, L.; Moeller, F.; Gotman, J. (2010). Independent component analysis reveals dynamic ictal BOLD responses in EEG-fMRI data from focal epilepsy patients. NeuroImage, Vol.49, No.1, (January 2010), pp. 366-378, ISSN 10538119

Liao, W., Ding, J., Marinazzo, D., Xu, Q., Wang, Z., Yuan, C., Zhang, Z., Lu, G., Chen, H. (2011). Small-world directed networks in the human brain: Multivariate Granger causality analysis of resting-state fMRI. *Neuroimage*, Vol.54, pp.2683-2694.

Lopes da Silva, F. H., van Hulten, K., Lommen, J. G., Storm van Leeuwen, W., van Veelen, C. W., and Vliegenthart, W. (1977). Automatic detection and localization of epileptic foci. Electroencephalogr. *Clin. Neurophysiol*. 43, 1–13.

Lu, Y., Bagshaw, A.P., Grova, C., Kobayashi, E., Dubeau, F., Gotman, J., (2006). Using voxel-specific hemodynamic response function in EEG-fMRI data analysis. NeuroImage, Vol.32, No. 1, (August 2006), pp. 238-247, ISSN 1053-8119.

Lu, Y., Grova, C., Kobayashi, E., Dubeau, F., Gotman, J., (2007). Using voxel-specific hemodynamic response function in EEG-fMRI data analysis: An estimation and detection model. NeuroImage, Vol.34, No.1, (January 2007), pp.195-203, ISSN 1053-8119.

Makni, S., Ciuciu, P., Idier, J., Poline, J.B. (2004). Semiblind deconvolution of neuronal impulse response in event-related fMRI using Gibbs sampler. *Proc. IEEE International Symposium on Biomedical Imaging,* (April 2004), pp.860-863.

Makni, S., Idier, J., Vincent, V., Thirion, B., Dehaene-Lambertz, G .and Ciuciu, P. (2008). A fully Bayesian approach to the parcel-based detection-estimation of brain activity in fMRI. Neuroimage, Vol.41, No.3, (July 2008), pp.941-969, ISSN 1053-8119.

Marrelec, G., Benali, H., Ciuciu ,P,. Pelegrini-Issac, M .and Poline. J.-B. (2003). Robust bayesian estimation of the hemodynamic response function in event-related BOLD MRI using basic physiological information. Hum Brain Mapp Vol.19, No.1, pp.1-17, ISSN 1097-0193.

Marrelec, G,. Bellec, P., Benali, H. (2006). Exploring Large-Scale Brain Networks in Functional MRI. Journal of Physiology-Paris, Vol. 100, pp.171-181.

Mars, N., and Lopes da Silva, F. (1983). Propagation of seizure activity in kindled dogs. Electroencephalogr. *Clin. Neurophysiol.* 56, 194–209.

McKeown, M.J.; Makeig, S.; Brown, G.G.; Jung, T.P.; Kindermann, S.S.; Bell, A.J.; Sejnowski, T.J. (1998) Analysis of fMRI data by blind separation into independent spatial components. Human Brain Mapping, Vol. 6, No.3, (December 1998), pp.160-88, ISSN 1097-0193

Mechelli, A., Henson, R.N.A., Price, C.J., Friston, K.J., (2003). Comparing event-related and epoch analysis in blocked design fMRI. NeuroImage Vol.18, pp. 806–810.

Moeller, F.; Siebner, H.; Wolff, S.; Muhle, H.; Boor, R.; Granert, O.; Jansen, O.; Stephani, U.; Siniatchkin, M. (2008): Changes in activity of striato-thalamo-cortical network precede generalized spike wave discharges. NeuroImage, Vol. 39, No.4, (February 2008), pp.1839–1849, ISSN 10538119

Moeller, F.; LeVan, P.; Gotman, J. (2011). Independent Component Analysis (ICA) of Generalized Spike Wave Discharges in fMRI: Comparison with General Linear Model-Based EEG-fMRI. Hum Brain Mapping, Vol. 32, No.2, (February 2011), pp. 209-217, ISSN 1097-0193

Penny, W.D., Stephan, K.E., Mechelli, A., Friston, K.J., (2004a). Modelling functional integration: a comparison of structural equation and dynamic causal models. NeuroImage, Vol. 23 (S1), pp. S264–S274.

Penny, W.D., Stephan, K.E., Mechelli, A., Friston, K.J., (2004a). Comparing dynamic causal models. NeuroImage Vol.22, pp.1157–1172, ISSN 10538119

Razavi, M., Grabowski, T.J., Vispoel, W.P., Monahan, P., Mehta, S., Eaton, B., Bolinger, L., (2003). Model assessment and model building in fMRI. Hum. Brain Mapp. Vol.20, No.4, pp.227–238, ISSN 1097-0193 .

Rodionov, R.; De Martino, F.; Laufs, H.; Carmichael, D.W.; Formisano, E.; Walker, M.; Duncan, J.S.; Lemieux, L. (2007). Independent component analysis of interictal fMRI in focal epilepsy: comparison with general linear model-based EEG-correlated fMRI. NeuroImage, Vol 38, No.3, (November 2007), pp. 488–500, ISSN 10538119

Roebroeck A, Formisano E, Goebel R (2005). Mapping directed influence over the brain using Granger causality and fMRI. Neuroimage Vol. 25, pp.230-242.

Roebroeck, A., Formisano, E., Goebel, R., (2009). The identification of interacting networks in the brain using fMRI: Model selection, causality and deconvolution. Neuroimage, in press. ISSN 1053-8119.

Salek-Haddadi, A.; Merschhemke, M.; Lemieux, L.; Fish, D.R. (2002), Simultaneous EEG correlated ictal fMRI. NeuroImage, Vol. 16, No.1, (May 2002), pp. 32- 40, ISSN 1053-8119

Sato, J.R., Junior, E.A., Takahashi, D.Y., Felix, M., Brammer, M.J., Morettin, P.A. (2006). A method to produce evolving functional connectivity maps during the course of an fMRI experiment using wavelet-based time-varying Granger causality. *Neuroimage,* Vol. 31, No.1, (May 2006), pp.187-196, ISSN1053-8119.

Sato, J.R., Takahashi, D.Y., Arcuri, S.M., Sameshima, K., Morettin, P.A., Baccalà, L.A. (2009). Frequency Domain Connectivity Identification: An Application of Partial Directed Coherence in fMRI. *Human Brain Mapping,* Vol.30, No.2, (February 2009), pp.452-461, ISSN 1097-0193.

Sato, J.R., Fujita, A., Cardoso, E.F., Thomaz, C.E., Brammer, M.J., Amaro, E. Jr (2010). Analyzing the connectivity between regions of interest: An approach based on cluster Granger causality for fMRI data analysis. *Neuroimage* Vol.5, No.4, (October 2010), pp.1444-1455, ISSN 1053-8119.

Schippers, M.B., Keysers, C. (2011). Mapping the flow of information within the putative mirror neuron system during gesture observation. *Neuroimage,* in press.

Seger, C.A., Dennison, C.S., Lopez-Paniagua, D., Peterson, E.J., Roark, A.A. (2011). Dissociating hippocampal and basal ganglia contributions to category learning using stimulus novelty and subjective judgments. *Neuroimage,* in press.

Stam, C. J., Breakspear, M., van Cappellen van Walsum, A. M., and van Dijk, B. W. (2003). Nonlinear synchronization in EEG and whole-head MEG recordings of healthy subjects. *Human Brain Mapping,* Vol.19, pp. 63–78.

Stephan, K.E., Penny, W.D., Daunizeau, J., Moran, R.J., Friston K.J. Bayesian model selection for group studies, NeuroImage, Vol. 46, No. 4, (July 2009), pp. 1004-1017, ISSN 1053-8119.

Stilla, R., Deshpande, G., Laconte, S., Hu, X., Sathian, K. (2007). Posteromedial parietal cortical activity and inputs predict tactile spatial acuity. *Journal of Neuroscience,* Vol.27, No.41, (October 2007), pp.11091–11102.

Stilla, R., Hanna, R., Mariola, E., Deshpande, G., Hu, X., Sathian, K. (2008):Neural processing underlying tactile microspatial discrimination in the blind: a functional magnetic resonance imaging study, J. Vis. 8(10):13.1–13.19.

Tana, M.G., Bianchi ,A.M., Vitali P., Villani F., Cerutti S. (2007). The Haemodynamic response to interictal epileptic spikes. Proc, IEEE EMBS Annual International Conference. (22-26 Aug. 2007), pp. 5223 - 5226, ISSN 1557-170X.

Tana, M.G., Bianchi, A.M., Sclocco, R., Franchin, T., Cerutti, S., Leal, A. (2011) Parcel-based connectivity of fMRI data for the study of epileptic seizure propagation. Submitted

Theiler, J., Eubank, S., Longtin, A., Galdrikian, B., Farmer, D. (1992). Testing for nonlinearity in time series: the method of surrogate data. *Physica D* , Vol. 58, pp. 77-94.

Vaudano, A. E., Laufs, H., Kiebel, S. J., Carmichael, D. W., Hamandi, K., Guye, M., Thornton, R., Rodionov, R., Friston, K. J., Duncan, J. S., and Lemieux, L. (2009). Causal hierarchy within the thalamo-cortical network in spike and wave discharges. PLoS ONE 4,

Wendling, F., and Bartolomei, F. (2001). Modeling EEG signals and interpreting measures of relationship during temporal-lobe seizures: an approach to the study of epileptogenic networks. Epileptic Disord. 3, 67–78.

Wendling, F., Ansari-Asl, K., Bartolomei, F., and Senhadji, L. (2009). From EEG signals to brain connectivity: a model-based evaluation of interdependence measures. J. Neurosci. Methods 183, 9–18.

Wendling F, Chauvel P, Biraben A and Bartolomei F (2010). From intracerebral EEG signals to brain connectivity: identification of epileptogenic networks in partial epilepsy. *Front. Syst. Neurosci.* Vol.4, No.154.

5

Investigations of Brain Network Alterations in Epilepsy Using Functional Magnetic Resonance Imaging

Victoria L. Morgan and Bassel Abou-Khalil
Vanderbilt University
USA

1. Introduction

Epilepsy is a chronic condition characterized by recurrent unprovoked seizures with potentially disabling effects. These seizures, even when generated from a single focus, are believed to involve an extensive network of regions across the brain (Norden & Blumenfeld 2002). The propagation across these networks is responsible for the complex events associated with seizures including altered consciousness and motor phenomena. Additionally, repeated seizures can also produce chronic deficits that persist in between seizures, mainly cognitive deficits, primarily of memory and language related functions (Helmstaedter, et al. 2003). It is likely that these cognitive effects can be related to measurable brain network alterations as well. The non-invasive quantification of alterations in brain networks related to epilepsy is critical in determining the mechanisms of epileptogenesis and its treatments. In addition, it may also identify imaging biomarkers of epilepsy which can be used to diagnose and monitor these patients.

Electroencephalography (EEG) is the most widely used method to quantify epileptic activity across the brain. The high temporal resolution of EEG measurements is advantageous in detecting the electrophysiological activity that defines the seizure focus and associated network. However, these techniques have relatively low spatial resolution when performed non-invasively, and can be corrupted by attenuation of the signal by bone or other tissue. Invasive EEG monitoring can measure electrical activity directly from the cortex, but the spatial resolution is still relatively low. The recording can only be obtained from preselected regions of the cortex. This method also involves more significant risk than non-invasive methods, but can be useful in detecting limited networks of epileptic activity (Blumenfeld, et al. 2004b, Englot, et al. 2008, Guye, et al. 2006).

Imaging methodologies make it possible to investigate networks across the whole brain without the need for identifying predefined regions. Some non-invasive, low spatial resolution techniques to detect epileptic networks include interictal positron emission tomography (PET) with [18F] fluoro-2-deoxy-glucose (FDG) (Cascino & Jack 1996, Spencer & Bautista 2000) and ictal single-photon emission computed tomography (SPECT) imaging (Cascino & Jack 1996, Spencer & Bautista 2000). In general, these methods attempt to detect regions of metabolic (PET) or perfusion (SPECT) changes during the interictal state or ictal events. Studies have detected widespread brain networks associated with seizures using these methods (Blumenfeld, et al. 2004a, Blumenfeld, et al. 2009, Wong, et al. 2010). One advantage of using ictal SPECT imaging is that different phases of the seizure can be probed in different seizures at different times (e.g. pregeneralization vs. post ictal) (Blumenfeld, et al. 2009). The disadvantages are that it requires injection of radiotracer at the time of the seizure prior to scanning and the spatial resolution is low. In addition, measurements cannot be made longitudinally with high temporal resolution in order to examine seizure propagation in the same event.

The objective of this chapter is to discuss how functional Magnetic Resonance Imaging (fMRI) can be used to examine brain network alterations in epilepsy. First, an introduction to the concepts of fMRI and functional connectivity will be presented. The main focus of the chapter will be a review of the current published work involving the investigations of changes in healthy resting-state brain networks caused by epilepsy and the identification of possible epileptogenic networks. In addition, the relationship of the network parameters to disease characteristics, diagnosis and treatment will be discussed in relation to the network alterations. Studies of quantification of causal influences across these networks using Granger causality and dynamic causal modeling will also be included. More novel methods of fMRI network analysis being applied to epilepsy will be described. Finally, the chapter will conclude with a brief overview of future research directions.

2. Functional MRI and functional connectivity mapping

Functional MRI is a widely used non-invasive neuroimaging technique that can detect and localize areas of the brain engaged in performing a specific task. This technique typically uses echo-planar image acquisition parameters that are sensitive to the changes in blood oxygenation occurring with neuronal activation (Blood Oxygenation Level Dependent or BOLD acquisitions) (Logothetis, et al. 2001, Ogawa, et al. 1990). Signal intensity in the BOLD images is increased when oxyhemoglobin concentrations increase due to neuronal activation. In conventional block-design fMRI studies, a series of images is collected during at least two different activation states (e.g. rest and stimulation) and their signal intensities are compared statistically on a voxel by voxel basis. The difference between these two image series indicates the location and intensity of neuronal activation in response to the given stimulation. In event-related fMRI, the images are collected following a repeated transient stimulus. Signal intensity following the stimuli is compared to the rest of the series. Therefore, in typical fMRI experiments, the timings of the various stimuli are known. The primary challenge in using fMRI in epilepsy is that interictal and ictal seizure activity is spontaneous and its timing cannot be controlled. There are two general approaches to attempt to overcome this problem. The first approach is to combine fMRI acquisitions with scalp EEG measurements (Gotman, et al. 2004). The EEG will provide the timing of the epileptic activity for conventional fMRI analysis. The second is to use a data-driven approach that identifies the interictal BOLD response in the fMRI data without EEG or other monitoring (Rodionov, et al. 2007).

Simple fMRI activation maps can determine the level of involvement of distinct regions of a network to perform a task at the time of acquisition. However, fMRI potentially can also reveal additional information about the functional coupling within this network using functional connectivity mapping. Functional connectivity uses linear correlations of low frequency (<0.1 Hz) fMRI BOLD signal oscillations usually at rest or during steady-state performance of a task (Rogers, et al. 2007). The resting state (awake with eyes closed) is a potentially interesting focus of attention because even at rest the brain accounts for approximately 20% of the total body oxygen consumption, primarily to maintain excitatory and inhibitory neurotransmission (Shulman, et al. 2004).

The two most commonly used methods of determining functional connectivity are seed based methods and independent component analysis (ICA). Both are based on temporal series of BOLD signals. The seed based approaches require the identification of a seed voxel or region, and the linear correlation across time of other voxels or regions to that seed is considered the measure of connectivity. This method is more suited for hypothesis testing due to its a priori identification of a seed. However, the most appropriate technique for defining a seed may be different for different applications. The ICA method attempts to transform the original data time series into individual components assuming that all of the signal sources and noise are statistically independent and are mixed linearly to create the observed signal. This technique has also been used successfully with fMRI data (Calhoun, et al. 2003, Moritz, et al. 2005). The advantage in applying these techniques to epilepsy is that all of the components of the signal (presumably from independent sources) are identified which can result in a large number of components. The primary disadvantages are (1) that these components will include many of those of no-interest due to shape or amplitude expectations, and separating the ones of interest becomes a significant task, and (2) the expected signal of interest may be relatively small.

3. Networks defined in healthy controls

There exists a set of functional brain networks that are consistently identified in the resting brain using fMRI time series data in healthy subjects. Typically these are identified as a group using an ICA analysis with varying numbers of components (Damoiseaux, et al. 2006, De Luca, et al. 2006). However, they can also be identified individually using seed region analysis of connectivity by placing a seed within an expected network (Biswal, et al. 1995, Xiong, et al. 1999), and also by using hierarchical clustering methods (Cordes, et al. 2002). While there are varying numbers of resting-state networks that have been described (based on varying degrees of specificity), they generally can be divided into approximately five overlapping spatial maps (De Luca, et al. 2006):

1. *Visual cortex network*- lateral and medial occipital cortex
2. *Default-mode network* - anterior cingulate, posterior cingulate, lateral inferior parietal cortex, hippocampus and prefrontal cortex
3. *Sensorimotor and auditory network* - pre and post-central gyrus, superior temporal gyrus, insula, thalamus and hippocampus
4. *Dorsal pathway* - lateral frontal regions and dorsal parietal cortex
5. *Ventral pathway* - lateral temporal, and inferior prefrontal cortex

These networks are reliable and reproducible within a scanning session and between sessions up to months apart (Zuo, et al. 2010). Several of these networks also seem to have unique electrophysiological signatures determined by EEG (Mantini, et al. 2007) and MEG (magnetoencephalography) (de Pasquale, et al. 2010) power. The networks similar to the visual, auditory and motor processing in adults have been detected in infants (Fransson, et al. 2007). This suggests the order of maturation of various networks in the brain, and may explain development of specific cognitive functions as a child ages. In order to understand how epilepsy and its treatment can affect normal cognitive function and behavior, it is useful to investigate the changes within the known resting-state networks of these patients.

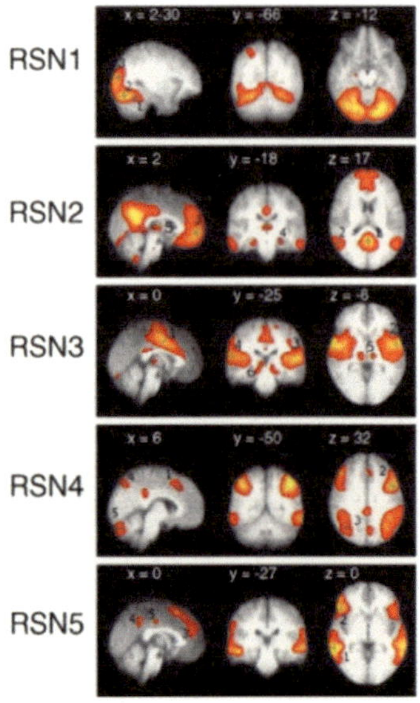

Fig. 1. Five resting state networks defined in healthy controls (Reprinted from NeuroImage, 29(4), De Luca, M et al., "fMRI resting state networks define distinct modes of long-distance interactions in the human brain" 1359-1367 (2006) with permission from Elsevier)

3.1 Language and memory networks

Chronic drug-resistant temporal lobe epilepsy (TLE) is associated with progressive memory impairment (Fisher, et al. 2000, Helmstaedter, et al. 2003) which is related to the structural damage of the epileptic hippocampus and other mesial temporal lobe structures in these patients (Kilpatrick, et al. 1997). In addition to the chronic epilepsy itself, the surgical treatment of TLE can also have a negative impact on language and memory functions. The fact that the seizures are generated from a specific focus in the mesial temporal lobe makes many drug-resistant mesial TLE patients good candidates for resective surgery. The success rate for seizure control following surgical resection is approximately 80% (Siegel 2004). In a randomized-control study of surgery vs. antiepileptic drug treatment for temporal lobe epilepsy, 58% of patients became seizure free with surgery vs. 8% on drug therapy (Wiebe, et al. 2001). The resulting seizure control can result in a significant increase in quality of life in these patients including employment or school attendance (Wiebe, et al. 2001). However, further declines in verbal memory and word finding after respective surgery to treat seizures are side effects occurring in as many as 40% of TLE patients (Langfitt & Wiebe 2008). If severe, these impairments can affect the individual's ability to perform in work and social situations. Langfitt et al. reported that in patients with good seizure outcome, quality of life improved even if some memory loss occurred; but, in patients without post-surgical seizure control, quality of life decreased when memory loss occurred (Langfitt, et al. 2007). These findings illustrate the importance of quantifying and understanding these cognitive functions, and using this information to accurately predict the risk of cognitive decline after resective surgery. It is likely that these impairments, both before and after surgery, involve alterations in long-range networks in language and memory. Functional MRI provides a way to probe the functional integrity of these networks, and allows quantification of the relationships between cognition and connectivity in order to address these issues.

To assess the utility of fMRI for prediction of post-surgical language and memory function, it must first be compared to the Intracarotid Amobarbital Test (IAT or Wada test) which was first developed by Wada in 1949. This test is used to determine hemisphere dominance for language and memory by an intra-arterial injection of an anesthetic agent to one hemisphere of the brain at a time while evaluating the patient's ability to perform language and memory tasks. The development of aphasia after injection indicates hemisphere dominance for language, and the lack of memory encoding suggests that the contralateral hippocampus cannot sustain memory function. The Wada test is an invasive and uncomfortable procedure with serious potential risks including carotid artery dissection, infection and stroke. One study reported almost 11% of patients had complications with 0.6% having residual deficits after three months (Loddenkemper, et al. 2008). In addition to risk, the cost of the Wada test can be high relative to fMRI (Medina, et al. 2004). Furthermore, even when successful, the Wada test lateralizes, but does not localize language and memory functions and their associated networks. As a result, the use of the Wada test in the presurgical evaluation of all TLE patients is decreasing (Baxendale, et al. 2008), while other non-invasive methods including fMRI are gaining acceptance (Abou-Khalil 2007, Pelletier, et al. 2007).

Functional MRI has been very successful for lateralizing language dominance as well as identifying and localizing language networks. There is a wide variety of stimulation tasks used for this purpose. Some of the more widely used tasks include word generation (Deblaere, et al. 2002, Ramsey, et al. 2001) for activating the inferior frontal language regions (Broca's Area), and tasks such as reading (Gaillard, et al. 2002, Rutten, et al. 2002b) and listening to speech (Binder, et al. 2008b, Bookheimer 2007) for identifying temporoparietal language regions (Wernicke's Area). The literature on this topic is vast, describing other potentially useful tasks. The concordance of these protocols with Wada test results is over 70% in many of these studies, but may be less in patients with atypical right-sided or bilateral dominance by Wada test. The combination of multiple fMRI tasks has been found to be more accurate than a single task (Arora, et al. 2009, Deblaere, et al. 2002, Ramsey, et al. 2001, Rutten, et al. 2002a), and these methods can also be modified for use in children (Arora, et al. 2009, Gaillard, et al. 2002). For these reasons, fMRI, when available, is quickly becoming the preferred technique for determining language lateralization and localization.

While the use of fMRI for language lateralization is gaining widespread acceptance, the assessment of memory functions with this method has been slower to develop. Some reasons for this disparity include the fact that fMRI memory paradigms are generally more complicated and require more trials to provide detectible signal changes than language paradigms. Also, the material being encoded in memory tasks can have a lateralizing effect itself (verbal vs. visual stimuli), (Golby, et al. 2001), and the interaction of this effect with the epilepsy can be difficult to interpret. Thus, memory paradigms have shown mixed success in lateralizing memory function in TLE compared to the Wada test (Deblaere, et al. 2005, Golby, et al. 2002, Jokeit, et al. 2001).

Some fMRI memory paradigms designed to activate the mesial temporal structures have been used with varying levels of success to predict post-surgical memory declines (Frings, et al. 2008b, Rabin, et al. 2004, Richardson, et al. 2006, Wagner, et al. 2007). Their general finding was that increased fMRI activation in the mesial temporal lobe ipsilateral to the surgical resection was correlated with increased post-surgical declines, thus supporting the "functional adequacy model" of hippocampal function. This model predicts that severity of decline depends on the function of the region resected and not on the ability of the contralateral region to support function after surgery ("functional reserve model") (Chelune 1995). These studies report positive predictive values of 56 to 100% (Richardson, et al. 2004) for fMRI to predict post-surgical change in memory neuropsychological scores. Interestingly, some more recent reports show that evaluating multiple regions of the language and memory networks, including those in the frontal and lateral temporal lobes, can improve this prediction (Binder, et al. 2008a, Binder, et al. 2010, Bonelli, et al. 2010, Everts, et al. 2010). Bonelli, et al. (Bonelli, et al. 2010) found that in their cohort the positive predictive value of memory fMRI activation asymmetry in the anterior temporal lobe was 20-35%, but when fMRI language lateralization, calculated using multiple regions across the frontal and temporal lobes, and pre-operative neuropsychological scores are included, the positive predictive value rose to 70-100%.

While fMRI activation of long range regions is informative, it is likely that probing the functional connectivity across language and/or memory networks may be a more direct measure of cognitive function or predictor of post-surgical function. However, the appropriate choices for regions and task paradigm (or none) remain unknown. Studies performed thus far have varied significantly in these study parameters, and so consistent results are few. One promising repeated finding is that the functional connectivity between the anterior cingulate and the left inferior frontal gyrus was found to be decreased in TLE compared to healthy controls during rest (Waites, et al. 2006) and during block-design performance of a word-generation task (Vlooswijk, et al. 2010). Similarly, the functional connectivity of the left hippocampus and other regions involved with memory was also decreased relative to controls (Addis, et al. 2007). Generally, these decreases in functional connectivity were associated with diminished cognitive performance as measured by the neuropsychological testing. In support of the functional adequacy model, higher fMRI connectivity of the ipsilateral hippocampus to the superior temporal gyrus was associated with greater decline of verbal memory performance after surgery (Wagner, et al. 2007).

While fMRI has great potential to identify noninvasive markers of language and memory cognition and post-surgical outcome, there are many possible sources of error and variability in fMRI methods. First, there can be much variability in task performance. Many patients have cognitive deficits which reduce their ability to cooperate, understand and remember the directions of the task. Including children in the patient population increases this variation even more. For many cognitive tasks, it is difficult to impossible to monitor externally how well the tasks are being performed. Also, fMRI analysis methods are not standard. Differences in statistical thresholds and regions of interest used to calculate laterality indices can also lead to uncertainty (Abbott, et al. 2010, Branco, et al. 2006, Sidtis 2007, Suarez, et al. 2008). Research focused on resolving these issues is required before it will be possible to utilize fMRI for assessing surgical risk of cognitive deficits.

3.2 The default-mode network

There are regions of the brain that have been regularly observed to reduce fMRI activity (deactivate) during performance of demanding cognitive tasks or goal directed behavior (Fox, et al. 2005). When studied in a wakeful resting state using positron emission tomography (PET), increases in cerebral metabolic rate for oxygen ($CMRO_2$) and cerebral blood flow (CBF) are detected in these regions over other regions of the brain (Raichle, et al. 2001). The data suggest the existence of a baseline activation level in these areas at rest above the mean level of the brain, which may reflect internal modes of cognition, such as mind wandering or daydreaming in this state. This collection of regions is commonly referred to as the "default-mode network" (DMN, network 2, Figure 1) and typically include the following regions (Buckner, et al. 2008): ventral medial prefrontal cortex, posterior cingulate/retrosplenial cortex, bilateral inferior parietal lobule, lateral temporal cortex, dorsal medial prefrontal cortex, and hippocampus.

In addition to being identified as a network of regions deactivated during goal-oriented cognitive tasks, this same network can reliably be identified by performing independent component analysis on resting state fMRI data (Damoiseaux, et al. 2006, De Luca, et al. 2006) and by seed region based functional connectivity analyses (Greicius, et al. 2003). Inter-subject variability in the functional connectivity across the DMN is influenced by factors such as age (Grady, et al. 2010), cognitive load (i.e. eyes open vs. eyes closed) (Yan, et al. 2009), genetics (Glahn, et al. 2010), level of consciousness (Greicius, et al. 2008) and sleep (Horovitz, et al. 2008). It has been directly correlated in part to EEG delta and beta power (Hlinka, et al. 2010). However, the robustness of this network and its implications on baseline cognitive function and consciousness make it a frequent focus of investigations of neurological disease (Broyd, et al. 2009).

The relationship between DMN and epilepsy was first reported in activation studies of generalized spike-and-wave (GSW) bursts in patients with idiopathic generalized epilepsy (IGE) (Archer, et al. 2003, Gotman, et al. 2005, Hamandi, et al. 2006, Laufs, et al. 2006, Salek-Haddadi, et al. 2003). In these studies, simultaneous measures of EEG and fMRI (Gotman, et al. 2004) were acquired in individual or groups of IGE patients with frequent GSW bursts on EEG. The EEG was used to determine the timing of any GSW bursts occurring during fMRI scanning. These times were then used to localize the regions of the brain in which the fMRI signal increased (activation) or decreased (deactivation) concurrently with the GSW bursts. While the results were somewhat variable across subjects, there was an overarching finding of positive activation located bilaterally in the thalamus and deactivation found in regions of the DMN. These findings suggest that the activation in the thalamus indicated this region's involvement in the generation or spread of generalized epileptic discharges. Furthermore, the authors propose that the combination of the activation of the thalamus with the deactivation of the DMN may lead to the lapse in responsiveness associated with absence seizures in IGE (Gotman, et al. 2005, Hamandi, et al. 2006). Conversely, there is evidence that the functional connectivity across the DMN assessed in IGE patients during time periods without GSW is not significantly different from healthy controls (Moeller, et al. 2011), indicating that this is primarily an ictal effect.

In order to verify the existence of a correlation between impaired consciousness and fMRI changes with GSW bursts, Berman et al. (Berman, et al. 2010) had a group of patients with typical childhood absence epilepsy perform a continuous performance task during the simultaneous EEG and fMRI acquisition. They used any interruption of task performance during the acquisition as an indicator of impaired consciousness. They then determined fMRI changes due to GSW bursts with interruption of the task and those without. During GSW bursts associated with interruption of the task, expected regions in the thalamus and cortex were activated and DMN regions were deactivated. However, when GSW bursts were not associated with task interruption, little fMRI change was detected. This suggests that the deactivation of the DMN and activation of the thalamus may be directly related to the impaired consciousness in absence seizures. On the other hand, in a case report of a study with similar methods, the expected fMRI activations and deactivations were detected in response to GSW bursts without task interruption (Moeller, et al. 2010b). The case study detected GSW bursts with an average duration of 4.2 seconds and with an fMRI temporal resolution of 2250 msec, whereas the group study included GSW bursts with an average duration of 6.2 sec and an fMRI temporal resolution of 1550 msec. One may expect that the increased temporal resolution and longer periods of GSW of the group study may increase detectability of fMRI signal changes even without task interruption, if they were present. Further study is required to clarify this issue.

More recent studies have attempted to resolve timing differences between fMRI changes in the DMN and other regions in response to GSW bursts (Carney, et al. 2010, Moeller, et al. 2010a). Both studies showed fMRI deactivations in DMN generally occurring prior to the increased thalamic response. In several instances fMRI signal change in the DMN started prior to the event onset on EEG. Another study (Szaflarski, et al. 2010) found parietal (but not necessarily DMN) activation occurring prior to thalamic activation and also detected similar causal links using Granger causality measures of fMRI data (Deshpande, et al. 2009, Goebel, et al. 2003). Another causal methodology, dynamic causal modeling (Friston, et al. 2003), can estimate the influence of one system on another. This method was used to determine which of three models including the ventromedial prefrontal cortex, the thalamus and the precuneus best fit the fMRI time series data when assuming the GSW bursts on EEG as the input (Vaudano, et al. 2009). The results over the group of IGE patients indicated that the GSW bursts initially influenced the precuneus and then the other two regions. These may infer the role of the DMN in the initiation of absence seizures, contradicting previous theories of thalamic generation of GSW bursts. Overall, the current literature provides convincing evidence for the potential link between function of the DMN and absence seizures and GSW bursts, but the direct mechanism of this relationship remains unknown.

There is a smaller, but growing, body of work linking activity in the DMN with focal epilepsy. Using the simultaneous EEG and fMRI protocol, deactivation has been detected in DMN regions in response to interictal EEG spiking (Kobayashi, et al. 2006, Laufs, et al. 2007). Using the data-driven method, 2dTCA (Morgan & Gore 2009, Morgan, et al. 2008), we have detected robust fMRI transient signal changes during resting, interictal periods in the DMN (Morgan, et al. 2007, Morgan, et al. 2010) in TLE patients.

Independent component analysis can assess the functional connectivity across the DMN in the interictal state, without temporally associating changes directly with interictal spiking. In unilateral TLE patients, this method has revealed decreased connectivity between the hippocampus (predominantly ipsilateral to the epilepsy) and the rest of the DMN as compared to healthy controls (Zhang, et al. 2010a). Similar finding were reported using a seed-based functional connectivity analysis in unilateral TLE patients performing a verbal memory task (Frings, et al. 2009). Linearly relating these changes in connectivity with epilepsy duration suggests that the mechanism of the disease is at least partly responsible for the dysfunction.

3.3 Perception and attention networks

While the language, memory and default-mode networks are the most commonly studied with fMRI in relation to epilepsy, this condition can have effects on other known networks across the brain that may possibly result in sensory or cognitive deficits. One such network is the auditory system in the bilateral superior temporal lobes including Heschl's gyrus, planum temporale and the temporal poles (part of network 3, Figure 1). Auditory function is integral in language (i.e. auditory sentence comprehension) and memory (i.e. verbal memory), which are known to be impaired in TLE (Fisher, et al. 2000, Helmstaedter, et al. 2003). However, auditory processing itself may also be impaired in these patients as suggested by increased errors, response times and latencies of electrical event-related potentials in response to auditory stimuli (more pronounced in IGE than TLE) in humans (Verleger, et al. 1997), and in auditory discrimination deficits in rat models of epilepsy (Neill, et al. 2005). These effects were explored in an fMRI functional connectivity study using independent component analysis that revealed decreased connectivity in auditory cortex networks in a group of bilateral mesial TLE patients as compared to healthy controls (Zhang, et al. 2009a). Furthermore, the decrease in connectivity across the auditory cortex was linearly correlated with increase in duration of disease (i.e. longer duration was associated with lower connectivity).

Network	Type of epilepsy	fMRI findings and uses (activation and connectivity)
Language	TLE	Language fMRI tasks are effective in lateralizing and potentially localizing dominant language regions; FC across this network is decreased compared to controls
Memory	TLE	Memory fMRI paradigms have mixed results in localizing memory functions; Memory and/or language tasks activating mesial temporal structures and beyond may be effective in predicting post-surgical memory deficits; Most studies show increased activation is associated with decreased post-surgical performance; Decreased FC compared to controls; Increased FC from ipsilateral hippocampus is correlated with decreased post-surgical verbal memory performance
Default-mode	IGE	Deactivation in response to GSW bursts; May be related to impaired consciousness; May be generator of GSW bursts
Default-mode	TLE	Deactivation in response to interictal spiking
Auditory	TLE	Decreases in FC across network positively compared to controls; Decrease correlated with duration of disease
Sensorimotor	TLE	Decreases in FC at rest compared to controls; Decrease correlated with duration of disease
Visual	TLE	Increases in FC in primary visual cortex, decreases in FC across higher order visual regions such as MT+ compared to controls at rest
Dorsal Attention	TLE	Decreases in FC at rest correlated with decreased scores on the Trail Making Test

TLE = temporal lobe epilepsy, IGE = idiopathic generalized epilepsy, FC = fMRI functional connectivity, GSW bursts = generalized spike-and-wave bursts on EEG

Table 1. Summary of effects of epilepsy on brain networks determined using fMRI

In the same fMRI study (Zhang, et al. 2009a), the authors also compared connectivity across the sensorimotor cortex (part of network 3, Figure 1) in the pre and post-central gyri in the frontal lobes between bilateral TLE patients and controls. Like the auditory network, the sensorimotor network connectivity was diminished in the TLE group as duration of disease increased.

In the visual cortex (network 1, Figure 1), the functional connectivity findings in the same study were mixed (Zhang, et al. 2009a). The results showed increases in connectivity in TLE in primary visual cortex, coupled with decreases in higher order visual processing regions such as MT+ when compared to controls that decreased with duration of disease. These findings may be consistent with behavioral results that showed no differences between reaction time or accuracy responding to visual stimuli in IGE (Verleger, et al. 1997) or TLE (Grant, et al. 2008); but deficits in processing of visual stimuli detected by EEG studies of visual evoked potentials (Lucking, et al. 1970) and event-related potentials (Verleger, et al. 1997).

The dorsal attention network is another set of regions that is repeatedly and reliably identified in healthy subjects (part of network 4, Figure 1). This network is made up of the intraparietal sulcus and the junction of the pre-central and superior frontal sulcus (or frontal eye field) in each hemisphere (Fox, et al. 2006) and is involved in attention orienting in searching for a target among non-targets (Shulman, et al. 2003). This function can be assessed using a neuropsychological test called the Trail Making Test (Reitan & Wolfson 1995) in which the subject connects numbers or letters in numerical or alphabetical order in a timed fashion. This and similar tests have been used in epilepsy to quantify the effects of different anti-epileptic drugs such as topiramate (negative effects) (Kockelmann, et al. 2003), zonisamide (negative effects) (Park, et al. 2008), lamotrigine (positive effects) and oxcarbazepine (positive effects) (Seo, et al. 2007) on cognition. Using the same ICA methods as in their previous work in perceptual networks above, Zhang et al. compared the resting functional connectivity in the dorsal attention network between patients with bilateral TLE and controls (Zhang, et al. 2009b). They found decreases across most of the network in TLE which correlated with decreased scores on the Trail Making Test. Interestingly, they also found an increase in the right superior frontal sulcus which also correlated with decreases in the Trail Making Test scores across patients.

4. Unique epilepsy related networks

In addition to the changes in known resting-state networks, epilepsy can alter connections between regions, thereby identifying networks unique to this condition. These networks may delineate seizure propagation, or impairment or compensatory mechanisms to structural and/or functional damage across the brain. The changes may be a result of the seizures or epilepsy, or may play a part in the underlying epileptogencity of a region. Furthermore, it may be more difficult to define these altered networks because they may be different even between patients with similar disease characteristics. Currently, most of the work in this area has focused on TLE and hippocampal networks.

4.1 Intrahemispheric mesial temporal lobe networks

It is known that the hippocampus and surrounding structures are most commonly the generators of seizures in mesial TLE. The networks that are comprised of these regions are potentially the most affected by the condition. Studies by Bettus et al. (Bettus, et al. 2010, Bettus, et al. 2009) have investigated intrahemispheric mesial temporal lobe networks in TLE at rest with the objective to determine whether resting-state functional connectivity can be used to determine the epileptogenic hemisphere. They identified five mesial temporal regions of interest in each hemisphere including the anterior and posterior hippocampus, amygdala, entorhinal cortex and the temporal pole. Intrahemispheric connectivity between these regions was compared to a group of healthy controls. Interestingly, there were decreases in connectivity between regions in both hemispheres in many subjects, but increases in connectivity compared to controls occurred primarily in the hemisphere contralateral to the seizures. This increase in resting functional connectivity, speculated to be a compensatory effect, was shown to have 63% sensitivity and 90% specificity in lateralizing the TLE.

4.2 Interhemispheric mesial temporal lobe networks

In addition to the intrahemispheric networks involving mesial temporal lobe structures in TLE, the network between the left and right hippocampus may very likely be one of the most susceptible to changes due to long term seizure propagation effects. However, the direct consequences of these effects on functional connectivity are not clear. In left TLE, the interhemispheric hippocampal network was found to be almost non-existent in a resting fMRI study of nine patients (Pereira, et al. 2010). In the same study, the connectivity between the hippocampi was stronger in a group of nine patients with right TLE than in left TLE, but both patient groups were significantly less than the strong interhemispheric hippocampal connectivity detected in the nine healthy controls. Another investigation quantified the interhemispheric connectivity in TLE during a spatial memory task which would utilize the network between these two regions (Frings, et al. 2008a). They found that hippocampal connectivity during the memory task significantly increased as age of onset of epilepsy increased; and that as disease duration increased hippocampal connectivity decreased. This suggests a negative effect of repeated seizures or hippocampal damage across this network during the task, which may be reflected in the poorer memory performance of TLE patients in general. However, the different behavioral states (resting vs. task) of the two studies and the lack of disease duration information in the resting study, make these difficult to interpret together.

In an attempt to reconcile these two studies, we recruited 15 TLE patients with left temporal ictal and interictal EEG, and 7 TLE patients with right temporal interictal and ictal EEG. We performed resting fMRI on a 3T MRI scanner using a 2 sec temporal sampling rate (compared to 2.0T MRI with a 2 sec sampling rate (Pereira, et al. 2010), and 1.5T MRI scanner with a 4 sec sampling rate (Frings, et al. 2008a)) and computed interhemispheric hippocampal connectivity using structurally defined hippocampal regions of interest similar to above. While no additional physiological noise corrections were performed in the two published studies, we linearly regressed motion and a global time course from the seed time courses before performing correlations. We compared connectivity to 12 healthy controls and found that there was no significant difference between the connectivity of controls and TLE patients, especially those patients with a shorter duration of disease (Figure 2, left). We also computed a linear correlation between connectivity and duration of disease. This revealed no significant correlation across the group of all TLE patients, but a significant decrease in connectivity as duration increased in the left TLE patients (correlation coefficient = -0.531, $p = 0.042$) (Figure 2, left).

Therefore, we were not able to duplicate the results of Pereira et al. to find decreased interhemispheric connectivity in the TLE patients, unless the patients in their study all had extensively long duration of disease (which is not stated). But, we were able to duplicate in left TLE at rest what Frings et al. showed during the memory task; that hippocampal connectivity decreased as duration of disease increased. However, it is clear that further study is required to fully understand this network and the effects of epilepsy on it. We believe that it is likely that the choice of hippocampal region of interest may have a significant effect on these results. To investigate this we identified functionally defined regions in the anterior left and right hippocampus that were about one-half the volume and completely within the structurally defined regions. The interhemispheric connectivity result from these regions was different from what was seen with anatomically defined regions (Figure 2, right). With the functionally-defined restricted regions, the connectivity across all TLE patients increased as duration of disease increased (correlation coefficient = 0.465, p = 0.029). However, the connectivity across the group was not different from that in controls, possibly because the epilepsy was greater than 20 years in duration in several patients. This suggests that the anterior and posterior portions of the hippocampus are functionally distinct and that, perhaps, the effects of TLE occur initially in the anterior portion of the hippocampus.

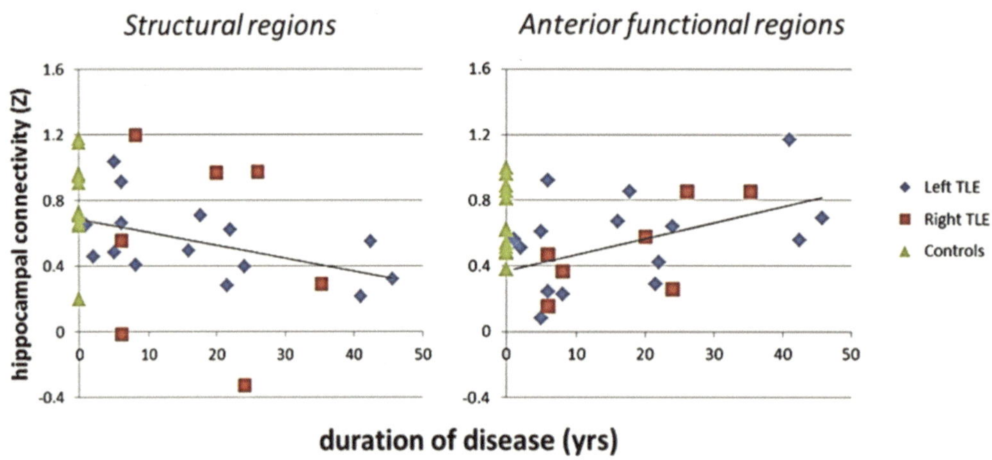

Fig. 2. Interhemispheric hippocampal connectivity at rest in TLE patients and controls correlated with duration of disease. (Left) Measures calculated with structurally defined regions between the entire left and right hippocampus. Connectivity in Left TLE decreased as duration of disease increased (p = 0.042). (Right) Measures calculated with functionally defined regions in the anterior portion of the left and right hippocampus. Connectivity across all TLE patients increased as duration of disease increased (p = 0.029). Functionally defined regions are about one-half the volume of the structurally defined regions.

Hippocampal connectivity measures calculated using correlation coefficients as above, do not yield information regarding the direction of influence across the network. This can be determined using Granger causality analyses of fMRI data (Goebel, et al. 2003, Roebroeck, et al. 2005, Rogers, et al. 2010), but are most effective using faster temporal sampling (Deshpande, et al. 2010). Therefore, we performed a Granger causality analysis on fMRI data with a 500 ms temporal sampling rate using the functionally defined anterior hippocampal regions discussed above (Morgan, et al. 2011). We also determined the hippocampal connectivity measures using the faster sampled data. The results revealed that during the interictal state the interhemispheric hippocampal connectivity initially is disrupted and then linearly increases with the epilepsy duration longer than 10 years. This increase in connectivity appears to be due to the hippocampus contralateral to the epileptogenic focus exerting more influence over the ipsilateral hippocampus. These findings may have implications in understanding the functional development of epileptic networks in mTLE.

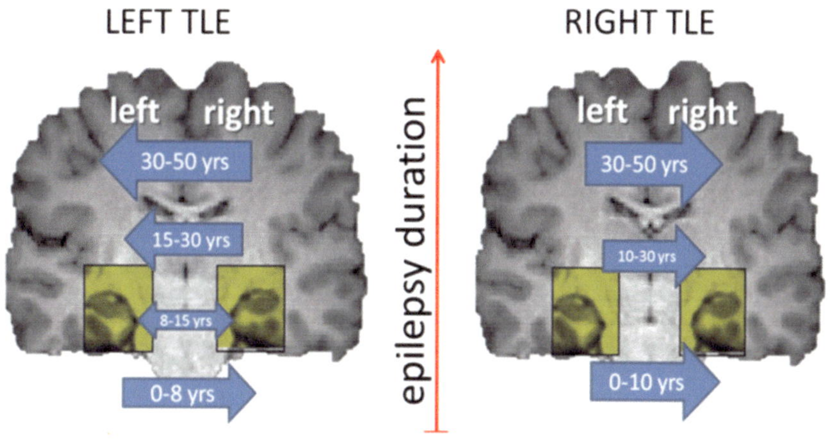

Fig. 3. Direction of hippocampal influence in TLE determined by Granger causality measures using high temporal resolution fMRI at rest. Direction and size of arrows represent direction and relative magnitude of influence between hippocampi at different periods of the epilepsy duration. At the longest duration, the hippocampus contralateral to the epileptogenic focus exerts more influence over the ipsilateral hippocampus.

5. Other fMRI analysis methods applied to epilepsy network investigation

5.1 Clustering methods

In addition to the ICA methods discussed, other types of data-driven techniques such as hierarchical clustering (Cordes, et al. 2002, Stanberry, et al. 2003) and fuzzy clustering (Baumgartner, et al. 2000, Dimitriadou, et al. 2004, Meyer-Baese, et al. 2004) use clustering of similar fMRI signal time courses to group and determine voxel time courses of interest. They are based on the assumption that BOLD stimuli will create a response in multiple voxels simultaneously. These techniques also are effective in fMRI data and have been applied to epilepsy data in animal models (Keogh, et al. 2005).

Temporal clustering analysis (TCA) is a method for determining times at which a significantly large number of voxels experience a similar response such as signal increase (Liu, et al. 2000, Lu, et al. 2006). This is done by creating a histogram of the number of voxels that individually reach their maximum (or contain some other shape of interest) at each time point of an imaging series. In other words, a plot of the number of voxels reaching a maximum or shape of interest (y-axis) versus time point in the series (x-axis) is created. Peaks in the histogram indicate the timing of many voxels experiencing the shape of interest indicating brain activity in response to whatever stimulus was present. The basis of this technique is that the probability of maximal signal intensity of each voxel is equal for all times unless the response to some stimulus occurs. Therefore, if no stimuli were present, the histogram would be relatively flat. Liu et al. first developed this method to identify time of maximal activation after eating (Liu, et al. 2000). The advantage of this technique is that it can detect specific time course characteristics of interest.

Any of the data-driven approaches above could be used to search for the BOLD responses of epileptic discharges in fMRI time series. When using ICA type methods, the results will include all components of the signal, regardless of amplitude or shape. Further investigations would be required to determine which of these components contain the signals of interest (De Martino, et al. 2007). In the case of interictal activity, the signal of interest is based on the hemodynamic response of the electrical spike activity. The TCA techniques can be "tuned" to this signal of interest. However, for success of any clustering algorithms we must assume that these discharges give rise to significant BOLD signal changes. This is supported by the work of Krakow et al. (Krakow, et al. 2001) in which they found, using EEG-triggered fMRI, that 34.9% of interictal spikes in a subject were associated with significant focal fMRI activation (signal intensity increases) consistent with results from several spikes averaged together. In fact, TCA has been used relatively successfully to localize epileptic discharges in animal models (Makiranta, et al. 2005) and in humans (Morgan, et al. 2004).

However, the original TCA methods map all signal changes of the desired shape into one histogram and therefore, they are highly sensitive to motion, physiological noise and other sources of signal change that may have the signal shape of interest (Hamandi, et al. 2005). Therefore, we have developed of a two-dimensional TCA technique (2dTCA) which creates separate histograms for groups of voxels with a similar timing of transient signal increases (epileptic spike). Using the 2dTCA technique we have developed, multiple histograms are created as columns on a two-dimensional grid. Thereby, groups of voxels with different timing patterns will be grouped in different "components". We evaluated the performance of 2dTCA in simulated functional MRI datasets (Morgan, et al. 2008). Comparisons were made with TCA and a freely-distributed ICA algorithm. The results suggest that the increased sensitivity of 2dTCA over TCA in detecting this particular signal of interest is comparable to detection with ICA, but with fewer other signals detected. We further validated it in healthy volunteers with controlled stimulus timing (Morgan & Gore 2009). Finally, we were able to implement this method to detect regions of activation in the left mesial temporal lobe, bilateral insula and default-mode network in a group of left TLE patients (Morgan, et al. 2007, Morgan, et al. 2010). Using the region of activation in the mesial temporal lobe as the seed, we were able to calculate functional connectivity to the rest of the brain to detect changes from healthy controls (Morgan, et al. 2010). This revealed a network including the thalamus, brainstem, frontal and parietal regions consistent with the "network inhibition hypothesis" (Norden & Blumenfeld 2002, Yu & Blumenfeld 2009). This theory proposes that complex partial seizures originating in the mesial temporal lobes may propagate to the medial thalamus and upper brain stem which inhibits function of the frontal and parietal cortices causing loss of consciousness.

5.2 Graph theory applied to fMRI network analysis

One method to model the complex structural and functional networks of the brain is by using graph theoretical analysis (He & Evans 2010). This method is described as a powerful mathematical framework for characterizing the organization of the complicated networks. He et al. (He & Evans 2010) describe how structural and functional brain networks can be modeled using various MRI and EEG techniques. This theory assumes that the brain consists of nodes (voxels or regions) and edges (the connections between the nodes). Characteristics about the nodes and edges are determined such as the presence of hubs, or highly connected nodes. Other characteristics include shortest path lengths and clustering parameters. Liao et al. (Liao, et al. 2010) used graph theory to compare fMRI data from TLE patients and controls by identifying 90 cortical and subcortical nodes across the brain. They found that the TLE patients had increased connectivity within the mesial temporal lobes and decreased connectivity in the frontal and parietal lobes, consistent with several other methodologies discussed in this chapter. They also found decreases in the number of connections in the DMN in the patients. Overall, this is a potentially powerful, quantitative method for assessing small-world properties and network robustness in the brain.

5.3 Regional homogeneity (ReHo) analysis

The regional homogeneity (ReHo) analysis is an fMRI analysis method to probe the most local connections in a given region of the brain first developed by Zang et al. (Zang, et al. 2004). The ReHo is measured by determining the local coherence of the fMRI time series of a given voxel to all of its directly neighboring voxels using Kendall's coefficient of concordance (Kendall & Gibbons 1990). The assumption is that increases in the ReHo value will reflect changes in neuronal activity, however the direct link is not known. This method has been used in numerous studies including those in autism (Shukla, et al. 2010), depression (Liu, et al. 2010) and intelligence in healthy controls (Wang, et al. 2011). In a group of non-lesional children with TLE, increased ReHo was found in the posterior cingulate and the right medial temporal lobe. Decreased ReHo was detected in right frontal gyrus and the cerebellum. There were also differences between those patients with abnormal EEG and those without. The significance of these ReHo changes are not known, but the authors suggest that this increased local synchronization aids in the spread of epileptiform activity (Mankinen, et al. 2011).

5.4 Amplitude of low frequency fluctuation (ALFF) analysis

It has been determined that the spontaneous fluctuations measured using functional connectivity analyses are in the low frequency range (0.01-0.08 Hz) (Cordes, et al. 2001). Therefore, it is possible that the power of these low frequency fluctuations can be informative regarding the characteristics of the underlying neuronal activity generating these signals (Duff, et al. 2008). From this idea, Zang et al. developed the "amplitude of low frequency fluctuation" (ALFF) analysis. The general method is to do a voxel-wise calculation of the low-frequency power, and to statistically compare this power across the brain or other series. This method has been used to compare visual states in healthy controls (Yang, et al. 2007) and to study schizophrenia (Hoptman, et al. 2010, Huang, et al. 2010) and attention deficit disorder (Zang, et al. 2007). The approach was used to compare a group of unilateral TLE patients to healthy controls (Zhang, et al. 2010b). Similar to other methods of connectivity, increases in the TLE patients were detected in the bilateral hippocampi, amygdala, temporal pole, midbrain and lateral temporal and parietal regions. Decreases in ALFF in TLE patients were detected in the DMN. The patients also showed an asymmetry in their ALFF measures in the mesial temporal lobes and thalamus, possibly indicating the epileptogenic region.

6. Conclusions and future directions

In this chapter we have discussed the numerous ways in which epilepsy can affect the functional networks of the brain and the various fMRI methods used to determine this. We also explained how these changes may be related to behavioral, cognitive or disease characteristics. In parallel to the functional connectivity work being pursued, a large effort has been devoted to examining the same issues in relation to MRI measured structural connectivity (Focke, et al. 2008). The comparison between functional and structural connectivity in epilepsy may provide answers that neither method can individually (Voets, et al. 2009). We believe that large scale neuroimaging studies that incorporate both structural and functional imaging with genetic, physiological and neuropsychological testing, like those for controls (The Human Connectome Project, www.humanconnectome.org) and Alzheimer's Disease (Alzheimer's Disease Neuroimaging Initiative (ADNI), University of California, San Francisco, USA) already underway, may provide the greatest potential in uncovering the mechanisms and effects of network alterations in the brain in epilepsy.

7. Abbreviations

ADNI - Alzheimer's Disease Neuroimaging Initiative
ALFF - amplitude of low frequency fluctuations
BOLD - blood oxygen level dependent
CBF - cerebral blood flow
CMRO2 - cerebral metabolic rate for oxygen
DMN - default mode network
EEG - electroencephalography
fMRI - functional Magnetic Resonance Imaging
GSW - generalize spike-and-wave
IAT - Intracarotid Amobarbital Test
ICA - independent component analysis
IGE - idiopathic generalized epilepsy
MEG - magnetoencephalography
PET - positron emission tomography
ReHo - regional homogeneity
SPECT - single photon emission tomography
TCA, 2dTCA - temporal clustering analysis, two-dimensional temporal clustering analysis
TLE - temporal lobe epilepsy

8. Acknowledgements

This work was supported in part by NIH R01 NS055822.

9. References

Abbott, D.F., Waites, A.B., Lillywhite, L.M. & Jackson, G.D. (2010) fMRI assessment of language lateralization: An objective approach. *Neuroimage* 50:1446-1455.

Abou-Khalil, B. (2007) An update on determination of language dominance in screening for epilepsy surgery: the Wada test and newer noninvasive alternatives. *Epilepsia* 48:442-455.

Addis, D.R., Moscovitch, M. & McAndrews, M.P. (2007) Consequences of hippocampal damage across the autobiographical memory network in left temporal lobe epilepsy. *Brain* 130:2327-2342.

Archer, J.S., Abbott, D.F., Waites, A.B. & Jackson, G.D. (2003) fMRI "deactivation" of the posterior cingulate during generalized spike and wave. *Neuroimage* 20:1915-1922.

Arora, J., Pugh, K., Westerveld, M., Spencer, S., Spencer, D.D. & Constable, R.T. (2009) Language lateralization in epilepsy patients: fMRI validated with the Wada procedure. *Epilepsia* 50:2225-2241.

Baumgartner, R., Ryner, L., Richter, W., Summers, R., Jarmasz, M. & Somorjai, R. (2000) Comparison of two exploratory data analysis methods for fMRI: fuzzy clustering vs. principal component analysis. *Magn Reson Imaging* 18:89-94.

Baxendale, S., Thompson, P.J. & Duncan, J.S. (2008) The role of the Wada test in the surgical treatment of temporal lobe epilepsy: An international survey. *Epilepsia* 49:715-720.

Berman, R., Negishi, M., Vestal, M., Spann, M., Chung, M.H., Bai, X.X., Purcaro, M., Motelow, J.E., Danielson, N., Dix-Cooper, L., Enev, M., Novotny, E.J., Constable, R.T. & Blumenfeld, H. (2010) Simultaneous EEG, fMRI, and behavior in typical childhood absence seizures. *Epilepsia* 51:2011-2022.

Bettus, G., Bartolomei, F., Confort-Gouny, S., Guedj, E., Chauvel, P., Cozzone, P.J., Ranjeva, J.P. & Guye, M. (2010) Role of resting state functional connectivity MRI in presurgical investigation of mesial temporal lobe epilepsy. *J. Neurol. Neurosurg. Psychiatry* 81:1147-1154.

Bettus, G., Guedj, E., Joyeux, F., Confort-Gouny, S., Soulier, E., Laguitton, V., Cozzone, P.J., Chauvel, P., Ranjeva, J.P., Bartolomei, F. & Guye, M. (2009) Decreased basal fMRI functional connectivity in epileptogenic networks and contralateral compensatory mechanisms. *Human brain mapping* 30:1580-1591.

Binder, J.R., Sabsevitz, D.S., Swanson, S.J., Hammeke, T.A., Raghavan, M. & Mueller, W.M. (2008a) Use of preoperative functional MRI to predict verbal memory decline after temporal lobe epilepsy surgery. *Epilepsia* 49:1377-1394.

Binder, J.R., Swanson, S.J., Hammeke, T.A. & Sabsevitz, D.S. (2008b) A comparison of five fMRI protocols for mapping speech comprehension systems. *Epilepsia* 49:1980-1997.

Binder, J.R., Swanson, S.J., Sabsevitz, D.S., Hammeke, T.A., Raghavan, M. & Mueller, W.M. (2010) A comparison of two fMRI methods for predicting verbal memory decline after left temporal lobectomy: Language lateralization versus hippocampal activation asymmetry. *Epilepsia* 51:618-626.

Biswal, B., Yetkin, F.Z., Haughton, V.M. & Hyde, J.S. (1995) Functional connectivity in the motor cortex of resting human brain using echo-planar MRI. *Magn Reson Med* 34:537-541.

Blumenfeld, H., McNally, K.A., Vanderhill, S.D., Paige, A.L., Chung, R., Davis, K., Norden, A.D., Stokking, R., Studholme, C., Novotny, E.J., Jr., Zubal, I.G. & Spencer, S.S. (2004a) Positive and negative network correlations in temporal lobe epilepsy. *Cereb Cortex* 14:892-902.

Blumenfeld, H., Rivera, M., McNally, K.A., Davis, K., Spencer, D.D. & Spencer, S.S. (2004b) Ictal neocortical slowing in temporal lobe epilepsy. *Neurology* 63:1015-1021.

Blumenfeld, H., Varghese, G.I., Purcaro, M.J., Motelow, J.E., Enev, M., McNally, K.A., Levin, A.R., Hirsch, L.J., Tikofsky, R., Zubal, I.G., Paige, A.L. & Spencer, S.S. (2009) Cortical and subcortical networks in human secondarily generalized tonic-clonic seizures. *Brain* 132:999-1012.

Bonelli, S.B., Powell, R.H.W., Yogarajah, M., Samson, R.S., Symms, M.R., Thompson, P.J., Koepp, M.J. & Duncan, J.S. (2010) Imaging memory in temporal lobe epilepsy: predicting the effects of temporal lobe resection. *Brain* 133:1186-1199.

Bookheimer, S. (2007) Pre-surgical language mapping with functional magnetic resonance imaging. *Neuropsychol. Rev.* 17:145-155.

Branco, D.M., Suarez, R.O., Whalen, S., O'Shea, J.P., Nelson, A.P., da Costa, J.C. & Golby, A.J. (2006) Functional MRI of memory in the hippocampus: Laterality indices may be more meaningful if calculated from whole voxel distributions. *Neuroimage* 32:592-602.

Broyd, S.J., Demanuele, C., Debener, S., Helps, S.K., James, C.J. & Sonuga-Barke, E.J.S. (2009) Default-mode brain dysfunction in mental disorders: A systematic review. *Neurosci. Biobehav. Rev.* 33:279-296.

Buckner, R.L., Andrews-Hanna, J.R. & Schacter, D.L. (2008) The brain's default network: anatomy, function, and relevance to disease. *Ann N Y Acad Sci* 1124:1-38.

Calhoun, V.D., Adali, T., Hansen, L.K., Larsen, J. & Pekar, J.J. (2003) ICA of functional MRI data: an overview. *4th International Symposium on ICA and BLind Separation*, Nara, Japan.

Carney, P.W., Masterton, R.A.J., Harvey, A.S., Scheffer, I.E., Berkovic, S.F. & Jackson, G.D. (2010) The core network in absence epilepsy Differences in cortical and thalamic BOLD response. *Neurology* 75:904-911.

Cascino, G.D. & Jack, C.R. (1996) Neuroimagingin Epilepsy: Principals and Practice. Butterworth-Heinemann, Boston, MA.

Chelune, G.J. (1995) Hippocampal adequacy versus functional reserve: predicting memory functions following temporal lobectomy. *Arch Clin Neuropsychol* 10:413-432.

Cordes, D., Haughton, V., Carew, J.D., Arfanakis, K. & Maravilla, K. (2002) Hierarchical clustering to measure connectivity in fMRI resting-state data. *Magnetic Resonance Imaging* 20:305-317.

Cordes, D., Haughton, V.M., Arfanakis, K., Carew, J.D., Turski, P.A., Moritz, C.H., Quigley, M.A. & Meyerand, M.E. (2001) Frequencies contributing to functional connectivity in the cerebral cortex in "resting-state" data. *Ajnr* 22:1326-1333.

Damoiseaux, J.S., Rombouts, S.A.R.B., Barkhof, F., Scheltens, P., Stam, C.J., Smith, S.M. & Beckmann, C.F. (2006) Consistent resting-state networks across healthy subjects. *Proceedings of the National Academy of Sciences of the United States of America* 103:13848-13853.

De Luca, M., Beckmann, C.F., De Stefano, N., Matthews, P.M. & Smith, S.M. (2006) fMRI resting state networks define distinct modes of long-distance interactions in the human brain. *Neuroimage* 29:1359-1367.

De Martino, F., Gentile, F., Esposito, F., Balsi, M., Di Salle, F., Goebel, R. & Formisano, E. (2007) Classification of fMRI independent components using IC-fingerprints and support vector machine classifiers. *Neuroimage* 34:177-194.

de Pasquale, F., Della Penna, S., Snyder, A.Z., Lewis, C., Mantini, D., Marzetti, L., Belardinelli, P., Ciancetta, L., Pizzella, V., Romani, G.L. & Corbetta, M. (2010)

Temporal dynamics of spontaneous MEG activity in brain networks. *Proceedings of the National Academy of Sciences of the United States of America* 107:6040-6045.
Deblaere, K., Backes, W.H., Hofman, P., Vandemaele, P., Boon, P.A., Vonck, K., Boon, P., Troost, J., Vermeulen, J., Wilmink, J., Achten, E. & Aldenkamp, A. (2002) Developing a comprehensive presurgical functional MRI protocol for patients with intractable temporal lobe epilepsy: a pilot study. *Neuroradiology* 44:667-673.
Deblaere, K., Backes, W.H., Tieleman, A., Vandemaele, P., Defreyne, L., Vonck, K., Hofman, P., Boon, P., Vermeulen, J., Wilmink, J., Aldenkamp, A., Boon, P., Vingerhoets, G. & Achten, E. (2005) Lateralized anterior mesiotemporal lobe activation: Semirandom functional MR imaging encoding paradigm in patients with temporal lobe epilepsy-initial experience. *Radiology* 236:996-1003.
Deshpande, G., LaConte, S., James, G.A., Peltier, S. & Hu, X.P. (2009) Multivariate Granger Causality Analysis of fMRI Data. *Human brain mapping* 30:1361-1373.
Deshpande, G., Sathian, K. & Hu, X.P. (2010) Effect of hemodynamic variability on Granger causality analysis of fMRI. *Neuroimage* 52:884-896.
Dimitriadou, E., Barth, M., Windischberger, C., Hornik, K. & Moser, E. (2004) A quantitative comparison of functional MRI cluster analysis. *Artif. Intell. Med.* 31:57-71.
Duff, E.P., Johnston, L.A., Xiong, J.H., Fox, P.T., Mareels, I. & Egan, G.F. (2008) The power of spectral density analysis for mapping endogenous BOLD signal fluctuations. *Human brain mapping* 29:778-790.
Englot, D.J., Mishra, A.M., Mansuripur, P.K., Herman, P., Hyder, F. & Blumenfeld, H. (2008) Remote effects of focal hippocampal seizures on the rat neocortex. *J Neurosci* 28:9066-9081.
Everts, R., Harvey, A.S., Lillywhite, L., Wrennall, J., Abbott, D.F., Gonzalez, L., Kean, M., Jackson, G.D. & Anderson, V. (2010) Language lateralization correlates with verbal memory performance in children with focal epilepsy. *Epilepsia* 51:627-638.
Fisher, R.S., Vickrey, B.G., Gibson, P., Hermann, B., Penovich, P., Scherer, A. & Walker, S. (2000) The impact of epilepsy from the patient's perspective I. Descriptions and subjective perceptions. *Epilepsy research* 41:39-51.
Focke, N.K., Yogarajah, M., Bonelli, S.B., Bartlett, P.A., Symms, M.R. & Duncan, J.S. (2008) Voxel-based diffusion tensor imaging in patients with mesial temporal lobe epilepsy and hippocampal sclerosis. *Neuroimage* 40:728-737.
Fox, M.D., Corbetta, M., Snyder, A.Z., Vincent, J.L. & Raichle, M.E. (2006) Spontaneous neuronal activity distinguishes human dorsal and ventral attention systems. *Proceedings of the National Academy of Sciences of the United States of America* 103:10046-10051.
Fox, M.D., Snyder, A.Z., Vincent, J.L., Corbetta, M., Van Essen, D.C. & Raichle, M.E. (2005) The human brain is intrinsically organized into dynamic, anticorrelated functional networks. *Proceedings of the National Academy of Sciences of the United States of America* 102:9673-9678.
Fransson, P., Skiold, B., Horsch, S., Nordell, A., Blennow, M., Lagercrantz, H. & Aden, U. (2007) Resting-state networks in the infant brain. *Proceedings of the National Academy of Sciences of the United States of America* 104:15531-15536.
Frings, L., Schulze-Bonhage, A., Spreer, J. & Wagner, K. (2008a) Reduced interhemispheric hippocampal BOLD signal coupling related to early epilepsy onset. *Seizure* 18:153-157.

Frings, L., Schulze-Bonhage, A., Spreer, J. & Wagner, K. (2009) Remote effects of hippocampal damage on default network connectivity in the human brain. *Journal of neurology* 256:2021-2029.

Frings, L., Wagner, K., Halsband, U., Schwarzwald, R., Zentner, J. & Schulze-Bonhage, A. (2008b) Lateralization of hippocampal activation differs between left and right temporal lobe epilepsy patients and correlates with postsurgical verbal learning decrement. *Epilepsy research* 78:161-170.

Friston, K.J., Harrison, L. & Penny, W. (2003) Dynamic causal modelling. *Neuroimage* 19:1273-1302.

Gaillard, W.D., Balsamo, L., Xu, B., Grandin, C.B., Braniecki, S.H., Papero, P.H., Weinstein, S., Conry, J., Pearl, P.L., Sachs, B., Sato, S., Jabbari, B., Vezina, L.G., Frattali, C. & Theodore, W.H. (2002) Language dominance in partial epilepsy patients identified with an fMRI reading task. *Neurology* 59:256-265.

Glahn, D.C., Winkler, A.M., Kochunov, P., Almasy, L., Duggirala, R., Carless, M.A., Curran, J.C., Olvera, R.L., Laird, A.R., Smith, S.M., Beckmann, C.F., Fox, P.T. & Blangero, J. (2010) Genetic control over the resting brain. *Proceedings of the National Academy of Sciences of the United States of America* 107:1223-1228.

Goebel, R., Roebroeck, A., Kim, D.S. & Formisano, E. (2003) Investigating directed cortical interactions in time-resolved fMRI data using vector autoregressive modeling and Granger causality mapping. *Magnetic Resonance Imaging* 21:1251-1261.

Golby, A.J., Poldrack, R.A., Brewer, J.B., Spencer, D., Desmond, J.E., Aron, A.P. & Gabrieli, J.D.E. (2001) Material-specific lateralization in the medial temporal lobe and prefrontal cortex during memory encoding. *Brain* 124:1841-1854.

Golby, A.J., Poldrack, R.A., Illes, J., Chen, D., Desmond, J.E. & Gabrieli, J.D.E. (2002) Memory lateralization in medial temporal lobe epilepsy assessed by functional MRI. *Epilepsia* 43:855-863.

Gotman, J., Benar, C.G. & Dubeau, F. (2004) Combining EEG and FMRI in epilepsy: methodological challenges and clinical results. *J. Clin. Neurophysiol.* 21:229-240.

Gotman, J., Grova, C., Bagshaw, A., Kobayashi, E., Aghakhani, Y. & Dubeau, F. (2005) Generalized epileptic discharges show thalamocortical activation and suspension of the default state of the brain. *Proceedings of the National Academy of Sciences of the United States of America* 102:15236-15240.

Grady, C.L., Protzner, A.B., Kovacevic, N., Strother, S.C., Afshin-Pour, B., Wojtowicz, M., Anderson, J.A.E., Churchill, N. & McIntosh, A.R. (2010) A Multivariate Analysis of Age-Related Differences in Default Mode and Task-Positive Networks across Multiple Cognitive Domains. *Cereb Cortex* 20:1432-1447.

Grant, A.C., Donnelly, K.M., Chubb, C., Barr, W.B., Kuzniecky, R. & Devinsky, O. (2008) Temporal lobe epilepsy does not impair visual perception. *Epilepsia* 49:710-713.

Greicius, M.D., Kiviniemi, V., Tervonen, O., Vainionpaa, V., Alahuhta, S., Reiss, A.L. & Menon, V. (2008) Persistent default-mode network connectivity during light sedation. *Human brain mapping* 29:839-847.

Greicius, M.D., Krasnow, B., Reiss, A.L. & Menon, V. (2003) Functional connectivity in the resting brain: a network analysis of the default mode hypothesis. *Proceedings of the National Academy of Sciences of the United States of America* 100:253-258.

Guye, M., Regis, J., Tamura, M., Wendling, F., McGonigal, A., Chauvel, P. & Bartolomei, F. (2006) The role of corticothalamic coupling in human temporal lobe epilepsy. *Brain* 129:1917-1928.

Hamandi, K., Salek-Haddadi, A., Laufs, H., Liston, A., Friston, K., Fish, D.R., Duncan, J.S. & Lemieux, L. (2006) EEG-fMRI of idiopathic and secondarily generalized epilepsies. *Neuroimage* 31:1700-1710.

Hamandi, K., Salek Haddadi, A., Liston, A., Laufs, H., Fish, D.R. & Lemieux, L. (2005) fMRI temporal clustering analysis in patients with frequent interictal epileptiform discharges: comparison with EEG-driven analysis. *Neuroimage* 26:309-316.

He, Y. & Evans, A. (2010) Graph theoretical modeling of brain connectivity. *Current opinion in neurology* 23:341-350.

Helmstaedter, C., Kurthen, M., Lux, S., Reuber, M. & Elger, C.E. (2003) Chronic epilepsy and cognition: A longitudinal study in temporal lobe epilepsy. *Ann Neurol* 54:425-432.

Hlinka, J., Alexakis, C., Diukova, A., Liddle, P.F. & Auer, D.P. (2010) Slow EEG pattern predicts reduced intrinsic functional connectivity in the default mode network: An inter-subject analysis. *Neuroimage* 53:239-246.

Hoptman, M.J., Zuo, X.N., Butler, P.D., Javitt, D.C., D'Angelo, D., Mauro, C.J. & Milham, M.P. (2010) Amplitude of low-frequency oscillations in schizophrenia: A resting state fMRI study. *Schizophr. Res.* 117:13-20.

Horovitz, S.G., Fukunaga, M., de Zwart, J.A., van Gelderen, P., Fulton, S.C., Balkin, T.J. & Duyn, J.H. (2008) Low frequency BOLD fluctuations during resting wakefulness and light sleep: A simultaneous EEG-fMRI study. *Human brain mapping* 29:671-682.

Huang, X.Q., Lui, S., Deng, W., Chan, R.C.K., Wu, Q.Z., Jiang, L.J., Zhang, J.R., Jia, Z.Y., Li, F., Li, X.L., Chen, L., Li, T. & Gong, Q.Y. (2010) Localization of cerebral functional deficits in treatment-naive, first-episode schizophrenia using resting-state fMRI. *Neuroimage* 49:2901-2906.

Jokeit, H., Okujava, M. & Woermann, F.G. (2001) Memory fMRI lateralizes temporal lobe epilepsy. *Neurology* 57:1786-1793.

Kendall, M. & Gibbons, J.D. (1990) Rank Correlation Methods. Edward Arnold, New York.

Keogh, B.P., Cordes, D., Stanberry, L., Figler, B.D., Robbins, C.A., Tempel, B.L., Green, C.G., Emmi, A., Maravilla, K.M. & Schwartzkroin, P.A. (2005) BOLD-fMRI of PTZ-induced seizures in rats. *Epilepsy research* 66:75-90.

Kilpatrick, C., Murrie, V., Cook, M., Andrewes, D., Desmond, P. & Hopper, J. (1997) Degree of left hippocampal atrophy correlates with severity of neuropsychological deficits. *Seizure* 6:213-218.

Kobayashi, E., Bagshaw, A.P., Grova, C., Dubeau, F. & Gotman, J. (2006) Negative BOLD responses to epileptic spikes. *Human brain mapping* 27:488-497.

Kockelmann, E., Elger, C.E. & Helmstaedter, C. (2003) Significant improvement in frontal lobe associated neuropsychological functions after withdrawal of Topiramate in epilepsy patients. *Epilepsy research* 54:171-178.

Krakow, K., Messina, D., Lemieux, L., Duncan, J.S. & Fish, D.R. (2001) Functional MRI activation of individual interictal epileptiform spikes. *Neuroimage* 13:502-505.

Langfitt, J.T., Westerveld, M., Hamberger, M.J., Walczak, T.S., Cicchetti, D.V., Berg, A.T., Vickrey, B.G., Barr, W.B., Sperling, M.R., Masur, D. & Spencer, S.S. (2007) Worsening of quality of life after epilepsy surgery: effect of seizures and memory decline. *Neurology* 68:1988-1994.

Langfitt, J.T. & Wiebe, S. (2008) Early surgical treatment for epilepsy. *Current opinion in neurology* 21:179-183.

Laufs, H., Hamandi, K., Salek-Haddadi, A., Kleinschmidt, A.K., Duncan, J.S. & Lemieux, L. (2007) Temporal lobe interictal epileptic discharges affect cerebral activity in "Default mode" brain regions. *Human brain mapping* 28:1023-1032.

Laufs, H., Lengler, U., Hamandi, K., Kleinschmidt, A. & Krakow, K. (2006) Linking generalized spike-and-wave discharges and resting state brain activity by using EEG/fMRI in a patient with absence seizures. *Epilepsia* 47:444-448.

Liao, W., Zhang, Z.Q., Pan, Z.Y., Mantini, D., Ding, J.R., Duan, X.J., Luo, C., Lu, G.M. & Chen, H.F. (2010) Altered Functional Connectivity and Small-World in Mesial Temporal Lobe Epilepsy. *Plos One* 5:e8525.

Liu, Y., Gao, J.H., Liu, H.L. & Fox, P.T. (2000) The temporal response of the brain after eating revealed by functional MRI. *Nature* 405:1058-1062.

Liu, Z.F., Xu, C., Xu, Y., Wang, Y.F., Zhao, B., Lv, Y.T., Cao, X.H., Zhang, K.R. & Du, C.X. (2010) Decreased regional homogeneity in insula and cerebellum: A resting-state fMRI study in patients with major depression and subjects at high risk for major depression. *Psychiatry Res. Neuroimaging* 182:211-215.

Loddenkemper, T., Morris, H.H. & Moddel, G. (2008) Complications during the Wada test. *Epilepsy Behav* 13:551-553.

Logothetis, N.K., Pauls, J., Augath, M., Trinath, T. & Oeltermann, A. (2001) Neurophysiological investigation of the basis of the fMRI signal. *Nature* 412:150-157.

Lu, N., Shan, B.C., Li, K., Yan, B., Wang, W. & Li, K.C. (2006) Improved temporal clustering analysis method for detecting multiple response peaks in fMRI. *Journal of Magnetic Resonance Imaging* 23:285-290.

Lucking, C.H., Creutzfe.Od & Heineman.U. (1970) Visual Evoked Potenials of Patients With Epilepsy and of a Control Group. *Electroencephalogr. Clin. Neurophysiol.* 29:557-&.

Makiranta, M., Ruohonen, J., Suominen, K., Niinimaki, J., Sonkajarvi, E., Kiviniemi, V., Seppanen, T., Alahuhta, S., Jantti, V. & Tervonen, O. (2005) BOLD signal increase preceeds EEG spike activity - a dynamic penicillin induced focal epilepsy in deep anesthesia. *Neuroimage* 27:715-724.

Mankinen, K., Long, X.-Y., Paakki, J.-J., Harila, M., Rytky, S., Tervonen, O., Nikkinen, J., Starck, T., Remes, J., Rantala, H., Zang, Y.-F. & Kiviniemi, V. (2011) Alterations in regional homogeneity of baseline brain activity in pediatric temporal lobe epilepsy. *Brain Res.* 1373:221-229.

Mantini, D., Perrucci, M.G., Del Gratta, C., Romani, G.L. & Corbetta, M. (2007) Electrophysiological signatures of resting state networks in the human brain. *Proceedings of the National Academy of Sciences of the United States of America* 104:13170-13175.

Medina, L.S., Aguirre, E., Bernal, B. & Altman, N.R. (2004) Functional MR imaging versus Wada test for evaluation of language lateralization: Cost analysis. *Radiology* 230:49-54.

Meyer-Baese, A., Wismueller, A. & Lange, O. (2004) Comparison of two exploratory data analysis methods for fMRI: unsupervised clustering versus independent component analysis. *IEEE Trans Inf Technol Biomed* 8:387-398.

Moeller, F., LeVan, P., Muhle, H., Stephani, U., Dubeau, F., Siniatchkin, M. & Gotman, J. (2010a) Absence seizures: Individual patterns revealed by EEG-fMRI. *Epilepsia* 51:2000-2010.

Moeller, F., Maneshi, M., Pittau, F., Gholipour, T., Bellec, P., Dubeau, F., Grova, C. & Gotman, J. (2011) Functional connectivity in patients with idiopathic generalized epilepsy. *Epilepsia* 52:515-522.

Moeller, F., Muhle, H., Wiegand, G., Wolff, S., Stephani, U. & Siniatchkin, M. (2010b) EEG-fMRI study of generalized spike and wave discharges without transitory cognitive impairment. *Epilepsy Behav.* 18:313-316.

Morgan, V.L. & Gore, J.C. (2009) Detection of irregular, transient fMRI activity in normal controls using 2dTCA: Comparison to event-related analysis using known timing. *Human brain mapping* 30:3393-3405.

Morgan, V.L., Gore, J.C. & Abou-Khalil, B. (2007) Cluster analysis detection of functional MRI activity in temporal lobe epilepsy. *Epilepsy research* 76:22-33.

Morgan, V.L., Gore, J.C. & Abou-Khalil, B. (2010) Functional epileptic network in left mesial temporal lobe epilepsy detected using resting fMRI. *Epilepsy research* 88:168-178.

Morgan, V.L., Li, Y., Abou-Khalil, B. & Gore, J.C. (2008) Development of 2dTCA for the detection of irregular, transient BOLD activity. *Human brain mapping* 29:57-69.

Morgan, V.L., Price, R.R., Arain, A., Modur, P. & Abou-Khalil, B. (2004) Resting functional MRI with temporal clustering analysis for localization of epileptic activity without EEG. *Neuroimage* 21:473-481.

Moritz, C.H., Carew, J.D., McMillan, A.B. & Meyerand, M.E. (2005) Independent component analysis applied to self-paced functional MR imaging paradigms. *Neuroimage* 25:181-192.

Morgan, V.L., Rogers, B.P., Sonmezturk, H.H., Gore, J.C. & Abou-Khalil, B. (2011) Cross hippocampal influence in mesial temporal lobe epilepsy measured with high temporal resolution functional Magnetic Resonance Imaging. *Epilepsia* in press.

Neill, J.C., Liu, Z., Mikati, M. & Holmes, G.L. (2005) Pilocarpine seizures cause age-dependent impairment in auditory location discrimination. *J. Exp. Anal. Behav.* 84:357-370.

Norden, A.D. & Blumenfeld, H. (2002) The role of subcortical structures in human epilepsy. *Epilepsy Behav* 3:219-231.

Ogawa, S., Lee, T.M., Nayak, A.S. & Glynn, P. (1990) Oxygenation-sensitive contrast in magnetic-resonance image of rodent brain at high magnetic-fields *Magnet Reson Med* 14:68-78.

Park, S.P., Hwang, Y.H., Lee, H.W., Suh, C.K., Kwon, S.H. & Lee, B.I. (2008) Long-term cognitive and mood effects of zonisamide monotherapy in epilepsy patients. *Epilepsy Behav.* 12:102-108.

Pelletier, I., Sauerwein, H.C., Lepore, F., Saint-Amour, D. & Lassonde, M. (2007) Non-invasive alternatives to the Wada test in the presurgical evaluation of language and memory functions in epilepsy patients. *Epileptic Disord* 9:111-126.

Pereira, F.R.S., Alessio, A., Sercheli, M.S., Pedro, T., Bilevicius, E., Rondina, J.M., Ozelo, H.F.B., Castellano, G., Covolan, R.J.M., Damasceno, B.P. & Cendes, F. (2010) Asymmetrical hippocampal connectivity in mesial temporal lobe epilepsy: evidence from resting state fMRI. *BMC Neuroscience* 11:66.

Rabin, M.L., Narayan, V.M., Kimberg, D.Y., Casasanto, D.J., Glosser, G., Tracy, J.I., French, J.A., Sperling, M.R. & Detre, J.A. (2004) Functional MRI predicts post-surgical memory following temporal lobectomy. *Brain* 127:2286-2298.

Raichle, M.E., MacLeod, A.M., Snyder, A.Z., Powers, W.J., Gusnard, D.A. & Shulman, G.L. (2001) A default mode of brain function. *Proceedings of the National Academy of Sciences of the United States of America* 98:676-682.

Ramsey, N.F., Sommer, I.E.C., Rutten, G.J. & Kahn, R.S. (2001) Combined analysis of language tasks in fMRI improves assessment of hemispheric dominance for language functions in individual subjects. *Neuroimage* 13:719-733.

Reitan, R.M. & Wolfson, D. (1995) Category Test and Trail Making Test as Measures of Frontal-Lobe Functions. *Clin. Neuropsychol.* 9:50-56.

Richardson, M.P., Strange, B.A., Duncan, J.S. & Dolan, R.J. (2006) Memory fMRI in left hippocampal sclerosis - Optimizing the approach to predicting postsurgical memory. *Neurology* 66:699-705.

Richardson, M.P., Strange, B.A., Thompson, P.J., Baxendale, S.A., Duncan, J.S. & Dolan, R.J. (2004) Pre-operative verbal memory fMRI predicts post-operative memory decline after left temporal lobe resection. *Brain* 127:2419-2426.

Rodionov, R., De Martino, F., Laufs, H., Carmichael, D.W., Formisano, E., Walker, M., Duncan, J.S. & Lemieux, L. (2007) Independent component analysis of interictal fMRI in focal epilepsy: comparison with general linear model-based EEG-correlated fMRI. *Neuroimage* 38:488-500.

Roebroeck, A., Formisano, E. & Goebel, R. (2005) Mapping directed influence over the brain using Granger causality and fMRI. *Neuroimage* 25:230-242.

Rogers, B.P., Katwal, S.B., Morgan, V.L., Asplund, C.L. & Gore, J.C. (2010) Functional MRI and multivariate autoregressive models. *Magnetic Resonance Imaging* 28:1058-1065.

Rogers, B.P., Morgan, V.L., Newton, A.T. & Gore, J.C. (2007) Assessing functional connectivity in the human brain by fMRI. *Magn Reson Imaging* 25:1347-1357.

Rutten, G.J.M., Ramsey, N.F., van Rijen, P.C., Alpherts, W.C. & van Veelen, C.W.M. (2002a) fMRI-determined language lateralization in patients with unilateral or mixed language dominance according to the Wada test. *Neuroimage* 17:447-460.

Rutten, G.J.M., Ramsey, N.F., van Rijen, P.C., Noordmans, H.J. & van Veelen, C.W.M. (2002b) Development of a functional magnetic resonance imaging protocol for intraoperative localization of critical temporoparietal language areas. *Ann Neurol* 51:350-360.

Salek-Haddadi, A., Lemieux, L., Merschhemke, M., Friston, K.J., Duncan, J.S. & Fish, D.R. (2003) Functional magnetic resonance imaging of human absence seizures. *Ann Neurol* 53:663-667.

Seo, J.G., Lee, D.I., Hwang, Y.H., Lee, H.W., Jung, D.K., Suh, C.K., Kwon, S.H. & Park, S.P. (2007) Comparison of cognitive effects of lamotrigine and oxcarbazepine in epilepsy patients. *J. Clin. Neurol.* 3:31-37.

Shukla, D.K., Keehn, B. & Muller, R.A. (2010) Regional homogeneity of fMRI time series in autism spectrum disorders. *Neuroscience letters* 476:46-51.

Shulman, G.L., McAvoy, M.P., Cowan, M.C., Astafiev, S.V., Tansy, A.P., d'Avossa, G. & Corbetta, M. (2003) Quantitative analysis of attention and detection signals during visual search. *J. Neurophysiol.* 90:3384-3397.

Shulman, R.G., Rothman, D.L., Behar, K.L. & Hyder, F. (2004) Energetic basis of brain activity: implications for neuroimaging. *Trends Neurosci.* 27:489-495.

Sidtis, J.J. (2007) Some problems for representations of brain organization based on activation in functional imaging. *Brain Lang.* 102:130-140.

Siegel, A.M. (2004) Presurgical evaluation and surgical treatment of medically refractory epilepsy. *Neurosurgical review* 27:1-18; discussion 19-21.

Spencer, S.S. & Bautista, R.E. (2000) Functional neuroimaging in localization of the ictal onset zone. *Advances in neurology* 83:285-296.

Stanberry, L., Nandy, R. & Cordes, D. (2003) Cluster analysis of fMRI data using dendrogram sharpening. *Human brain mapping* 20:201-219.

Suarez, R.O., Whalen, S., O'Shea, J.P. & Golby, A.J. (2008) A Surgical Planning Method for Functional MRI Assessment of Language Dominance: Influences from Threshold, Region-of-Interest, and Stimulus Mode. *Brain Imaging Behav.* 2:59-73.

Szaflarski, J.P., DiFrancesco, M., Hirschauer, T., Banks, C., Privitera, M.D., Gotman, J. & Holland, S.K. (2010) Cortical and subcortical contributions to absence seizure onset examined with EEG/fMRI. *Epilepsy Behav.* 18:404-413.

Vaudano, A.E., Laufs, H., Kiebel, S.J., Carmichael, D.W., Hamandi, K., Guye, M., Thornton, R., Rodionov, R., Friston, K.J., Duncan, J.S. & Lemieux, L. (2009) Causal Hierarchy within the Thalamo-Cortical Network in Spike and Wave Discharges. *Plos One* 4.

Verleger, R., Lefebre, C., Wieschemeyer, R. & Kompf, D. (1997) Event-related potentials suggest slowing of brain processes in generalized epilepsy and alterations of visual processing in patients with partial seizures. *Cognit. Brain Res.* 5:205-219.

Vlooswijk, M.C.G., Jansen, J.F.A., Majoie, H.J.M., Hofman, P.A.M., de Krom, M.C.T.F.M., Aldenkamp, A.P. & Backes, W.H. (2010) Functional connectivity and language impairment in cryptogenic localization-related epilepsy. *Neurology* 75:395-402.

Voets, N.L., Adcock, J.E., Stacey, R., Hart, Y., Carpenter, K., Matthews, P.M. & Beckmann, C.F. (2009) Functional and Structural Changes in the Memory Network Associated with Left Temporal Lobe Epilepsy. *Human brain mapping* 30:4070-4081.

Wagner, K., Frings, L., Halsband, U., Everts, R., Buller, A., Spreer, J., Zentner, J. & Schulze-Bonhage, A. (2007) Hippocampal functional connectivity reflects verbal episodic memory network integrity. *Neuroreport* 18:1719-1723.

Waites, A.B., Briellmann, R.S., Saling, M.M., Abbott, D.F. & Jackson, G.D. (2006) Functional connectivity networks are disrupted in left temporal lobe epilepsy. *Ann Neurol* 59:335-343.

Wang, L.Q., Song, M., Jiang, T.Z., Zhang, Y.T. & Yu, C.S. (2011) Regional homogeneity of the resting-state brain activity correlates with individual intelligence. *Neuroscience letters* 488:275-278.

Wiebe, S., Blume, W.T., Girvin, J.P. & Eliasziw, M. (2001) A randomized, controlled trial of surgery for temporal-lobe epilepsy. *The New England journal of medicine* 345:311-318.

Wong, C.H., Bleasel, A., Wen, L.F., Eberl, S., Byth, K., Fulham, M., Somerville, E. & Mohamed, A. (2010) The topography and significance of extratemporal hypometabolism in refractory mesial temporal lobe epilepsy examined by FDG-PET. *Epilepsia* 51:1365-1373.

Xiong, J., Parsons, L.M., Gao, J.H. & Fox, P.T. (1999) Interregional connectivity to primary motor cortex revealed using MRI resting state images. *Human brain mapping* 8:151-156.

Yan, C.G., Liu, D.Q., He, Y., Zou, Q.H., Zhu, C.Z., Zuo, X.N., Long, X.Y. & Zang, Y.F. (2009) Spontaneous Brain Activity in the Default Mode Network Is Sensitive to Different Resting-State Conditions with Limited Cognitive Load. *Plos One* 4.

Yang, H., Long, X.Y., Yang, Y.H., Yan, H., Zhu, C.Z., Zhou, X.P., Zang, Y.F. & Gong, Q.Y. (2007) Amplitude of low frequency fluctuation within visual areas revealed by resting-state functional MRI. *Neuroimage* 36:144-152.

Yu, L. & Blumenfeld, H. (2009) Theories of Impaired Consciousness in Epilepsy. *Disorders of Consciousness* 1157:48-60.

Zang, Y.F., He, Y., Zhu, C.Z., Cao, Q.J., Sui, M.Q., Liang, M., Tian, L.X., Jiang, T.Z. & Wang, Y.F. (2007) Altered baseline brain activity in children with ADHD revealed by resting-state functional MRI. *Brain Dev.* 29:83-91.

Zang, Y.F., Jiang, T.Z., Lu, Y.L., He, Y. & Tian, L.X. (2004) Regional homogeneity approach to fMRI data analysis. *Neuroimage* 22:394-400.

Zhang, Z., Lu, G., Zhong, Y., Tan, Q., Liao, W., Chen, Z., Shi, J. & Liu, Y. (2009a) Impaired perceptual networks in temporal lobe epilepsy revealed by resting fMRI. *Journal of neurology* 256:1705-1713.

Zhang, Z., Lu, G., Zhong, Y., Tan, Q., Yang, Z., Liao, W., Chen, Z., Shi, J. & Liu, Y. (2009b) Impaired attention network in temporal lobe epilepsy: a resting FMRI study. *Neuroscience letters* 458:97-101.

Zhang, Z.Q., Lu, G.M., Zhong, Y., Tan, Q.F., Liao, W., Wang, Z.G., Wang, Z.Q., Li, K., Chen, H.F. & Liu, Y.J. (2010a) Altered spontaneous neuronal activity of the default-mode network in mesial temporal lobe epilepsy. *Brain Res.* 1323:152-160.

Zhang, Z.Q., Lu, G.M., Zhong, Y.A., Tan, Q.F., Chen, H.F., Liao, W., Tian, L., Li, Z.H., Shi, J.X. & Liu, Y.J. (2010b) FMRI Study of Mesial Temporal Lobe Epilepsy Using Amplitude of Low-Frequency Fluctuation Analysis. *Human brain mapping* 31:1851-1861.

Zuo, X.N., Kelly, C., Adelstein, J.S., Klein, D.F., Castellanos, F.X. & Milham, M.P. (2010) Reliable intrinsic connectivity networks: Test-retest evaluation using ICA and dual regression approach. *Neuroimage* 49:2163-2177.

Part 4

Evaluation of Epilepsy

6

Blood-Brain Barrier Permeability: From Bench to Bedside

Svetlana M. Stamatovic[1], Nikola Sladojevic[1], Richard F. Keep[2] and Anuska V. Andjelkovic[1,2]
[1]Department of Pathology and
[2]Neurosurgery, University of Michigan, Ann Arbor, Michigan, United States of America

1. Introduction

The concept of the blood-brain barrier (termed hematoencephalic barrier) was first introduced by Lina Stern in 1921, although the early work by Paul Ehrlich and Edwin Goldmann suggested the compartmentalization between blood and brain and a role of blood vessels in maintaining these compartments (Ehrlich, 1885; Goldmann, 1913; Vein, 2008). However, actual proof of the existence of a BBB came in the 1960s. Since then, significant progress has been made in defining the functions and properties of that barrier.
The BBB is a highly specialized structural and biochemical barrier that regulates the entry of blood-borne molecules and cells into brain and preserves ionic homeostasis within the brain microenvironment (Pardridge, 2007; Rubin & Staddon, 1999; Ueno, 2007). Formed at the interface between blood and brain parenchyma, the BBB is composed of a tightly sealed monolayer of brain endothelial cells at the brain capillary surface and adjacent perivascular cells, including astrocytes and pericytes. Both astrocytic endfeet and pericyte processes wrap the abluminal capillary surface and through indirect or direct synapse-like "peg-socket" interactions provide physical support and stability to the BBB (Abbott, 2002; Armulik et al, 2010; Kim et al, 2006; Williams et al, 2001). In recent years, the concept of a BBB has been significantly extended to the concept of a neurovascular unit, which best describes the dynamic communication between brain endothelium, neurons, astrocytes, pericytes, vascular smooth muscle cells, microglia and perivascular macrophages at the interface between the blood and brain parenchyma compartments (Hawkins & Davis, 2005; Wolburg et al, 2009). A healthy brain relies on all of the cells of the neurovascular unit to function properly and communicate with each other in order for neuronal synapses and circuitries to maintain normal cognitive functions (Fig. 1).

2. Blood-brain barrier junctional complexes

The structural properties of the BBB are primarily determined by the endothelial junctional complexes, consisting of tight junctions (TJ) and adherens junctions (AdJ). The interactions between brain endothelial cells provide high endothelial electrical resistance barrier, in the range of 1500-2000 $\Omega.cm^2$ (pial vessels), as compared to 3-33 $\Omega.cm^2$ endothelial barrier in other tissues (Butt et al., 1990; Crone & Christensen, 1981). The TJ complexes seal the interendothelial cleft and regulates BBB paracellular permeability, while the AdJ is important for initiating and maintaining endothelial cell-cell contact (Denker &Nigam, 1998; Huber et al, 2001; Gonzalez-Mariscal et al, 2003). Structurally both complexes are composed of transmembrane proteins, which physically interact with their counterparts on the plasma membrane of adjacent cells, and cytoplasmic plaque proteins, which provide a link between transmembrane TJ/AdJ proteins and the actin cytoskeleton and participate in intracellular signaling (Fig. 2).

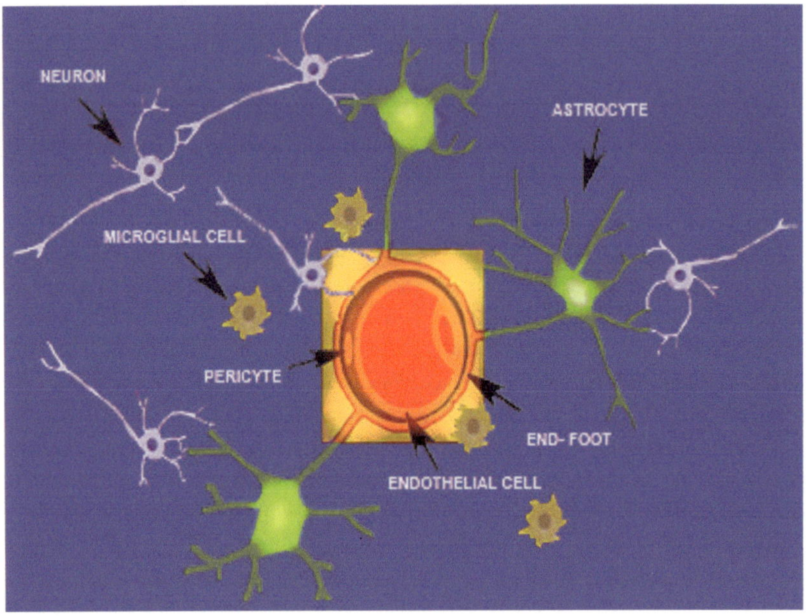

Fig. 1. Blood Brain barrier: neurovascular units.

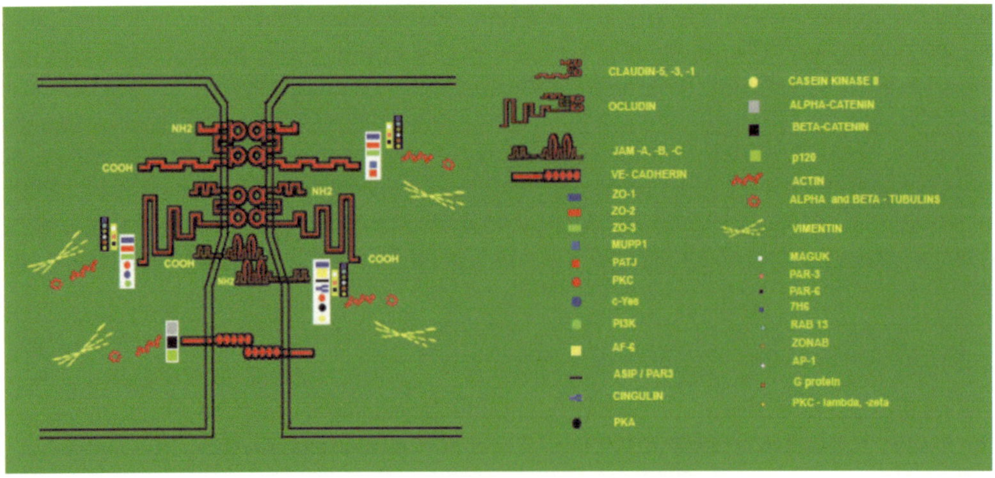

Fig. 2. Blood brain barrier: Tight and adherenst junction complex

The TJ transmembrane proteins include occludin, claudins (for example, claudin-5, -3, -12, -1) and junctional adhesion molecule (JAM) -A, -B and -C (Martin-Padura et al, 1998; Mitic & Aderon, 1998; Staddon and Rubin, 1996). Occludin (MW ~65kDa) was one of the first TJ transmembrane proteins to be described. It has four transmembrane spanning regions, two extracellular loops responsible for intercellular adhesion and maintaining transendothelial electrical resistance, and N- and C- terminal sites through which occludin can fully oligomerize or directly interact with scaffolding TJ [zonula occludens -1, -2, -3 (ZO-1, -2- 3)] and regulatory proteins [protein kinase C (PKC), tyrosine kinase c-Yes and Phosphatidylinositol 3-kinases (PI3K)] (Clump et al, 2005; Feldman et al 2005; Suzukiet al, 2002). The C-terminus of occludin plays a critical role in paracellular channel formation, mediating endocytosis and trafficking of occludin (Li et al, 2005; Nusrat et al, 2005). It is also involved in the integration and function of occludin within the TJ complex.

Claudins (MW 20 to 27 kDa) are the principal barrier-forming proteins. They belong to the PMP22/EMP/MP20/claudin family of proteins (Koval, 2006). Until now, twenty different claudins have been discovered and each of them shows a unique pattern of tissue expression and interactions. Claudins have a similar structural pattern to occludin: four membrane-spanning regions, two extracellular loops and two cytoplasmic termini (Morita et al, 1999; Nitta et al, 2003; Ruffer & Gerke, 2004; Soma et al, 2004). The first extracellular loop influences paracellular charge selectivity, while the second loop is known as a receptor for a bacterial toxin. Similar to occludin, the C-terminal site of claudins possesses a binding site (domain) for cytoplasmic proteins (ZO-1, ZO-2, ZO-3, MUPP1, PATJ) through a PDZ motif (Koval, 2006; Morita et al, 1999; Ruffer & Gerke, 2004). The role of the N-terminal site is still unclear. Brain endothelial cells express the cell specific claudin-5, which plays pivotal role in interendothelial occlusion and size selective permeability (Nitta et al, 2003; Ohtsuki et al, 2007). Besides claudin-5, recent data suggest the BBB possesses claudin-3, mostly during vasculogenesis, claudin-1, during adult brain angiogenesis and barrier genesis, and claudin-12 (Belanger et al, 2007; Lampugnani et al, 2010). However, there is little information on the interaction between these claudins and their role at the BBB.

JAM-A, -B, and -C (MW 32 kDa) are members of the immunoglobulin superfamily of proteins (Martin-Padura et al 1998). Similar to other immunoglobulins, these molecules are composed of a single membrane spanning domain, an extracellular domain, and two termini, an extracellular N-terminus and a short cytoplasmic tail C-terminus (Sobocki et al, 2006; Williams et al, 1999). The extracellular region of JAMs consists of two IgG-like domains and it appears to be subject to glycosylation, although the function of that glycosylation is still unknown. The short cytoplasmatic tail (40 amino acids) contains a binding domain which facilitates interactions with TJ associated scaffold proteins such as ZO-1, AF-6, ASIP/Par3, and cingulin (Bazzoni et al 2000; Bazzoni & Dejana, 2004; Williams et al, 1999). It also has phosphorylation sites for PKC, PKA and casein kinase II (Williams et al, 1999). JAMs display different patterns of homophilic and heterophilic cis- and trans-interactions. While they interact with JAM on adjacent cells, they can also act as adhesion molecules for interacting with integrins on leukocytes to regulate leukocyte trafficking (Bazzoni et al, 2000; Lamagna et al, 2005).

The cytoplasmic plaque proteins of TJ are divided into PDZ containing proteins (family membrane-associated guanylate-kinase (MAGUK) homologues (ZO-1, ZO-2, ZO-3), partitioning-defective proteins Par-3, Par-6, afadin/Af-6) and PDZ lacking proteins (cingulin, 7H6, Rab13, ZONAB, AP-1, PKCζ, PKCλ, heterotrimeric G protein) (Gonzalez-Mariscal et al, 2000, 2003; Ponting et al, 1999). The PDZ containing TJ proteins act as scaffolds that bring together cytoskeleton, signaling and integral proteins at specific regions of the plasma membrane and, via the PDZ domain, have a critical role in clustering and anchoring transmembrane proteins (Fanning et al, 2007; Hamazaki et al, 2002; McNeil et al, 2006). For example, ZO-1 functions as a multidomain scaffold that coordinates assembly of transmembrane and cytosolic proteins, including components of the cortical cytoskeleton, into TJs and/or regulates the activity of these proteins once they are assembled. Thus, ZO-1 is required for the normal kinetics of TJ assembly, for TJ specific localization and unique organization of transmembrane proteins (Gonzalez-Mariscal et al, 2000; McNeil et al, 2006; Utepbergenov et al, 2006).

PDZ lacking proteins have a variety functions at the TJ complex. For example, cingulin acts as a cross-link between TJ proteins (ZO-2, ZO-3, AF-6, JAM) and the actin-myosin cytoskeleton. Rab proteins (Rab13, Rab3b) have a role in the docking and fusion of transport vesicles at the TJ complex, while PKCζ and PKCλ have roles in regulating polarization and in TJ assembly (Andreeva et al, 2006; Suzuki et al, 2002; Terai et al, 2006; Yamanaka et al, 2001;). G proteins (Gα-i0, Gα-i2, Gα12, Gαs) co-immunoprecipitate with ZO-1 and play a role in accelerating TJ assembly and maintaining transendothelial electrical resistance (Citi &Cordenonsi, 1998; Meyer et al, 2003).

The major AdJ transmembrane protein in endothelial cells is vascular endothelium (Ve)-cadherin. The AdJ cytoplasmic plaque proteins include catenin family members (α-, β-catenin, p120) (Bazzoni & Dejana, 2004; Nagafuchi, 2001). Ve-cadherin is an important determinant of microvascular integrity both *in vitro* and *in vivo*. Together with the catenins, it forms a complex that functions as an early recognition mechanism between endothelial cells (Vorbrodt & Dobrogowska, 2004). In that complex, β-catenin and p120 are linked with cadherin and to α-catenin, and this provides a functional interaction for Ve-cadherin with the actin microfilament network of the cell cytoskeleton. A p120 binds Ve-cadherin with high affinity suggesting that it may be engaged in regulating vascular permeability (Hatzfeld, 2005; Tao et al, 1996; Vorbrodt & Dobrogowska, 2004).

The actin cytoskeleton is also a critical component for establishing brain endothelial barrier integrity. The cytoskeleton is composed of three primary elements: actin microfilaments, intermediate filaments and microtubules. Actin microfilaments are focally linked to multiple membrane adhesive proteins such as cadherin, occludin, zonula occludens, catenins and focal adhesion complex, forming a structure known as the actin-rich adhesion belt and providing physical support to the junctional complexes (Lai et al, 2005; Small et al, 1999; Tao et al, 1996). In addition, actin microfilaments are involved in generating tension via myosin light chain phosphorylation and actin stress fiber formation during the unsealing of the junctional complex (Small et al, 1999; Stamatovic et al, 2003; Wang et al, 1983). A second major element of the cytoskeleton is the microtubules, polymers of α- and β-tubulins, which participate in rapid assembly of actin filaments and focal adhesion, isometric cellular contraction and/or increased transendothelial leucocyte migration (Honore et al, 2005; Tzima, 2006). A third major element of the cytoskeletal machinery is the intermediate filaments (predominantly vimentin) which have a role in reorganization of actin filaments and microtubules (Dudek& Garcia, 2001).

3. Blood-brain barrier transport systems

3.1 Transcellular transport

Due to the restrictive angioarchitecture of the BBB, brain endothelial cells have developed specific transport systems which allow the controlled exchange of proteins, nutrients and waste products between blood and brain. In this way, while impeding the general influx of hydrophilic intravascular substances from blood to brain, carrier- and receptor-mediated transport systems promote the transport into brain of select compounds important for cerebral function. In addition, active efflux transport systems promote the clearance of select compounds (e.g. waste products) from brain to blood. There is some 'non-selective' transport of compounds across the BBB through nonspecific vesicular transport (fluid phase endocytosis or adsorptive endocytosis) (Lossinsky et al, 1983; Lossinsky & Shivers, 2004).

Fluid phase endocytosis, adsorptive endocytosis and caveolae are some of the systems involved in the transcytosis of compounds across the brain endothelium. Transcytosis describes the vectorial movement of molecules within endocytotic vesicles across the cerebral endothelium (primarily from the luminal cell side to the abluminal side) where exocytosis occurs (Lossinsky & Shivers, 2004). Brain capillary endothelial cells contain two kinds of vesicles that are open to the luminal blood capillary space: caveolae and clathrin-coated pits/vesicles. Clathrin is a self-assembling protein whose polymerization into a polyhedral network promotes membrane vesiculation and budding of selected receptors (Miwako et al, 2003; Mukherjee et al, 1997). Compared to peripheral endothelia, the brain capillary endothelium is particularly enriched in clathrin-coated pits/vesicles (Lossinsky & Shivers, 2004). These are predominantly expressed on the luminal side suggesting that clathrin-dependent transcytosis is primarily from blood to brain. Clathrin-coated pits recruit cell-surface receptors and then, through a series of highly regulated steps, pinch off to form clathrin-coated vesicles, which further may fuse with a transcytotic endosome (Miwako et al, 2003; Mukherjee et al, 1997).

Caveolae are bud-like invaginations formed by the concentration of the caveolin proteins. These vesicles are enriched in cholesterol and glycosphingolipids on cellular membranes as well as glycosyl phosphatidyl inositol (GPI)-anchored proteins, not present in the coated pits (Hommelgaard et al, 2005; Kirkham & Parton, 2005). Caveolae are found on both luminal and abluminal plasma membranes of cerebral endothelial cells indicating bidirectional transcytosis from blood to brain and from brain to blood (Lossinsky & Shivers, 2004). Caveolae contain an abundance of membrane receptors, transporters and signaling molecules, suggesting their involvement in various important cellular processes in addition to their role in the endocytosis/transcytosis. Recent findings regarding the process of endocytosis have pinpointed the merging endosomes for both types of endocytotic pathways (see for review Hommelgaard et al, 2005) .

In fluid-phase transcytosis, invagination of caveolae entraps bulk plasma and soluble plasma molecules. The vesicles are then transported across the cerebral endothelium. In this transport process, there is a lack of interaction between the transported molecules and the caveolar vesicular membrane (Lossinsky & Shivers, 2004; Predescu et al, 2007). A very small portion fluid-phase transcytosis can occur via clathrin-coated pits/vesicles.

Adsorptive transcytosis can be *specific* (receptor-mediated transcytosis) and *nonspecific* (adsorptive-mediated transcytosis) processes. Receptor-mediated transcytosis is triggered by a specific interaction of a molecule with receptors expressed on capillary brain endothelial cells and it is limited to transport of proteins and peptides across the BBB. Examples of this type of adsorptive transcytosis are insulin, iron-transferrin and LDL-cholesterol (Broadwell et al, 1996; Hervé et al, 2008; Simionescu & Simionescu, 1985) This type of transport is very limited in brain endothelium with small amounts of insulin and transferrin being delivered into brain sufficient to maintain BBB and brain homeostasis. Clathrin-type vesicles are predominantly involved in receptor-mediated transcytosis.

Non-specific adsorptive transcytosis does not involve specific plasma membrane receptors and endocytosis is initiated through charge-charge interaction between polycationic substances and negative charges on the endothelial surface. Molecules that penetrate the brain via this mechanism include, but are not limited to, various cationic proteins. Clathrin-coated pits along the luminal surface of ECs are negatively charged and thus capable of binding positively charged substances (Hervé et al, 2008; Villegas et al, 1993). A few studies have, however, demonstrated that caveolae are involved in adsorptive endocytosis by transferring of cationized $F(ab')_2$ antibody fragments across the BBB (Girod et al, 1999).
Brain uptake via non-specific and specific adsorptive transcytosis is time- and concentration-dependent, and requires energy. Uptake via these types of endocytosis is slow compared with carrier-mediated transport of nutrients (e.g. glucose), taking minutes to occur. Both non-specific and specific adsorptive endocytosis/transcystosis are also saturable processes with the main difference being that non-specific adsorptive transcytosis becomes saturated at higher concentrations (micromolar level) while specific adsorptive transcytosis becomes saturated at a low nanomolar range (Hervé et al, 2008).

3.2 Carrier mediated: blood-to-brain influx systems

BBB possesses a wide array of carrier-mediated transport systems for small molecules to support and protect CNS function. For example, the blood-to-brain influx transport systems supply nutrients, such as glucose and amino acids.
D-glucose in the primary energy source for the brain and the BBB has very high levels of the facilitative (Na^+-independent) glucose transporter, GLUT1 (SLC2A1) which transports D- but not L-glucose (Cornford et al, 1993; Pardridge et al, 1990). GLUT1 is localized on both the luminal and abluminal sides of the BBB. As well as transporting D-glucose, GLUT1 transports hexoses and an oxidized form of L-ascorbic acid, L-dehydroascorbic acid. It is considered to have role in maintaining the high concentration of L-ascorbic acid in the brain compared with plasma (McAllister et al 2001; Vemula et al, 2009). In addition, GLUT1 can transport some glycosylated peptides (e.g. L-serinyl-β-D-glucoside analogues of Met^5 enkephalin) (Masand et al, 2006).
Amino acids like L-tyrosine, L-tryptophan, and L-histidine are transported from the blood to the brain via a Na^+-independent neutral amino acid transporter (system L) (Boado et al, 1999, Ohtsuki, 2004). This is a heteromeric transporter with a light chain (LAT1; SLC7A5) and a heavy chain (4F2hc; SLC3A2)(Omidi et al, 2008). As with GLUT1, it is facilitative and present on both the luminal and abluminal membranes. Same transporters is involved in transports L-leucine, L-isoleucine, L-valine, L-methionine, L-threonine, and L-phenylalanine (Audus & Borchardt, 1986; Omidi et al, 2008; Reichel et al, 1996; Xiang et al, 2003). Several amino acid-mimetic drugs, alkylating agent melphalan, the antiepileptic drug gabapentin, and the muscle relaxant baclofen use a System L for the influx form blood to brain (Luer et al, 1999; Sakaeda et al, 2000). Thus a high-protein diet reduces the concentration of these drugs in the brain due to competitive inhibition at the BBB.
The basic amino acids, such as L-lysine and l-arginine have a CAT1 (SCL7A2) transporter which expression is concentrated in brain capillaries (Lyck et al, 2009; Umeki et al, 2002). TAUT (SLC6A6) mediates taurine transport at the BBB, and due to neuroprotective effect of taurine the therapeutic manipulation of this transporter is important strategy in the treatment of neurodegenerative disorders (Kang et al, 2002; Lyck et al, 2009).
MCT1 (SCL16A1) mediates influx transport of monocarboxlic acids, such as lactate and pyruvate. MCT1 in the brain and the brain uptake rate of lactate are particularly increased

during the suckling period allowing brain the use lactate from milk (Batrakova et al, 2004; Kido et al 2000; Umeki et al, 2002).

CNT1 (SCL28A1) mediates transport of nucleosides and their analogues while Oatp2 (SLCO1B1; SLC21A6) mediates transport of organic anions and opioids (Bourasset et al, 2003; Cansev, 2006; Gao et al, 2000; Li et al, 2001). Both of these blood-to-brain influx transport systems are candidates to enhance drug delivery to the brain.

Creatine is important in energy storage in the brain and it is uptaken via CRT [SLC6A8] transporter (Braissant et al, 2001; Ohtsuki et al, 2002; Tachikawa et al, 2009;). This transporter is expressed on both luminal and an abluminal membrane of brain capillary endothelial cells and for this transporter is documented to mediate creatine supply to the brain (Braissant et al, 2001; Ohtsuki et al, 2002). Due to the fact that creatine has a neuroprotective effect, targeting CRT at BBB is the strategy to increase brain creatine levels and to prevent neurodegeneration (Fig. 3).

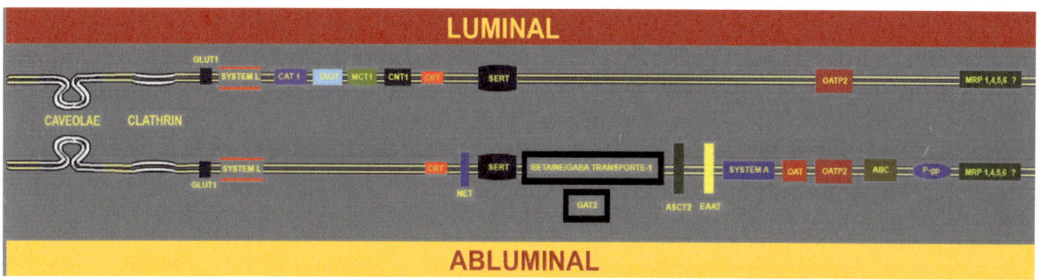

Fig. 3. Blood brain barrier transport system.

3.3 BBB efflux transporters: brain-to-blood efflux system

The BBB is involved in the brain-to-blood efflux transport of hydrophilic small molecules generated in the brain, such as neurotransmitters, neuromodulators, end-metabolites of neurotransmitters, uremic toxins, and also peptides, such as immunoglobulins.

Brain endothelial cells contain the norepinephrine transporter (NET), localized at the abluminal membrane and serotonin transporter (SERT), localized at both the abluminal and luminal membrane. In this way the brain microvasculature could receive signals and be regulated by monoamines released from adrenergic and serotonergic neurons (Ohtsuki, 2004; Wakayama et al, 2002). The abluminally localized NET and SERT is thought to be an inactivation system for neurotransmitters around the brain capillaries. The presence of luminal SERT is thought to play a role in serotonin clearance from the intravascular space (mostly secreted by platelets) to maintain cerebral blood flow (Nakatani et al, 2008; Olivier et al, 2000). Besides monoamines, brain endothelial cells are also involved in the efflux transport of GABA via Betaine/GABA transporter-1 (BGT-1; SLC6A12) or murine GABA transporter 2 (GAT2) present on the abluminal membrane (Gibbs et al, 2004; Kakee et al, 2001; Takanaga et al, 2001).

Brain endothelial cells exhibit stereo-selective efflux transport of aspartic acid (Asp), via ASC transporter ASCT2, selectively transporting the L-isomer of Asp (Tetsuka et al, 2003). In addition, excitatory amino acid transporters, EAATs, have been detected on the abluminal membrane of brain endothelial cells having a role in transport of both L- and D-Asp isomers and L-glutamate (Ennis et al, 1998; O'Kane et al, 1999; Tetsuka et al, 2003). System A is a transport system (ATA1, ATA2, ATA3) for small neutral amino acids that accepts L-alanine, L-proline and glycine (Hatanaka et al, 2001; Ling et al, 2001). Present on the abluminal membrane of brain endothelial cells, this system also may contribute to the regulation of the osmolarity in the brain and cell volume (Hatanaka et al, 2001; Ohtsuki, 2004).

The organic anion transporter (OAT) family is also involved in efflux transport at the BBB. These transporters are involved in the efflux of various neurotransmitter metabolites and act as a CNS detoxification system (Ohtsuki et al, 2004). For example, OAT3 (SLC22A8), localized at the abluminal membrane, transports homovanillic acid (HVA) from brain to blood (Mori et al, 2003; Ohtsuki et al, 2002). OAT3-mediated HVA transport is inhibited by various neurotransmitter metabolites such as 3,4-dihydroxyphenylacetic acid (dopamine metabolite), vanillylmandelic acid, 3,4-dihydroxymandelic acid and 4-hydroxy-3-methoxyphenylglycol (norepinephrine and epinephrine metabolites), 5-hydroxyindole acetic acid and 5-methoxytryptophol (serotonin metabolites), and imidazole-4-acetic acid and 1-methyl-4-imidazolic acid (histamine metabolites) (Duan & Wang, 2010; Ohtsuki et al, 2002). Thus it appears that OAT3 mediates the clearance of a wide range of neurotransmitter metabolites from brain. In addition, OAT3 mediates the brain-to-blood efflux of indoxyl sulfate, a uremic toxin (Ohtsuki et al, 2002). The brain concentration of under normal conditions is 3.4 times lower than that in serum and this limited distribution could be due to OAT3-mediated BBB efflux (Ohtsuki et al, 2002).

Another transporter of organic anions, Oatp2, is localized on both the luminal and abluminal membrane of brain endothelial cells and plays a role in the efflux of dehydroepiandrosterone sulfate, a neurosteroid that can interact with GABA type A receptors and σ receptors to increase memory and learning ability and to protect neurons against excitatory amino acid-induced neurotoxicity (Asaba et al, 2000; Gao et al, 1999; Ose et al, 2010). Oatp2 is also responsible for estrone-3-sulfate efflux transport (Asaba et al, 2000).

BBB active drug efflux transporters know as ATP-binding cassette (ABC) efflux transporters are increasingly recognized as important determinants of drug distribution to, and elimination from, the brain, minimizing or avoiding in this way neurotoxic adverse effects of drugs that otherwise would penetrate into the brain (Begley, 2004). Until now the best characterized of the BBB ABC efflux transporters are P-glycoprotein (Pgp, ABCB1), the multidrug resistance associated protein MRP (ABCC2) family and breast cancer resistance protein (BCRP) (Eisenblätter et al, 2003; Virgintino et al, 2002; Zhang et al, 2003).

P-glycoprotein (P-gp/MDR1/ABCB1) is a well-characterized efflux transporter of xenobiotics (Löscher et al, 2005). P-gp is a primary active transporter of relatively lipophilic compounds, such as the anticancer drug, vinblastine, cyclosporin A, and the cardiac glycoside, digoxin, by direct consumption of ATP (Hembury et al, 2008; Löscher et al, 2005; Quezada et al, 2008; van der Sandt et al, 2001). In addition, P-gp contributes to efflux of such as amyloid-beta proteins from the brain into the blood as well as many drugs such as anti-cancer drugs (Cirrito et al, 2005; Nazer et al, 2008; Piwnica-Worms et al, 2006). P-gp expressed on the luminal side of brain endothelial cells plays a very important role in restricting the entry of xenobiotics from the circulating blood into the brain (Matsuoka et al, 1999, Warren et al, 2009). Thus, for example, ivermectin reaches 20-fold higher concentrations in the brains of mice without P-gp (Lespine et al, 2006).

The multidrug resistance-associated protein (MRP) 1, 4, 5, and 6 has been detected in primary cultured bovine brain endothelial cells and the bovine brain capillary-enriched fraction (Nies et al, 2004; Yu et al, 2007; Zhang et al, 2000). MRP1 and 5 are predominantly localized on the luminal membrane fraction while MRP4 is localized almost equally on the luminal and abluminal membrane fractions (Nies et al, 2004; Yu et al, 2007). However, the localization of these subtypes is still unclear. Although the full functions of MRPs are still unknown (and the relative importance still debated), one recent study indicated that Mrp1 contributes in part to the efflux transport of Estradiol-17-β-D-glucuronide ($E_2 17\beta G$) at the BBB (Sugiyama et al, 2003) (Fig. 3).

4. BBB and epilepsy

Epilepsy is a chronic neurological disease that is characterized by spontaneous recurrent seizures and sometimes-untreatable seizures. In addition, epileptogenesis can occur after brain insults such as trauma, ischemia and infection. Several clinical and experimental studies have reported that BBB malfunction can trigger chronic seizures or an acute seizure (Friedman et al, 2009; Oby & Janigro, 2006; Tomkins et al 2011). Furthermore, transient BBB disruption is a consequence of epileptic seizures and multiple changes in BBB transporters have been reported in epilepsy patients/models. BBB obviously play an important multifaceted role in epileptic seizures as discussed below (Dombrowski et al, 2001; Löscher et al, 2002; Łotowska et al, 2008).

Pathological and immunohistochemical studies in human epileptic tissue as well as animal models of epilepsy consistently demonstrate structural evidence for an abnormal "leaky" BBB with an accumulation of serum albumin within the neuropil and cellular elements as functional evidence for abnormal vessels permeability to large hydrophilic molecules (Oby & Janigro, 2006; Stewart et al, 1987). A substantial increase in BBB permeability was found in approximately 2/3 of capillaries and perivascular astroglial processes.

4.1 Blood Brain Barrier permeability and epilepsy

Increased BBB permeability is associated with remodeling of interendothelial junctional complex and gap formation between brain endothelial cells (paracellular pathway) and/or intensive pinocytotic vesicular transport between the apical and basal side of brain endothelial cells (transcellular pathway) (Bazzoni, 2006; Garcia & Schaphorst, 1995; Lossinsky & Shivers, 2004). These two pathways display differences in cellular and molecular components as well as in physical properties. The transcellular pathway can be either passive or active, and is characterized by low conductance and high selectivity in either apical to basal or basal to apical directions. In contrast, the paracellular pathway is exclusively passive, being driven by electrochemical and osmotic gradients, and it shows a higher conductance and lower selectivity, although it can display charge and size selectivity (Bazzoni, 2006). There is evidence that both types of pathway are involved in the development and progression of epilepsy seizures. Ultrastructural studies on human epileptic tissue clearly demonstrated BBB abnormalities, including increased micropinocytosis and fewer mitochondria in endothelial cells, a thickening of the basal membrane, and the presence of abnormal tight junctions (Cornford & Hyman, 1999; Cornford & Oldendorf, 1986).

Increased BBB permeability could be an etiological factor contributing to seizure development. Both clinical and animal studies pinpoint that primary vascular lesions and, specifically an opening of the BBB (i.e. significant and long-lasting BBB breakdown in cortical injury), trigger a chain of events leading to epilepsy (Marchi et al, 2007; Oby and Janigro, 2006; Seiffert et al, 2004; Tomkins et al, 2007; Tomkins et al, 2008; van Vliet et al,

2007). Increased BBB permeability was found in 77% of patients with posttraumatic epilepsy and these patents had a larger cerebral cortex volume with BBB disruption (Tomkins et al, 2008). In 70% of patients, slow (delta band) activity was co-localized, by sLORETA, with regions showing BBB disruption (Tomkins et al, 2011). A consequence of increased para- and transcellular permeability is extravasation of albumin into the brain neuropil. This may be sufficient for the induction of epileptogenesis. It has been suggested that accumulated albumin binds to transforming growth factor beta receptor 2 (TGFbetaR2) in astrocytes and induces rapid astrocytic transformation and dysfunction (Cacheaux et al, 2009; David et al, 2009; Ivenset al, 2007;) In addition, leakage of some other serum-derived components into the extracellular space may also result in hyperexcitability and seizure onset. For example, it has been recently shown that the serum protein, thrombin, via receptors protease-activated receptor 1 (PAR1), produces a long-lasting enhancement of the reactivity of CA1 neurons to afferent stimulation (Maggio et al, 2008). It should also be noted that in many cases of epilepsy, that BBB breakdown has been associated with early or delayed neuronal damage (Rigau et al, 2007; Tomkins et al, 2007; van Vliet et al, 2007).

Furthermore, BBB dysfunction may not only trigger epileptic seizures, it may also contribute to the progression of epilepsy (Seiffert et al, 2004, van Vliet et al, 2007; Uva et al, 2008). Recently, a role for BBB opening in the progression of temporal epilepsy was suggested based on the finding of positive immunocytochemistry staining for accumulated albumin and a positive correlation between the extent of BBB opening and the number of seizures (van Vliet et al, 2007). In the line with that evidence, application of bile salts causes long-lasting BBB opening caused by application of bile salts and the delayed appearance of robust hypersynchronous epileptiform activity (Greenwood et al, 1991). Predictors of seizures during the BBB breakdown are elevation of serum S100beta (an astrocyte marker) levels and computed tomography (CT) scans (Marchi et al, 2007).

Vasogenic brain edema is one the best example of association between BBB dysfunction and epilepsy. In experimental epilepsy models (kainate- and pilocarpine-epilepsy models, layers II and III of the piriform cortex are vulnerable to brain edema and they have been shown to play a role in generation and propagation of paroxysmal activity (Gale, 1992, Löscher and Ebert, 1996, McIntyre and Kelly, 2000). In contrast to the piriform cortex, the hippocampus shows vacuolized CA1 astrocytes and neuronal death without vasogenic edema (Kim et al, 2009, Kim et al, 2010).

Many studies have reported an increased permeability of the BBB during epileptic activity (Öztas and Kaya, 1991, Ruth, 1984; Ilbay et al, 2003, Ates et al, 1999). A fast and significant increase in systemic blood pressure, particularly during tonic epileptic seizures, induces marked vasodilation of large cerebral arteries and an increase in blood pressure in capillaries, small arteries, and veins, leading to leakage of the BBB (Mayhan, 2001). Indeed, an acute increase in blood pressure or epileptic activity causes increased pinocytosis in the cerebral endothelium (Cornford and Oldendorf, 1986).

The loss of BBB integrity, however, is not only due to an abrupt increase in intraluminal pressure but also influenced by the properties of cerebral tissues, particularly in the perivascular area (Nitsch et al, 1985). The most notable changes are on perivascular astrocytes. Several recent studies have pinpointed alterations in astrocytic dystrophin expression during epileptogenesis, which may directly influence brain endothelial barrier permeability. Dystrophin, an actin-binding protein, is primarily localized in the astrocyte end-feet near capillaries where this anchor protein is responsible for maintenance of polarized expression of astrocytic aquaporin 4 (AQP4; a water channel) (Nico et al, 2003;

Sheen et al, 2011). Since astrocytes selectively control exchange between blood and neural tissue by induction of the morphological and biochemical features of endothelial cells to form TJ and of its enzymatic systems and transporters, it is likely that dystrophin plays a role in establishment of endothelial polarity and regulating vascular permeability (Anderson et al, 1989; Nico et al, 2003). However, some dystrophin isoforms are also present in brain endothelial cells where, as an actin binding protein, dystrophin may regulate the actin machinery associated with the TJ complex (Nico et al, 2004). During epileptogenesis, there is down-regulation of dystrophin immunoreactivity in perivascular astrocytes and endothelial cells and this was also accompanied by impaired AQP4 expression in perivascular astroglial end-feet. The perturbed expression of AQP4 and dystrophin furthermore may be one factor underlying loss of ion and water homeostasis in the epileptic brain tissue, leading to impaired buffering of extracellular K^+ and an increased propensity for seizures (Lee et al, 2004, Eid et al, 2005).

SMI-7 is an endothelial barrier antigen expressed on the luminal membrane at the rat BBB (Sternberger & Sternberger, 1987). SMI-71 immunoreactivity is also significantly reduced in blood vessels at day 1 after epileptogenesis when the neuronal damage is also present (Lu et al, 2010). However, the down-regulation of SMI-71 is also associated with widening of intercellular junctions between endothelial cells and swelling of perivascular astrocytic processes and this was caused by impaired interaction between endothelial cells and perivascular astrocytes (Ghabriel et al, 2002; Lawrenson et al, 1995).

4.2 Angiogenesis, blood brain barrier and epilepsy

In humans, there is evidence that cerebral vascularization (vessel density) is significantly higher in temporal lobe epilepsy (Rigau et al, 2007). This was neither dependent on etiology nor on the degree of neuronal loss, but was positively correlated with seizure frequency. Vascular endothelial growth factor (VEGF) and the VEGF receptors were detected in different types of cells suggesting a role of this growth factor in the increased vascularization. In that study, an impairment of the BBB was demonstrated by a loss of TJs and by immunoglobulin G (IgG) leakage and accumulation in neurons. In a rat model of temporal lobe epilepsy, VEGF over-expression and BBB impairment also occurred early after status epilepticus (Croll et al; 2004 Nicoletti et al, 2008). This was followed by a progressive increase in vascularization. In both humans and rodents, the processes of angiogenisis and BBB disruption were still obvious in the chronic focus, probably the result of recurrent seizures (Marcon et al, 2009; Ndode-Ekane et al, 2010).

4.3 Inflammation, blood brain barrier and epilepsy

Several proinflammatory signals are rapidly induced in rodent brain during epileptic activity. These include cytokines, chemokines, prostaglandins, toll-like receptors, signal-transduction pathways that recruit nuclear factor-κB (NF-κB), complement factors and cell-adhesion molecules (Alapirtti et al, 2009; Avignone et al, 2008; Gorter et al, 2006; Manley et al, 2007; Natoli et al, 2000; Oliveira et al, 2008; Sinha et al, 2008; Zattoni et al, 2011). Seizures induce a massive inflammatory response in parenchymal cells, involving both microglia and neurons (Riazi et al, 2008, Zattoni et al, 2011).

Inflammation might either contribute to epileptogenesis or be a response that develops after seizures. There is substantial evidence supporting both CNS and intravascular inflammation as being seizure promoting or pro-epileptogenic. BBB damage is known to directly cause seizures and to increase spontaneous seizure frequency (Rossi et al, 2011; Riazi et al, 2008; Vezzani et al, 2011,; Zattoni et al, 2011). Blockade of CNS or systemic inflammation pathways (e.g., via inhibition of interleukin [IL]-1β signaling with IL1-receptor antagonist or via blockade of IL-1β production with caspase-1 inhibitors) reduces status epilepticus and seizure frequency (Alapirtti et al, 2009; Gorter et al, 2006; Kim et al, 2010; Vezzani et al, 2010). Glia, neurons, and endothelial cells express cytokines following seizures in experimental models in human epileptogenic tissue and after brain injury (Rossi et al, 2011; Sinha et al, 2008). These findings point to a prominent role for cytokines in the pathogenesis of seizures. Elucidation of the mechanisms underlying the effects of cytokines in seizures highlights nonconventional modes of action involving direct effects on neuronal excitability or a direct action on BBB integrity.

Seizures also, however, induce elevated expression of vascular cell adhesion molecules and enhance leukocyte rolling and arrest in brain vessels, effects mediated by the leukocyte mucin P-selectin glycoprotein ligand-1 (PSGL-1, encoded by *Selplg*) and leukocyte integrins (Fabene et al, 2008; Gorter et al, 2006; Librizzi et al, 2007). Inhibition of leukocyte-vascular interactions, either with blocking antibodies, depletion of neutrophils or by genetically interfering with PSGL-1 function in mice, markedly reduced acute seizures and chronic spontaneous recurrent seizures (Fabene et al, 2008, Zattoni et al, 2011). Consistent with this experimental data there are also some clinical studies showing more abundant leukocytes in epileptic brains than in controls, pinpointing a potential leukocyte involvement (Zattoni et al, 2011). This, suggest that leukocyte-endothelial interaction could be a potential target for the prevention and treatment of epilepsy.

Taking into consideration all of these data, there is a need for the development of strategies to detect BBB permeability changes for diagnosis (i.e. to identify the epileptic region prior to surgery) and for targeting populations at risk of developing epilepsy. A diagnostic tool for measuring BBB permeability should give reliable, objective and quantitative information with high spatial resolution. Qualitative evaluation of BBB disruption in humans accompanied with analysis of the cerebrospinal fluid for serum proteins or peripheral blood for brain constituents (e.g. S100β) could be promising strategies (Marchi et al., 2003).

4.4 Blood Brain Barrier transporters and epilepsy

Changes in BBB transporter systems also play an important role in epilepsy. It is estimated that 20-25% of epileptic patients fail to achieve good control with the different antiepileptic drugs treatments, developing so-called refractory epilepsy. Changes in ABC transporters like P-gp, MRPs (MRP1 and MRP2) and BCRP are directly related with the refractoriness (Abbott et al, 2007; Dombrowski et al, 2001; Lazarowski et al, 2007; Liu et al, 2000; Löscher &Potschka, 2002). These transporters are overexpressed in the brains of patients with refractory epilepsy, with implications for active drug efflux from brain. The progressive neuronal P-gp expression, depending on intensity and time-constancy of seizure-injury, is in agreement with the development of "P-gp-positive seizure-axis" proposed by Kwan & Brodie, who also showed that the development of refractory epilepsy directly correlated with the number and frequency of seizures before initiation of drug therapy (Kwan & Brodie, 2005). Furthermore two recent studies highlighted a possible underlying mechanism of the increased Pgp protein expression during the seizures. The studies by Bauer and colleagues and Hartz and colleagues have indicated that NMDA receptor, cyclooxygenase-2 (COX-2) prostaglandin E2and NFκB are involved in increase expression of Pgp on brain

microvascular endothelial cells and subsequently with that specific COX-2 inhibitor, NMDA receptor antagonist and E2 receptor antagonist abolished seizers dependent increase in Pgp expression (Bauer et al, 2008; Hartz et al, 2006). Therefore, modulation of ABC efflux transporters at the BBB forms a novel strategy to enhance the penetration of drugs into the brain and may yield new therapeutic options for drug-resistant CNS diseases.
Another transporter prominent expressed in epilepsy is GLUT-1. GLUT-1 immunoreactivity is increased in blood vessels after status epilepticus and after kainic acid- or pentylenetetrazole-induced seizures (Cornford et al, 2000; Gronlund et al, 1996). As there is a rapid increase in neuronal metabolic energy demands during seizures (Gronlund et al, 1996), this indicates that GLUT-1 may be upregulated under conditions of elevated brain glucose metabolism. Alternatively, alteration in GLUT-1 expression may be relevant to angiogenesis, which contributes to epileptogenesis and/or ictogenesis in experimental and human epilepsy (Ndode-Ekane et al, 2010, Marcon et al, 2009).

5. Conclusion

The data from experimental animals and human clinical studies indicate that studying mechanisms underlying epileptogenesis and epileptic seizures must consider variety of interactions within the "neurovascular unit". Significant changes occur in the vascular system, astrocytes and microglia cells which contribute significantly to the pathogenesis of the disease. Recent advances in imaging indicate that identification and quantification of such events are in hand and call for large-scale prospective studies to explore the role of BBB breakdown in the epileptogenic process. Valuable information on the time resolution and extent of BBB permeability changes, the role of astrocytes, inflammation and specific molecular pathways in human epileptogenesis, may allow a better design of anti-epileptogenic and anti-epileptic treatments for specific populations.

6. References

Abbott, N.J. (2002). Astrocyte-endothelial interactions and blood-brain barrier permeability. *Journal of Anatomy*, Vol.200, No.6, pp. 629-638.

Abbott, N.J., Khan, E.U., Rollinson, C.M., Reichel, A., Janigro, D., Dombrowsk,i S.M., Dobbie, M.S., Begley, D.J. (2002). Drug resistance in epilepsy: the role of the blood-brain barrier. *Novartis Found Symposium*, vol. 243, pp. 38-47.

Alapirtti, T., Rinta, S., Hulkkonen, J., Mäkinen, R., Keränen, T., Peltola, J. (2009) Interleukin-6, interleukin-1 receptor antagonist and interleukin-1beta production in patients with focal epilepsy: A video-EEG study. *Journal of Neurological Science*, Vol. 280, No.1-2, pp. 94-97.

Anderson, P.N., Woodham, P., Turmaine, M. (1989). Peripheral nerve regeneration through optic nerve grafts. *Acta Neuropathologicaogica*, Vol. 77, No.5, pp. 525-534.

Andreeva, A.Y., Piontek, J., Blasig, I.E., Utepbergenov, D.I. (2006). Assembly of tight junction is regulated by the antagonism of conventional and novel protein kinase C isoforms. *Int. J. Biochem. Cell Biol.*, Vol.38, No.2, pp. 222-233.

Armulik, A., Genové, G., Mäe, M., Nisancioglu, M.H., Wallgard, E., Niaudet, C., He, L., Norlin, J., Lindblom, P., Strittmatter, K., Johansson, B.R., Betsholtz, C. (2010). Pericytes regulate the blood-brain barrier. *Nature*, Vol. 468, No. 7323, pp.557-561.

Asaba, H., Hosoya, K., Takanaga, H., Ohtsuki, S., Tamura, E., Takizawa, T., Terasaki, T. (2000). Blood-brain barrier is involved in the efflux transport of a neuroactive steroid, dehydroepiandrosterone sulfate, via organic anion transporting polypeptide 2. *Journal of Neurochemistry,*Vol. 75, No.5, 1907-1916.

Ates, N., Esen, N., Ilbay, G. (1999). Absence epilepsy and regional blood-brain barrier permeability: the effects of pentylenetetrazole-induced convulsions. *Pharmacological Research,* Vol. 39, No. 4, pp. 305-310.

Avignone, E., Ulmann, L., Levavasseur, F., Rassendren, F., Audinat, E. (2008). Status epilepticus induces a particular microglial activation state characterized by enhanced purinergic signaling. *Journal of Neuroscience.* Vol. 28. No.37, pp. 9133-9144.

Audus, K.L., Borchardt, R.T. (1986). Characteristics of the large neutral amino acid transport system of bovine brain microvessel endothelial cell monolayers. *Journal of Neurochemistry.* Vol. 47, No. 2, pp. 484-488.

Batrakova, E.V., Zhang, Y., Li, Y., Li, S., Vinogradov, S.V., Persidsky, Y., Alakhov, V.Y., Miller, D.W., Kabanov, A.V. (2004). Effects of pluronic P85 on GLUT1 and MCT1 transporters in the blood-brain barrier. *Pharmacological Research.* Vol. 21, No.11, pp. 1993-2000.

Bauer, B., Hartz, A.M., Pekcec, A., Toellner, K., Miller, D.S., Potschka, H. (2008). Seizure-induced up-regulation of P-glycoprotein at the blood-brain barrier through glutamate and cyclooxygenase-2 signaling. *Molecular Pharmacology.* Vol. 73, No.5, pp. 1444-53.

Bazzoni, G., Dejana, E. (2004). Endothelial cell-to-cell junctions: molecular organization and role in vascular homeostasis. *Physiol. Rev.,* Vol. 84, No.3, pp. 869-901.

Bazzoni, G., Martinez-Estrada, O.M., Mueller, F., Nelboeck, P., Schmid, G., Bartfai, T., Dejana, E., Brockhaus, M. (2000). Homophilic interaction of junctional adhesion molecule. *Journal of Biological Chemistry.* Vol. 274, No.40, pp. 30970-30976.

Bazzoni, G. (2006). Endothelial tight junctions: permeable barriers of the vessel wall. *Thromb. Haemost.,* Vol. 95, No.1, pp. 36-42.

Begley, D.J. (2004). ABC transporters and the blood-brain barrier. *Curr Pharm Des.* Vol.10, No.12, pp.1295-312.

Belanger, M., Asashima, T., Ohtsuki, S., Yamaguchi, H., Ito S., Terasaki, T. (2007). Hyperammonemia induces transport of taurine and creatine and suppresses claudin-12 gene expression in brain capillary endothelial cells in vitro. *Neurochem. Int.,* Vol.50, No.1, pp. 95-101.

Boado, R.J., Li, J.Y., Nagaya, M., Zhang, C., Pardridge W.M. (1999). Selective expression of the large neutral amino acid transporter at the blood-brain barrier. *Proceedings of the National Academy of Sciences of the USA* ., Vol. 96, No. 21, pp. 12079-12084.

Bourasset, F., Cisternino, S., Temsamani, J., Scherrmann, J.M. (2003). Evidence for an active transport of morphine-6-beta-d-glucuronide but not P-glycoprotein-mediated at the blood-brain barrier. *Journal of Neurochemistry.* Vol. 86, No. 6, pp. 1564-7.

Braissant, O., Henry, H., Loup, M., Eilers, B., Bachmann, C. (2001). Endogenous synthesis and transport of creatine in the rat brain: an in situ hybridization study. *Brain Research Mol Brain Research.* Vol. 86, No. 1-2, pp.193-201.

Broadwell, R.D., Baker-Cairns, B.J., Friden, P.M., Oliver, C., Villegas, J.C. (1996). Transcytosis of protein through the mammalian cerebral epithelium and endothelium. III. Receptor-mediated transcytosis through the blood-brain barrier of blood-borne transferrin and antibody against the transferrin receptor. *Experimental Neurology*. Vol. 142, No.1, pp.47-65.

Butt, A.M., Jones, H.C., Abbott, N.J. (1990). Electrical resistance across the blood-brain barrier in anaesthetized rats: a developmental study. *Journal of Physiology*. Vol. 429, pp. 47-62.

Cacheaux, L.P., Ivens, S., David, Y., Lakhter, A.J., Bar-Klein, G., Shapira, M., Heinemann, U., Friedman, A., Kaufer, D. (2009). Transcriptome profiling reveals TGF-beta signaling involvement in epileptogenesis. *Journal of Neuroscience*. Vol. 29, No. 28, pp. 8927-35.

Cansev, M. (2006). Uridine and cytidine in the brain: their transport and utilization. *Brain Research Review*. Vol. 52, No. 2, pp. 389-97.

Cornford, E.M., Nguyen, E.V., Landaw, E.M. (2000). Acute upregulation of blood-brain barrier glucose transporter activity in seizures. *American Journal of Physiology-Heart and Circulatory Physiology*. Vol. 279, No. 3, pp.H1346-54.

Croll, S.D., Goodman, J.H., Scharfman, H.E. (2004). Vascular endothelial growth factor (VEGF) in seizures: a double-edged sword. *Advances in Experimental Medicine and Biology* . Vol. 548, pp. 57-68.

Cirrito, J.R., Deane, R., Fagan, A.M., Spinner, M.L., Parsadanian, M., Finn, M.B., Jiang, H., Prior, J.L., Sagare, A., Bales, K.R., Paul, S.M., Zlokovic, B.V., Piwnica-Worms, D., Holtzman, D.M. (2005). P-glycoprotein deficiency at the blood-brain barrier increases amyloid-beta deposition in an Alzheimer disease mouse model. *Journal of Clinical Investigation*. Vol. 115, No.11, pp.3285-90.

Citi, S., Cordenonsi, M. (1998). Tight junction proteins. *Biochimica et Biophysica Acta*, Vol. 1448, No. 1, pp.1-11.

Clump, D.A., Qazi, I.H., Sudol, M., Flynn D.C. (2005). c-Yes response to growth factor activation. *Growth Factors*, Vol. 23, No. 4, pp. 263-72

Cornford, E.M., Oldendorf, W.H. (1986). Epilepsy and the blood-brain barrier. *Advance Neurology*. Vol. 44, pp. 787-812.

Cornford, E.M., Hyman, S. (1999). Blood-brain barrier permeability to small and large molecules. *Advanced Drug Delivery Reviews*. Vol. 36, No. 2-3, pp. 145-163.

Cornford, E.M., Young, D., Paxton, J.W., Hyman, S., Farrell, C.L., Elliott, R.B. (1993). Blood-brain glucose transfer in the mouse. *Neurochemistry Research*. Vol. 18, No. 5, pp. 591-7.

Crone, C., Christensen, O. (1981). Electrical resistance of a capillary endothelium. *Journal of General Physiology*. Vol. 77, No. 4, pp. 349-71.

David, Y., Cacheaux, L.P., Ivens, S., Lapilover, E., Heinemann, U., Kaufer, D., Friedman, A. (2009). Astrocytic dysfunction in epileptogenesis: consequence of altered potassium and glutamate homeostasis? *Journal of Neuroscience*. Vol. 29, No. 34, pp. 10588-99.

Denker, B.M., Nigam, S.K. (1998). Molecular structure and assembly of the tight junction. *Am. J. Physiol*. Vol. 274, pp. F1-F9.

Dombrowski, S.M., Desai, S.Y., Marroni, M., Cucullo, L., Goodrich, K., Bingaman, W., Mayberg, M.R., Bengez, L., Janigro, D. (2001). Overexpression of multiple drug resistance genes in endothelial cells from patients with refractory epilepsy. *Epilepsia*. Vol. 42, No. 12, pp. 1501-6.

Duan H, Wang J. (2010). Selective transport of monoamine neurotransmitters by human plasma membrane monoamine transporter and organic cation transporter 3. *Journal of Pharmacology and Experimental Therapeutics*. Vol. 335, No. 3, pp. 743-53.

Dudek, S.M., Garcia, J.G. (2001). Cytoskeletal regulation of pulmonary vascular permeability. *J Appl Physiol*. Vol. 91, No. 4, pp. 1487-500.

Eid, T., Lee, T.S., Thomas, M.J., Amiry-Moghaddam, M., Bjørnsen, L.P., Spencer, D.D., Agre, P., Ottersen, O.P., de Lanerolle, N.C. (2005). Loss of perivascular aquaporin 4 may underlie deficient water and K+ homeostasis in the human epileptogenic hippocampus. *Proceedings of the National Academy of Sciences of the United States of America*. Vol. 102, No. 4, pp. 1193-8.

Eisenblätter, T., Hüwel, S., Galla, H.J. (2003). Characterisation of the brain multidrug resistance protein (BMDP/ABCG2/BCRP) expressed at the blood-brain barrier. *Brain Research*. Vol. 971, No. 2, pp. 221-31.

Ehrlich, P. (1885) Das sauerstufbudurfnis des organismus, in Eine Farbenanalytische Studie, Hirschwald, Berlin.

Ennis, S.R., Kawai, N., Ren, X.D., Abdelkarim, G.E., Keep, R.F. (1998). Glutamine uptake at the blood-brain barrier is mediated by N-system transport. *Journal of Neurochemistry*. Vol. 71, No. 6, pp. 2565-73.

Fabene, P.F., Navarro Mora, G., Martinello, M., Rossi, B., Merigo, F., Ottoboni, L., Bach, S., Angiari, S., Benati, D., Chakir, A., Zanetti, L., Schio, F., Osculati, A., Marzola, P., Nicolato, E., Homeister, J.W., Xia, L., Lowe, J.B., McEver, R.P., Osculati, F., Sbarbati, A., Butcher, E.C., Constantin, G. (2008). A role for leukocyte-endothelial adhesion mechanisms in epilepsy. *Nature Medicine*. Vol. 14, No. 12, pp. 1377-83.

Fanning, A.S., Little, B.P., Rahner, C., Utepbergenov, D., Walther, Z., Anderson, J.M. (2007). The unique-5 and -6 motifs of ZO-1 regulate tight junction strand localization and scaffolding properties. *Molecular Biology of the Cell*, Vol. 18, No. 3, pp. 721-731.

Feldman, G.J., Mullin, J.M., Ryan, M.P. (2005) Occludin: structure, function and regulation. *Adv. Drug Deliv. Rev.*, Vol. 57, No. 6, pp. 883-917.

Friedman, A., Kaufer, D., Heinemann, U. (2009). Blood-brain barrier breakdown-inducing astrocytic transformation: novel targets for the prevention of epilepsy. *Epilepsy Research*. Vol. 85, No. 2-3, pp. 142-9.

Gale, K. (1992). Subcortical structures and pathways involved in convulsive seizure generation. *Journal of Clinical Neurophysiology*. Vol. 9, No. 2, pp.264-77.

Gao, B., Hagenbuch, B., Kullak-Ublick, G.A., Benke, D., Aguzzi, A., Meier, P.J. (2000). Organic anion-transporting polypeptides mediate transport of opioid peptides across blood-brain barrier. *Journal of Pharmacology and Experimental Therapeutics*. Vol. 294, No. 1, pp. 73-9.

Gao, B., Stieger, B., Noé, B., Fritschy, J.M., Meier, P.J. (1999). Localization of the organic anion transporting polypeptide 2 (Oatp2) in capillary endothelium and choroid plexus epithelium of rat brain. *Journal of Histochemistry & Cytochemistry*. Vol. 47, No. 10, pp. 1255-64.

Garcia, J.G. and Schaphorst, K.L. (1995). Regulation of endothelial cell gap formation and paracellular permeability. *Journal of Investigative Medicine.*, Vol. 43, pp. 117-126.
Gibbs, J.P., Adeyeye, M.C., Yang, Z., Shen, D.D. (2004). Valproic acid uptake by bovine brain microvessel endothelial cells: role of active efflux transport. *Epilepsy Research*. Vol. 58, No. 1, pp. 53-66.
Girod, J., Fenart, L., Régina, A., Dehouck, M.P., Hong, G., Scherrmann, J.M., Cecchelli, R., Roux, F. (1999). Transport of cationized anti-tetanus Fab'2 fragments across an in vitro blood-brain barrier model: involvement of the transcytosis pathway. *Journal of Neurochemistry*. Vol. 73, No. 5, pp. 2002-8.
Goldmann, E.E. (1913). Vitalfarbung am zentralnervensystem. Abhandl Konigl preuss Akad Wiss 1: 1-60.
Gonzalez-Mariscal, L., Betanzos, A., Avila-Flores, A. (2000). MAGUK proteins: structure and role in the tight junction. *Seminars in Cell and Developmental Biology*. Vol. 11, No. 4, pp.315-324.
Gonzalez-Mariscal, L., Betanzos, A., Nava, P., Jaramillo, B.E. (2003). Tight junction proteins. *Progress in Biophysics and Molecular Biology.*, Vol. 81, No. 1, pp. 1-44.
Gorter, J.A., van Vliet, E.A., Aronica, E., Breit, T., Rauwerda, H., Lopes da Silva, F.H., Wadman, W.J. (2006). Potential new antiepileptogenic targets indicated by microarray analysis in a rat model for temporal lobe epilepsy. *Journal of Neuroscience*. Vol. 26, No. 43, pp. 11083-110.
Ghabriel, M.N., Zhu, C., Leigh, C. (2002). Electron microscope study of blood-brain barrier opening induced by immunological targeting of the endothelial barrier antigen. *Brain Research*. Vol. 934, No. 2, pp.140-51.
Greenwood, R.S., Meeker, R.B., Hayward, J.N. (1991). Amygdala kindling elevates plasma vasopressin. *Brain Research*. Vol. 538, No. 1, pp. 9-14.
Gronlund, K.M., Gerhart, D.Z., Leino, R.L., McCall, A.L., Drewes, L.R. (1996). Chronic seizures increase glucose transporter abundance in rat brain. *Journal of Neuropathology & Experimental Neurology*. Vol. 55, No. 7, pp. 832-40
Hamazaki, Y., Itoh, M., Sasaki, H., Furuse, M., Tsukita, S. (2002). Multi-PDZ domain protein 1 (MUPP1) is concentrated at tight junctions through its possible interaction with claudin-1 and junctional adhesion molecule. *Journal of Biological Chemistry*. Vol. 277, No. 1, pp. 455-461.
Hartz, A.M., Bauer, B., Fricker, G., Miller, D.S. (2006). Rapid modulation of P-glycoprotein-mediated transport at the blood-brain barrier by tumor necrosis factor-alpha and lipopolysaccharide. *Molecular Pharmacology*. Vol. 69, No. 2, pp. 462-70.
Hatanaka, T., Huang, W., Martindale, R.G., Ganapathy, V. (2001). Differential influence of cAMP on the expression of the three subtypes (ATA1, ATA2, and ATA3) of the amino acid transport system A. *FEBS Letters*. Vol. 505, No. 2, pp. 317-20.
Hatzfeld, M. (2005). The p120 family of cell adhesion molecules. *The European Journal of Cell Biolog.*, Vol. 84, No. 2-3, pp. 205-214.
Hawkins, B.T., Davis, T.P. (2005). The blood-brain barrier/neurovascular unit in health and disease. *Pharmacological Reviews*. Vol. 57, No. 2, pp. 173-85.

Hembury, A., Mabondzo, A. (2008). Endothelin-1 reduces p-glycoprotein transport activity in an in vitro model of human adult blood-brain barrier. *Cellular and Molecular Neurobiology*. Vol. 28, No. 7, pp. 915-21.

Hervé, F., Ghinea, N., Scherrmann, J.M. (2008). CNS delivery via adsorptive transcytosis. *AAPS Journal*. Vol. 10, No. 3, pp. 455-72.

Hommelgaard, A.M., Roepstorff, K., Vilhardt, F., Torgersen, M.L., Sandvig, K., van Deurs, B. (2005). Caveolae: stable membrane domains with a potential for internalization. *Traffic*. Vol. 6, No. 9, pp. 720-4.

Honore, S., Pasquier, E., Braguer, D. (2005) Understanding microtubule dynamics for improved cancer therapy. *Cell Mol. Life Sci.*, Vol. 62, No. 24, pp. 3039-3056.

Huber, J.D., Egleton, R.D., Davis, T.P. (2001). Molecular physiology and pathophysiology of tight junctions in the blood-brain barrier. *Trends in Neuroscience*. Vol. 24, No. 12, pp. 719-725.

Ilbay, G., Sahin, D., Ates, N. (2003). Changes in blood-brain barrier permeability during hot water-induced seizures in rats. *Neurological Science*. Vol. 24, No. 4, pp. 232-5.

Ivens, S., Kaufer, D., Flores, L.P., Bechmann, I., Zumsteg, D., Tomkins, O., Seiffert, E., Heinemann, U., Friedman, A. (2007). TGF-beta receptor-mediated albumin uptake into astrocytes is involved in neocortical epileptogenesis. *Brain*. Vol. 130, No.2, pp. 535-47.

Kakee, A., Takanaga, H., Terasaki, T., Naito, M., Tsuruo, T., Sugiyama, Y. (2001). Efflux of a suppressive neurotransmitter, GABA, across the blood-brain barrier. *Journal of Neurochemistry*. Vol. 79, No. 1, pp. 110-8.

Kang, Y.S., Ohtsuki, S., Takanaga, H., Tomi, M., Hosoya, K., Terasaki, T. (2002). Regulation of taurine transport at the blood-brain barrier by tumor necrosis factor-alpha, taurine and hypertonicity. *Journal of Neurochemistry*. Vol. 83, No. 5, pp. 1188-95.

Kido, Y., Tamai, I., Okamoto, M., Suzuki, F., Tsuji, A. (2000). Functional clarification of MCT1-mediated transport of monocarboxylic acids at the blood-brain barrier using in vitro cultured cells and in vivo BUI studies. *Pharmaceutical Research*. Vol. 17, No. 1, pp. 55-62.

Kim, J.E., Choi, H.C., Song, H.K., Jo, S.M., Kim, D.S., Choi, S.Y., Kim, Y.I., Kang, T.C. (2010). Levetiracetam inhibits interleukin-1 beta inflammatory responses in the hippocampus and piriform cortex of epileptic rats. *Neurosci Lett*. Vol. 471, No. 2, pp. 94-9.

Kim, J.H., Kim, J.H., Park, J.A., Lee, S.W., Kim, W.J., Yu, Y.S., Kim, K.W. (2006). Blood-neural barrier: intercellular communication at glio-vascular interface. *J Biochemistry Molecular Biology*. Vol. 39, No. 4, pp. 339-45.

Kim, D.W., Lee, S.K., Nam, H., Chu, K., Chung, C.K., Lee, S.Y., Choe, G., Kim, H.K. (2010) Epilepsy with dual pathology: surgical treatment of cortical dysplasia accompanied by hippocampal sclerosis. *Epilepsia*. Vol. 51, No. 8, pp. 1429-35.

Kim, J.E., Ryu, H.J., Yeo, S.I., Seo, C.H., Lee, B.C., Choi, I.G., Kim, D.S., Kang, T.C. (2009). Differential expressions of aquaporin subtypes in astroglia in the hippocampus of chronic epileptic rats. *Neuroscience*. Vol. 163, No. 3, pp. 781-9.

Kirkham, M., Parton, R.G. (2005). Clathrin-independent endocytosis: new insights into caveolae and non-caveolar lipid raft carriers. *Biochimica et Biophysica Acta*. Vol. 1745, No. 3, pp. 273-86.

Koval, M. (2006). Claudins--key pieces in the tight junction puzzle. *Cell Communication & Adhesion*. Vol. 13, No. 3, pp. 127-38.

Kwan, P., Brodie, M.J. (2005). Potential role of drug transporters in the pathogenesis of medically intractable epilepsy. *Epilepsia*. Vol. 46, No. 2, pp. 224-3.

Lai, C.H., Kuo, K.H., Leo, J.M. (2005). Critical role of actin in modulating BBB permeability. *Brain Research, Brain Research Review*. Vol. 50, No. 1, pp. 7-13.

Lamagna, C., Meda, P., Mandicourt, G., Brown, J., Gilbert, R.J., Jones, E.Y., Kiefer, F., Ruga, P., Imhof, B.A., Aurrand-Lions, M. (2005). Dual interaction of JAM-C with JAM-B and alpha(M)beta2 integrin: function in junctional complexes and leukocyte adhesion. *Molecular Biology of the Cell*. Vol. 16, No. 10, pp. 4992-5003.

Lampugnani, M.G., Orsenigo, F., Rudini, N., Maddaluno, L., Boulday, G., Chapon, F., Dejana, E. (2010). CCM1 regulates vascular-lumen organization by inducing endothelial polarity. *Journal of Cell Science*, Vol. 123, Pt 7, pp. 1073-1080.

Lawrenson, J.G., Ghabriel, M.N., Reid, A.R., Gajree, T.N., Allt, G. (1995). Differential expression of an endothelial barrier antigen between the CNS and the PNS. *Journal of Anatomy*, Vol. 186, Pt 1, pp. 217-221.

Lazarowski, A., Czornyj, L., Lubienieki, F., Girardi, E., Vazquez, S., D'Giano, C. (2007). ABC transporters during epilepsy and mechanisms underlying multidrug resistance in refractory epilepsy. *Epilepsia*, Vol. 48 , Suppl 5, pp. 140-149.

Lee, T.S., Eid, T., Mane, S., Kim, J.H., Spencer, D.D., Ottersen, O.P., de Lanerolle, N.C. (2004). Aquaporin-4 is increased in the sclerotic hippocampus in human temporal lobe epilepsy. *Acta Neuropathologica*, Vol. 108, No. 6, pp. 493-502..

Lespine, A., Dupuy, J., Orlowski, S., Nagy, T., Glavinas, H., Krajcsi, P., Alvinerie, M. (2006). Interaction of ivermectin with multidrug resistance proteins (MRP1, 2 and 3). *Chemico-Biological Interactions*, Vol. 159, No. 3, pp. 169-179.

Li, J.Y., Boado, R.J., Pardridge, W.M. (2001). Cloned blood-brain barrier adenosine transporter is identical to the rat concentrative Na+ nucleoside cotransporter CNT2. *Journal of Cerebral Blood Flow & Metabolism*. Vol. 21, No. 8, 929-936.

Li, Y., Fanning, A.S., Anderson, J.M., Lavie, A. (2005). Structure of the conserved cytoplasmic C-terminal domain of occludin: identification of the ZO-1 binding surface. *Journal of Molecular Biology*. Vol. 352, No. 1, pp. 151-164.

Librizzi, L., Regondi, M.C., Pastori, C., Frigerio, S., Frassoni, C., de Curtis, M. (2007). Expression of adhesion factors induced by epileptiform activity in the endothelium of the isolated guinea pig brain in vitro. *Epilepsia*. Vol. 48, No. 4, pp. 743-751.

Ling, R., Bridges, C.C., Sugawara, M., Fujita, T, Leibach, F.H., Prasad, P.D., Ganapathy, V. (2001). Involvement of transporter recruitment as well as gene expression in the substrate-induced adaptive regulation of amino acid transport system A. *Biochimica et Biophysica Acta*. Vol. 1512, No. 1, pp. 15-21.

Liu, Y., Hu, M. (2000). P-glycoprotein and bioavailability-implication of polymorphism. *Clinical Chemistry and Laboratory Medicine*, Vol. 38, No. 9, pp. 877-881.

Löscher, W., Ebert, U. (1996). The role of the piriform cortex in kindling. *Progress in Neurobiology*. Vol. 50, No. 5-6, pp. 427-481.

Löscher, W., Potschka, H. (2002). Role of multidrug transporters in pharmacoresistance to antiepileptic drugs. *Journal of Pharmacology and Experimental Therapeutics*. Vol. 301, No. 1, pp. 7-14

Löscher, W., Potschka, H. (2005). Blood-brain barrier active efflux transporters: ATP-binding cassette gene family. *NeuroRx Research*. Vol. 2, No. 1, pp. 86-98.

Lossinsky, A.S., Shivers R.R. (2004). Structural pathways for macromolecular and cellular transport across the blood-brain barrier during inflammatory conditions. *Histology and Histopathology*. 19(2), 535-564.

Lossinsky, A.S., Vorbrodt, A.W., Wisniewski, H.M. (1983) Ultracytochemical studies of vesicular and canalicular transport structures in the injured mammalian blood-brain barrier. *Acta Neuropathologica* (Berlin), Vol. 61, No. 3-4, pp. 239-245.

Łotowska, J.M., Sobaniec-Łotowska, M.E., Sendrowski, K., Sobaniec, W., Artemowicz, B. (2008). Ultrastructure of the blood-brain barrier of the gyrus hippocampal cortex in an experimental model of febrile seizures and with the use of a new generation antiepileptic drug--topiramate. *Folia Neuropathologica*, Vol. 46. No. 1, pp. 57-68.

Lu, H., Demny, S., Zuo, Y., Rea, W., Wang, L., Chefer, S.I., Vaupel, D.B., Yang, Y., Stein, E.A. (2010). Temporary disruption of the rat blood-brain barrier with a monoclonal antibody: a novel method for dynamic manganese-enhanced MRI. *Neuroimage*. Vol. 50, No. 1, pp. 7-14.

Luer, M.S., Hamani, C., Dujovny, M., Gidal, B., Cwik, M., Deyo, K., Fischer, J.H. (1999). Saturable transport of gabapentin at the blood-brain barrier. *Neurology Research*, Vol. 21, No. 6, pp. 559-562.

Lyck, R., Ruderisch, N., Moll, A.G., Steiner, O., Cohen, C.D., Engelhardt, B., Makrides, V., Verrey, F. (2009). Culture-induced changes in blood-brain barrier transcriptome: implications for amino-acid transporters in vivo. *Journal of Cerebral Blood Flow & Metabolism*. Vol. 29, No. 9, pp. 1491-1502.

Maggio, N., Shavit, E., Chapman, J., Segal, M. (2008). Thrombin induces long-term potentiation of reactivity to afferent stimulation and facilitates epileptic seizures in rat hippocampal slices: toward understanding the functional consequences of cerebrovascular insults. *Journal of Neuroscience*, Vol. 28, No. 3, pp. 732-736.

Manley, N.C., Bertrand, A.A., Kinney, K.S., Hing, T.C., Sapolsky, R.M. (2007). Characterization of monocyte chemoattractant protein-1 expression following a kainate model of status epilepticus. *Brain Research*, Vol. 1182, pp. 138-143.

Marchi, N., Angelov, L., Masaryk, T., Fazio, V., Granata, T., Hernandez, N., Hallene, K., Diglaw, T., Franic, L., Najm, I., Janigro, D. (2007). Seizure-promoting effect of blood-brain barrier disruption. *Epilepsia*, Vol. 48, No. 4, pp. 732-742.

Marcon, J., Gagliardi, B., Balosso, S., Maroso, M., Noé, F., Morin, M., Lerner-Natoli, M., Vezzani, A., Ravizza, T. (2009). Age-dependent vascular changes induced by status epilepticus in rat forebrain: implications for epileptogenesis. *Neurobiology of Disease*. Vol. 34, No. 1, pp.121-132.

Martin-Padura, I., Lostaglio, S., Schneemann, M., Williams, L., Romano, M., Fruscella, P., Panzeri, C., Stoppacciaro, A., Ruco, L., Villa, A., Simmons, D., Dejana, E. (1998).

Junctional adhesion molecule, a novel member of the immunoglobulin superfamily that distributes at intercellular junctions and modulates monocyte transmigration. *Journal of Cell Biology* Vol. 142, No. 1, pp. 117-127

Masand, G., Hanif, K., Sen, S., Ahsan, A., Maiti, S., Pasha, S. (2006). Synthesis, conformational and pharmacological studies of glycosylated chimeric peptides of Met-enkephalin and FMRFa. *Brain Research Bullten*. Vol. 68, No. 5, pp. 329-334.

Matsuoka, Y., Okazaki, M., Kitamura, Y., Taniguchi, T. (1999). Developmental expression of P-glycoprotein (multidrug resistance gene product) in the rat brain. *Journal of Neurobiology*. Vol. 39, No. 3, pp. 383-392.

Mayhan, W.G (2001). Regulation of blood-brain barrier permeability. *Microcirculation*, Vol.8, No. 2, pp. 89-104.

McAllister, M.S., Krizanac-Bengez, L., Macchia, F., Naftalin, R.J., Pedley, K.C., Mayberg, M.R., Marroni, M., Leaman, S., Stanness, K.A., Janigro, D. (2001). Mechanisms of glucose transport at the blood-brain barrier: an in vitro study. *Brain Research*, Vol. 904, No. 1, pp. 20-30.

McIntyre, D.C., Kelly, M.E. (2000). The parahippocampal cortices and kindling. *Annals of the New York Academy of Sciences*. Vol. 911, pp. 343-354.

McNeil, E., Capaldo, C.T., Macara, I.G. (2006). Zonula occludens-1 function in the assembly of tight junctions in Madin-Darby canine kidney epithelial cells. *Molecular Biology of the Celll*. Vol. 17, No. 4, pp. 1922-1932.

Meyer, T.N., Hunt, J., Schwesinger, C., Denker, B.M. (2003). Galpha12 regulates epithelial cell junctions through Src tyrosine kinases. *American Journal of Physiology - Cell Physiology*. Vol. 285, No. 5, pp. C1281-1293.

Mitic, L.L., Aderon, J.M. (1998). Molecular architecture of tight junctions. *Annual Review of Physiology*, Vol. 60, pp. 121-142.

Miwako, I., Schroter, T., Schmid, S.L. (2003). Clathrin- and dynamin-dependent coated vesicle formation from isolated plasma membranes. *Traffic*. Vol. 4, No. 6, pp. 376-89.

Mori, S., Takanaga, H., Ohtsuki, S., Deguchi, T., Kang, Y.S., Hosoya, K., Terasaki, T. (2003). Rat organic anion transporter 3 (rOAT3) is responsible for brain-to-blood efflux of homovanillic acid at the abluminal membrane of brain capillary endothelial cells. *Journal of Cerebral Blood Flow & Metabolism*. Vol. 23, No. 4, pp. 432-440.

Morita, K., Sasaki, H., Furuse, M., Tsukita, S. (1999). Endothelial claudin: claudin-5/TMVCF constitutes tight junction strands in endothelial cells. *Journal of Cell Biology*, Vol. 147, No. 1, pp.185-194.

Mukherjee, S., Ghosh, R.N., Maxfield, F.R. (1997). Endocytosis. *Physiological Reviews*. Vol. 77, No. 3, pp. 759-803.

Nagafuchi, A. (2001). Molecular architecture of adherens junctions. *Current Opinion in Cell Biology, Vol.* 13, pp. 600-603.

Nakatani, Y., Sato-Suzuki, I., Tsujino, N., Nakasato, A., Seki, Y., Fumoto, M., Arita, H. (2008). Augmented brain 5-HT crosses the blood-brain barrier through the 5-HT transporter in rat. *European Journal of Neuroscience*, Vol. 27, No. 9, pp. 2466-2472.

Natoli, M., Montpied, P., Rousset, M.C., Bockaert, J., Rondouin, G. (2000). NFkappaB by hippocampal cells in excitotoxicity and experimental epilepsy. *Epilepsy Research*. Vol. 41, No. 2, pp. 141-154.

Nazer, B., Hong, S., Selkoe, D.J. (2008). LRP promotes endocytosis and degradation, but not transcytosis, of the amyloid-beta peptide in a blood-brain barrier in vitro model. *Neurobiology of Disease*, Vol. 30, No. 1, pp. 94-102.

Nico, B., Frigeri, A., Nicchia, G.P., Corsi, P., Ribatti, D., Quondamatteo, F., Herken, R., Girolamo, F., Marzullo, A., Svelto, M., Roncali, L. (2003). Severe alterations of endothelial and glial cells in the blood-brain barrier of dystrophic mdx mice. *Glia*, Vol. 42, No. 3, pp. 235-251.

Nico, B., Paola- Nicchia, G., Frigeri, A., Corsi, P., Mangieri, D., Ribatti, D., Svelto, M., Roncali, L. (2004). Altered blood-brain barrier development in dystrophic MDX mice. *Neuroscience*, Vol. 125, No. 4, pp. 921-935.

Nicoletti, J.N., Shah, S.K., McCloskey, D.P., Goodman, J.H., Elkady, A., Atassi, H, Hylton, D., Rudge, J.S., Scharfman, H.E., Croll, S.D. (2008). Vascular endothelial growth factor is up-regulated after status epilepticus and protects against seizure-induced neuronal loss in hippocampus. *Neuroscience*. Vol. 151, No. 1, pp. 232-241.

Nies, A.T., Jedlitschky, G., König, J., Herold-Mende, C., Steiner, H.H., Schmitt, H.P., Keppler, D. (2004). Expression and immunolocalization of the multidrug resistance proteins, MRP1-MRP6 (ABCC1-ABCC6), in human brain. *Neuroscience*. Vol. 129, No. 2, pp. 349-60.

Nitsch, C., Suzuki, R, Fujiwara, K., Klatzo, I. (1985). Incongruence of regional cerebral blood flow increase and blood-brain barrier opening in rabbits at the onset of seizures induced by bicuculline, methoxypyridoxine, and kainic acid. *Journal of Neurological Science*, Vol. 67, No. 1, pp. 67-79.

Nitta, T., Hata, M., Gotoh, S., Seo, Y., Sasaki, H., Hashimoto, N., Furuse, M., Tsukita, S. (2003). Size-selective loosening of the blood-brain barrier in claudin-5-deficient mice. *Journal of Cell Biology*. Vol. 161, No. 3, pp. 653-660.

Nusrat, A., Brown, G.T., Tom, J., Drake, A., Bui, T.T., Quan, C., Mrsny, R.J. (2005). Multiple protein interactions involving proposed extracellular loop domains of the tight junction protein occludin. *Molecular Biology of the Cell*. Vol. 16, No. 4, pp. 1725-1734.

Ndode-Ekane, X.E., Hayward, N., Gröhn, O., Pitkänen, A. (2010). Vascular changes in epilepsy: functional consequences and association with network plasticity in pilocarpine-induced experimental epilepsy. *Neuroscience*. Vol. 166, No. 1, pp. 312-32.

Oby, E., Janigro, D. (2006). The blood-brain barrier and epilepsy. *Epilepsia*. Vol. 47, No. 11, pp. 1761-1774.

Ohtsuki, S. (2004). New aspects of the blood-brain barrier transporters; its physiological roles in the central nervous system. *Biological & Pharmaceutical Bulletin*. Vol. 27, No. 10, pp. 1489-1496.

Ohtsuki, S., Asaba, H., Takanaga, H., Deguchi, T., Hosoya, K., Otagiri, M., Terasaki, T. (2002). Role of blood-brain barrier organic anion transporter 3 (OAT3) in the efflux of indoxyl sulfate, a uremic toxin: its involvement in neurotransmitter metabolite clearance from the brain. *Journal of Neurochemistry*, Vol. 83, No. 1, pp. 57-66.

Ohtsuki, S., Sato, S., Yamaguchi, H., Kamoi, M., Asashima, T., Terasaki, T. (2007). Exogenous expression of claudin-5 induces barrier properties in cultured rat brain capillary endothelial cells. *Journal of Cellular Physiology*. Vol. 210, No. 1, pp. 81-86.

Ohtsuki, S., Takizawa, T., Takanaga, H., Hori, S., Hosoya, K., Terasaki, T. (2004). Localization of organic anion transporting polypeptide 3 (oatp3) in mouse brain parenchymal and capillary endothelial cells. *Journal of Neurochemistry*, Vol. 90, No. 3, 743-749.

Ohtsuki, S., Tachikawa, M., Takanaga, H., Shimizu, H., Watanabe, M., Hosoya, K., Terasaki, T. (2002). The blood-brain barrier creatine transporter is a major pathway for supplying creatine to the brain. *Journal of Cerebral Blood Flow & Metabolism*. Vol. 22, No. 11, pp. 1327-1335.

O'Kane, R.L., Martínez-López, I., DeJoseph, M.R., Viña, J.R., Hawkins, R.A. (1999). Na(+)-dependent glutamate transporters (EAAT1, EAAT2, and EAAT3) of the blood-brain barrier. A mechanism for glutamate removal. *Journal of Biological Chemistry*, Vol. 274, No. 45, pp. 31891-31895.

Olivier, B., Soudijn, W., van Wijngaarden, I. (2000). Serotonin, dopamine and norepinephrine transporters in the central nervous system and their inhibitors. *Progress in Drug Research*, Vol. 54, pp. 59-119.

Oliveira, M.S., Furian, A.F., Royes, L.F., Fighera, M.R., Fiorenza, N.G., Castelli, M., Machado, P., Bohrer, D., Veiga, M., Ferreira, J., Cavalheiro, E.A., Mello CF. (2008). Cyclooxygenase-2/PGE2 pathway facilitates pentylenetetrazol-induced seizures, *Epilepsy Research*, Vol. 79, No. 1, pp. 14-21.

Omidi, Y., Barar, J., Ahmadian, S., Heidari, H.R., Gumbleton, M. (2008). Characterization and astrocytic modulation of system L transporters in brain microvasculature endothelial cells. *Cell Biochemistry and Function*, Vol. 26, No. 3, pp. 381-391.

Ose, A., Kusuhara, H., Endo, C., Tohyama, K., Miyajima, M., Kitamura, S., Sugiyama, Y. (2010). Functional characterization of mouse organic anion transporting peptide 1a4 in the uptake and efflux of drugs across the blood-brain barrier. *Drug Metabolism and Disposition*. Vol. 38. No.1, pp. 168-176.

Oztaş, B., Kaya, M. (1991). The effect of acute hypertension on blood-brain barrier permeability to albumin during experimentally induced epileptic seizures. *Pharmacological Research*. Vol. 23. No. 1, pp. 41-6.

Pardridge, W.M. (2007). Blood-brain barrier delivery. *Drug Discovery Today*. Vol. *12*, No. 1-2, pp. 54-61.

Pardridge, W.M., Boado, R.J., Farrell, C.R. (1990). Brain-type glucose transporter (GLUT-1) is selectively localized to the blood-brain barrier. Studies with quantitative western blotting and in situ hybridization. *Journal of Biological Chemistry*. Vol. 265, No.29, pp. 18035-18040.

Piwnica-Worms, D., Kesarwala, A.H., Pichler, A., Prior, J.L., Sharma, V. (2006). Single photon emission computed tomography and positron emission tomography imaging of multi-drug resistant P-glycoprotein--monitoring a transport activity important in cancer, blood-brain barrier function and Alzheimer's disease. *Neuroimaging Clinics of North America*. Vol. 16, No.4, pp. 575-589, viii.

Ponting, C..P., Phillips, C., Davies, K.E., Blake, D.J. (1997). PDZ domains: targeting signalling molecules to sub-membranous sites. *Bioessays*. Vol. 19, No. 6, 469-479.

Predescu, S.A., Predescu, D.N., Malik, A.B. (2007). Molecular determinants of endothelial transcytosis and their role in endothelial permeability. *American Journal of Physiology - Lung Cellular and Molecular Physiology*. Vol. 293, No. 4, L823-842.

Quezada, C.A., Garrido, W.X., González-Oyarzún, M.A., Rauch, M.C., Salas, M.R., San Martín, R.E., Claude, A.A., Yañez, A.J., Slebe, J.C., Cárcamo, J.G. (2008). Effect of tacrolimus on activity and expression of P-glycoprotein and ATP-binding cassette transporter A5 (ABCA5) proteins in hematoencephalic barrier cells. *Biological & Pharmaceutical Bulletin*. Vol. 31. No. 10, pp. 1911-1916.

Reichel, A., Begley, D.J., Ermisch, A. (1996). Arginine vasopressin reduces the blood-brain transfer of L-tyrosine and L-valine: further evidence of the effect of the peptide on the L-system transporter at the blood-brain barrier. *Brain Research*, Vol. 713, No. 1-2, pp. 232-239.

Riazi, K., Galic, M.A., Kuzmiski, J.B., Ho, W., Sharkey, K.A., Pittman, Q.J. (2008). Microglial activation and TNFalpha production mediate altered CNS excitability following peripheral inflammation. *Proceedings of the National Academy of Sciences of the United States of America*, Vol.105, No. 44, pp. 17151-17156.

Rigau, V., Morin, M., Rousset, M.C., de Bock, F., Lebrun, A., Coubes, P., Picot, M.C., Baldy-Moulinier, M., Bockaert, J., Crespel, A., Lerner-Natoli, M. (2007). Angiogenesis is associated with blood-brain barrier permeability in temporal lobe epilepsy. *Brain*, Vol. 130, Pt 7, pp. 1942-1956.

Rossi, B., Angiari, S., Zenaro, E., Budui S.L., Constantin, G. (2011). Vascular inflammation in central nervous system diseases: adhesion receptors controlling leukocyte-endothelial interactions. *Journal of Leukocyte Biology*, Vol. 89. No.4, pp. 539-556.

Rubin, L.L. and Staddon, J.M. (1999). The cell biology of the blood brain barrier. *The Annual Review of Neuroscience*. Vol. 22, pp. 11-28.

Ruffer, C., Gerke, V. (2004). The C-terminal cytoplasmic tail of claudins 1 and 5 but not its PDZ-binding motif is required for apical localization at epithelial and endothelial tight junctions. *European Journal of Cell Biology*, Vol. 83, No. 4, 135-144

Ruth, R.E. (1984). Increased cerebrovascular permeability to protein during systemic kainic acid seizures. *Epilepsia*, Vol. 25, No. 2, pp. 259-268.

Sakaeda, T., Siahaan, T.J., Audus, K.L., Stella, V.J. (2000). Enhancement of transport of D-melphalan analogue by conjugation with L-glutamate across bovine brain microvessel endothelial cell monolayers. *Journal of Drug Targeting*, Vol. 8, No. 3, pp. 195-204.

Seiffert, E., Dreier, J.P., Ivens, S., Bechmann, I., Tomkins, O., Heinemann, U., Friedman, A. (2004). Lasting blood-brain barrier disruption induces epileptic focus in the rat somatosensory cortex. *Journal of Neuroscience*, Vol. 24. No. 36, 7829-7836.

Sierralta, J., Mendoza, C. (2004). PDZ-containing proteins: alternative splicing as a source of functional diversity. *Brain Research Brain Research Review*, Vol. 47, No. 1-3, 105-115.

Simionescu, N., Simionescu, M. (1985). Interactions of endogenous lipoproteins with capillary endothelium in spontaneously hyperlipoproteinemic rats. *Microvascular Research*. Vol. 30, No. 3, pp. 314-332.

Sinha, S., Patil, S.A., Jayalekshmy, V., Satishchandra, P. (2008). Do cytokines have any role in epilepsy? *Epilepsy Research*, Vol. 82, No. 2-3, pp. 171-176.

Sheen, S.H., Kim, J.E., Ryu, H.J., Yang, Y., Choi, K.C., Kang, T.C. (2011). Decrease in dystrophin expression prior to disruption of brain-blood barrier within the rat piriform cortex following status epilepticus. *Brain Research*, Vol. 1369, pp. 173-183.

Small, V.J., Rottner, K. and Kaverina, I. (1999). Functional design in the actin cytoskeleton. *Current Opinion in Cell Biology*, Vol. 11, pp. 54-60.

Sobocki, T., Sobocka, M.B., Babinska, A., Ehrlich, Y.H., Banerjee, P., Kornecki, E. (2006). Genomic structure, organization and promoter analysis of the human F11R/F11 receptor/junctional adhesion molecule-1/JAM-A. *Gene*, Vol. 366, No. 1, pp. 128-144.

Soma, T., Chiba, H., Kato-Mori, Y., Wada, T., Yamashita, T., Kojima T., Sawada N. (2004). Thr(207) of claudin-5 is involved in size-selective loosening of the endothelial barrier by cyclic AMP. *Experimental Cell Research*, Vol. 300, No. 1, pp. 202-212.

Staddon, J.M. and Rubin, L.L. (1996). Cell adhesion, cell junctions and the blood-brain barrier. *Current Opinion in Neurobiology*, Vol. 6, pp. 622-627.

Stamatovic, S.M., Keep, R.F., Kunkel, S.L., Andjelkovic, A.V. (2003). Potential role of MCP-1 in endothelial cell tight junction 'opening': signaling via Rho and Rho kinase. *Journal of Cell Science*, Vol. 116, pp. 4615-4628.

Sternberger, N.H., Sternberger, L.A. (1987). Blood-brain barrier protein recognized by monoclonal antibody. *Proceedings of the National Academy of Sciences of the United States of America*, Vol. 84, No. 22, pp. 8169-8173.

Stewart, P.A., Magliocco, M., Hayakawa, K., Farrell, C.L., Del Maestro, R.F., Girvin, J., Kaufmann, J.C., Vinters, H.V., Gilbert, J. (1987). A quantitative analysis of blood-brain barrier ultrastructure in the aging human. *Microvascular Research*. Vol. 33, No. 2, pp. 270-282.

Sugiyama, D., Kusuhara, H., Lee, Y.J., Sugiyama, Y. (2003). Involvement of multidrug resistance associated protein 1 (Mrp1) in the efflux transport of 17beta estradiol-D-17beta-glucuronide (E217betaG) across the blood-brain barrier. *Pharmaceutical Research*. Vol. 20, No. 9, pp. 1394-1400.

Suzuki, A., Ishiyama, C., Hashiba, K., Shimizu, M., Ebnet, K., Ohno, S. (2002). aPKC kinase activity is required for the asymmetric differentiation of the premature junctional complex dur ing epithelial cell polarization. *Journal of Cell Science*, Vol. 115, pp. 3565-3573.

Tachikawa, M., Kasai, Y., Yokoyama, R., Fujinawa, J., Ganapathy, V., Terasaki, T., Hosoya, K. (2009). The blood-brain barrier transport and cerebral distribution of guanidinoacetate in rats: involvement of creatine and taurine transporters. *Journal of Neurochemistry*. Vol. 111, No. 2, pp. 499-509.

Takanaga, H., Ohtsuki, S., Hosoya, K., Terasaki, T. (2001). GAT2/BGT-1 as a system responsible for the transport of gamma-aminobutyric acid at the mouse blood-brain barrier. *Journal of Cerebral Blood Flow & Metabolism*, Vol. 21, No. 10, pp.1232-1239.

Tao, Y.S., Edwards, R.A., Tubb, B., Wang, S., Bryan, J., McCrea, P.D. (1996). beta-Catenin associates with the actin-bundling protein fascin in a noncadherin complex. *Journal of Cell Biology*, Vol. 134, No. 5, pp. 1271-1281.

Terai, T., Nishimura, N., Kanda, I., Yasui, N., Sasaki, T. (2006). JRAB/MICAL-L2 is a junctional Rab13-binding protein mediating the endocytic recycling of occludin. *Molecular Biology of the Cell,* Vol. 17, No. 5, pp. 2465-2475.

Tetsuka, K., Takanaga, H., Ohtsuki, S., Hosoya, K., Terasaki, T. (2003). The l-isomer-selective transport of aspartic acid is mediated by ASCT2 at the blood-brain barrier. *Journal of Neurochemistry,* Vol. 87. No.4, pp. 891-901.

Tinsley, J.M., Blake, D.J., Zuellig, R.A., Davies, K.E. (1994). Increasing complexity of the dystrophin-associated protein complex. *Proceedings of the National Academy of Sciences of the United States of America,* Vol. 91, No.18, pp. 8307-8013.

Tomkins, O., Feintuch, A., Benifla, M., Cohen, A., Friedman, A., Shelef, I. (2011). Blood-brain barrier breakdown following traumatic brain injury: a possible role in posttraumatic epilepsy. *Cardiovascular Psychiatry and Neurology.* 2011:765923

Tomkins, O., Friedman, O., Ivens, S., Reiffurth, C., Major, S., Dreier, J.P., Heinemann, U., Friedman, A. (2007). Blood-brain barrier disruption results in delayed functional and structural alterations in the rat neocortex. *Neurobiology of Disease,* Vol. 25, No. 2, pp. 367-377.

Tomkins, O., Shelef, I., Kaizerman, I., Eliushin, A., Afawi, Z., Misk, A., Gidon, M., Cohen, A., Zumsteg, D., Friedman, A.J. (2008). Blood-brain barrier disruption in post-traumatic epilepsy. *Journal of Neurology, Neurosurgery & Psychiatry,* Vol. 79, No. 7, pp. 774-777.

Tzima, E. (2006). Role of small GTPases in endothelial cytoskeletal dynamics and the shear stress response. *Circulation Research.* Vol. 98, No. 2, pp.176-185.

Ueno, M. (2007). Molecular anatomy of the brain endothelial barrier: an overview of the distributional features. *Current Medicinal Chemistry.* Vol. 14, No. 11, pp. 1199-1206.

Umeki, N., Fukasawa, Y., Ohtsuki, S., Hori, S., Watanabe, Y., Kohno, Y., Terasaki, T. (2002). mRNA expression and amino acid transport characteristics of cultured human brain microvascular endothelial cells (hBME). *Drug Metabolism and Pharmacokinetics,* Vol. 17, No. 4, pp. 367-73.

Utepbergenov, D.I., Fanning, A.S., Anderson, J.M. (2006). Dimerization of the scaffolding protein ZO-1 through the second PDZ domain. *Journal of Biological Chemistry.* Vol. 281, No. 34, pp. 24671-24677.

Uva, L., Librizzi, L., Marchi, N., Noe, F., Bongiovanni, R., Vezzani, A., Janigro, D., de Curtis, M. (2008). Acute induction of epileptiform discharges by pilocarpine in the in vitro isolated guinea-pig brain requires enhancement of blood-brain barrier permeability. *Neuroscience.* Vol. 151, No.1, pp. 303-12.

van der Sandt, I.C., Gaillard, P.J., Voorwinden, H.H., de Boer, A.G., Breimer, D.D. (2001). P-glycoprotein inhibition leads to enhanced disruptive effects by anti-microtubule cytostatics at the in vitro blood-brain barrier. *Pharmaceutical Research.* Vol. 18, No. 5, pp.587-592.

van Vliet, E.A., da Costa Araújo, S., Redeker, S., van Schaik, R., Aronica, E., Gorter, J.A. (2007). Blood-brain barrier leakage may lead to progression of temporal lobe epilepsy. *Brain.* Vol. 130,Pt 2, pp.521-534.

Vein, A.A. (2008). Science and fate: Lina Stern (1878-1968), a neurophysiologist and biochemist. *Journal of the History of the Neurosciences, Vol.* 17, No. 2, pp. 195–206.

Vemula, S., Roder, K.E., Yang, T., Bhat, G.J., Thekkumkara, T.J., Abbruscato, T.J. (2009). A functional role for sodium-dependent glucose transport across the blood-brain barrier during oxygen glucose deprivation. *Journal of Pharmacology and Experimental Therapeutics*, Vol. 328, No. 2, pp. 487-95.

Vezzani, A., Balosso, S., Maroso, M., Zardoni, D., Noé, F., Ravizza, T. (2010). ICE/caspase 1 inhibitors and IL-1beta receptor antagonists as potential therapeutics in epilepsy. *Current Opinion in Investigational Drugs*, Vol. 11, No. 1, pp. 43-50.

Vezzani, A., French, J., Bartfai, T., Baram, T.Z. (2011). The role of inflammation in epilepsy. *Nature Reviews Neurology*, Vol. 7, No. 1, pp. 31-40.

Villegas, J.C., Broadwell, R.D. (1993). Transcytosis of protein through the mammalian cerebral epithelium and endothelium. II. Adsorptive transcytosis of WGA-HRP and the blood-brain and brain-blood barriers. *Journal of Neurocytology.*, Vol. 22, No. 2, pp.67-80.

Virgintino, D., Robertson, D., Errede, M., Benagiano, V., Girolamo, F, Maiorano, E., Roncali, L., Bertossi, M. (2002). Expression of P-glycoprotein in human cerebral cortex microvessels. *Journal of Histochemistry & Cytochemistry*, Vol. 50. No. 12, pp. 1671-6.

Vorbrodt, A.W., Dobrogowska, D.H. (2004). Molecular anatomy of interendothelial junctions in human blood-brain barrier microvessels. *Folia Histochemica et Cytobiologica*, Vol. 42, No.2, pp. 67-75.

Wakayama, K., Ohtsuki, S., Takanaga, H., Hosoya, K., Terasaki, T. (2002). Localization of norepinephrine and serotonin transporter in mouse brain capillary endothelial cells. *Neuroscience Research*, Vol. 44, No. 2, pp.173-180.

Wang, A.J., Pollard, T.D. and Herman, I.M. (1983). Actin filaments stress fibers in vascular endothelial cells in vivo. *Science* Vol. 219, pp. 867-869

Warren, M.S., Zerangue, N., Woodford, K., Roberts, L.M., Tate, E.H., Feng, B., Li, C., Feuerstein, T.J., Gibbs, J., Smith, B., de Morais, S.M., Dower, W.J., Koller, K.J. (2009). Comparative gene expression profiles of ABC transporters in brain microvessel endothelial cells and brain in five species including human. *Pharmacological Research*, Vol. 59. No.6, pp.404-413.

Williams, K., Alvarez, X., Lackner, A.A. (2001). Central nervous system perivascular cells are immunoregulatory cells that connect the CNS with the peripheral immune system. *Glia*, Vol. 36. No. 2, pp. 156-164.

Williams, L.A., Martin-Padura, I., Dejana, E., Hogg N., Simmons, D.L. (1999). Identification and characterisation of human Junctional Adhesion Molecule (JAM). *Molecular Immunolology*. Vol. 36, No. 17, pp. 1175-1188.

Wolburg, H., Noell, S., Mack, A., Wolburg-Buchholz, K., Fallier-Becker, P. (2009). Brain endothelial cells and the glio-vascular complex. *Cell Tissue Research*. Vol. 335, No. 1, pp. 75-96.

Yamanaka, T., Horikoshi, Y., Suzuki, A., Sugiyama, Y., Kitamura, K., Maniwa, R., Nagai, Y., Yamashita, A., Hirose, T., Ishikawa, H., Ohno S. (2001). PAR-6 regulates aPKC activity in a novel way and mediates cell-cell contact-induced formation of the epithelial junctional complex. *Genes Cells*, Vol. 6, No. 8, pp. 721-731.

Yu, X.Q., Xue, C.C., Wang, G., Zhou, S.F. (2007). Multidrug resistance associated proteins as determining factors of pharmacokinetics and pharmacodynamics of drugs. *Current Drug Metabolism.* Vol. 8, No. 8, pp. 787-802.

Xiang, J., Ennis S.R., Abdelkarim, G.E., Fujisawa, M., Kawai, N., Keep, R.F. (2003). Glutamine transport at the blood-brain and blood-cerebrospinal fluid barriers. *Neurochemistry International,* Vol. 43, No. 4-5, pp. 279-288.

Zattoni, M., Mura, M.L., Deprez, F., Schwendener, R.A., Engelhardt, B., Frei, K., Fritschy, J.M. (2011). Brain infiltration of leukocytes contributes to the pathophysiology of temporal lobe epilepsy. *Journal of Neuroscience.* Vol. 31, No. 11, pp. 4037-4050.

Zhang, Y., Han, H., Elmquist, W.F., Miller, D.W. (2000). Expression of various multidrug resistance-associated protein (MRP) homologues in brain microvessel endothelial cells. *Brain Research,* Vol. 876, No. 1-2, pp. 148-153.

Zhang, W., Mojsilovic-Petrovic, J., Andrade, M.F., Zhang, H., Ball, M., Stanimirovic, D.B. (2003). The expression and functional characterization of ABCG2 in brain endothelial cells and vessels. *FASEB Journal.* Vol. 17, No. 14, pp.2085-2087.

7

The Use of Magnetoencephalography to Evaluate Febrile Seizures and Epilepsy in Children

A. Kotini[1], A. Tsalkidis[2], P. Anninos[1] and A. Chatzimichael[2]
[1]Lab of Medical Physics and
[2]Dept of Paediatrics, Medical School Democritus University of Thrace, Alex/polis, Greece

1. Introduction

The International League Against Epilepsy (ILAE) defined the febrile seizures as seizures occurring in childhood after one month of age, associated with a febrile illness not caused by an infection of the central nervous system, without previous neonatal seizures or a previous unprovoked seizure and not meeting the criteria for other acute symptomatic seizure (Østergaard, 2009). There is no evidence that electroencephalography (EEG) abnormalities help in the prediction of the development of subsequent epilepsy and are of limited value (American Academy of Pediatrics, 1996). Computed tomography (CT) and magnetic resonance imaging (MRI) is not indicated in children with simple febrile seizures, but may be useful in cases with prolonged or focal febrile seizures in order to reveal subtle underlying neurological diseases (Shinnar and Glauser, 2002).

The neuromagnetic field recordable outside of the head is a selective reflection of intracellular currents flowing in the apical dendrites of pyramidal cells parallel to the skull surface. The magnetic field generated by a single neuron is almost negligible. When several thousands of nearby cells are synchronously active, the summated extracranial magnetic field typically achieves a magnitude of a few hundred femto-Tesla ($1fT=10^{-15}$) where the strongest neuromagnetic signals like those associated with epileptic spikes are a few thousands femto-Tesla (Rose et al., 1987, Anninos et al., 1987; 1989a,b; 1991;1997; 1999a,b; 2000a-c; 2003; 2010;Anastasiadis et al., 1997, Kotini et al., 2007a-c). The magnetic activity of the brain is produced by cellular micro-currents, which emerge from ionic movements, due to the dynamical variations of the membrane potentials (Anninos and Raman, 1975; Anninos 1973).

The SQUID (Superconductive Quantum Interference Device) has the ability to detect magnetic fields of the order of 10^{-12}T which are much smaller than the magnetic fields of the earth which are $5X10^{-5}$ T. The SQUID is based on the Josephson effect of superconductivity (Josephson, 1962). Using multi-channel recordings the topography of the magnetic field can be recorded above the scalp with a temporal resolution of less than one millisecond (Braun, 2007). The signal measured by each channel of the SQUID is a time varying waveform voltage that reflects local changes in the magnetic flux as a function of time. This signal is called magnetoencephalography (MEG) if we measured the brain emitted magnetic fields

and it is very similar to the EEG if we measured the brain emitted electric fields. MEG is a non-invasive method for the study of electro-magnetic brain activity.
The major advantage of MEG over EEG, is that MEG has higher localization accuracy. This is due to the fact, that the different structures of the head influence the magnetic fields less than the volume current flow, that causes the EEG. MEG provides a high spatial density of recording points, which is difficult to obtain with EEG. The magnetic fields, are less distorted than electrical fields, because of the blurring effect of the skull, which acts as a low-pass filter for electrical potentials, providing, in this way, better conditions for the recording of fast activity. Moreover, inaccuracies in estimating the conductivities of the skull and other tissues of the head affect much more the interpretation of electrical than magnetic sources (Sobel et al., 2000; Wilson et al. 2007; Ramantani et al.,2006; RamachandranNai et al., 2007; Anninos et al., 2010; Kylliäinen et al.,2006; Elger et al., 1989) .
The MEG offers functional mapping information and measurement of brain activity in real time, unlike CT, MRI and functional magnetic resonance imaging (fMRI) which provide anatomical, structural and metabolic information. With the MEG the brain is seen in'action' rather than viewed as a still image. Finally, the MEG has far more superior ability to resolve millisecond temporal activity associated with the processing of information which is the main task of the brain. Thus, both normal spontaneous rhythms and pathological activities are readily identified in MEG waveforms as we do with the EEG waveforms. Whereas, MEG signals reflect current flow in the apical dentrites of pyramidal cells oriented tangential to the skull surface, EEG signals reflect both tangential and radial activities (Williamson and Kaufman, 1987; Cohen D and Cuffin, 1991; Lopes da Silva and Van Rotterdam,1987; Rose and Ducla-Soares, 1990; Hamalainen, 1993; Makela, 1996). For all of the above reasons we preferred the use of MEG for the evaluation of seizures.
In this study we investigated the possibility of any epileptic behavior caused by febrile seizures in 4 young sisters, by means of MEG. We utilized MEG to measure epileptic behavior because EEG abnormalities were not useful for the prediction of the development of subsequent epilepsy.

2. Methods

Four young sisters within the age range of 2 - 5 years were referred to our Lab by the Pediatric Department of our University General Hospital in order to be examined with MEG. There were no EEG, CT and MRI examinations in the patients' records. Informed consent for the methodology and the aim of the study was obtained from their parents prior to the procedure.
The MEG recordings were carried out in a magnetically shielded room with a whole head 122-channel-biomagnetometer (Neuromag-122, Helsinki, Finland) (Anninos et al., 2010; 2006; Kotini et al., 2010; 2008; 2005;2004; 2002; Tonoike et al., 1998; Antoniou et al., 2004) (**Figure 1**). All studies performed precisely 10 days after fever subsided for the purpose of comparison. The time duration of each MEG measurement was 3 min.
There was adequate head coverage for all children by the whole head helmet-shaped dewar. The MEG sensors were adjacent to the scalps. The sensors were consisted of rectangular pairs of planar-type gradiometers aligned in a helmet-shaped dewar vessel, into which the patient's head was inserted during the measurement. The pick-up-coils of the device are shaped like figure-of-eights to make them 'near-sighted', i.e. sensitive to sources in the brain, but insensitive to ambient noise fields. The device employs planar gradiometers that

record at each of the 61 measurement sites the magnetic field component normal to the helmet-shaped dewar bottom surface.

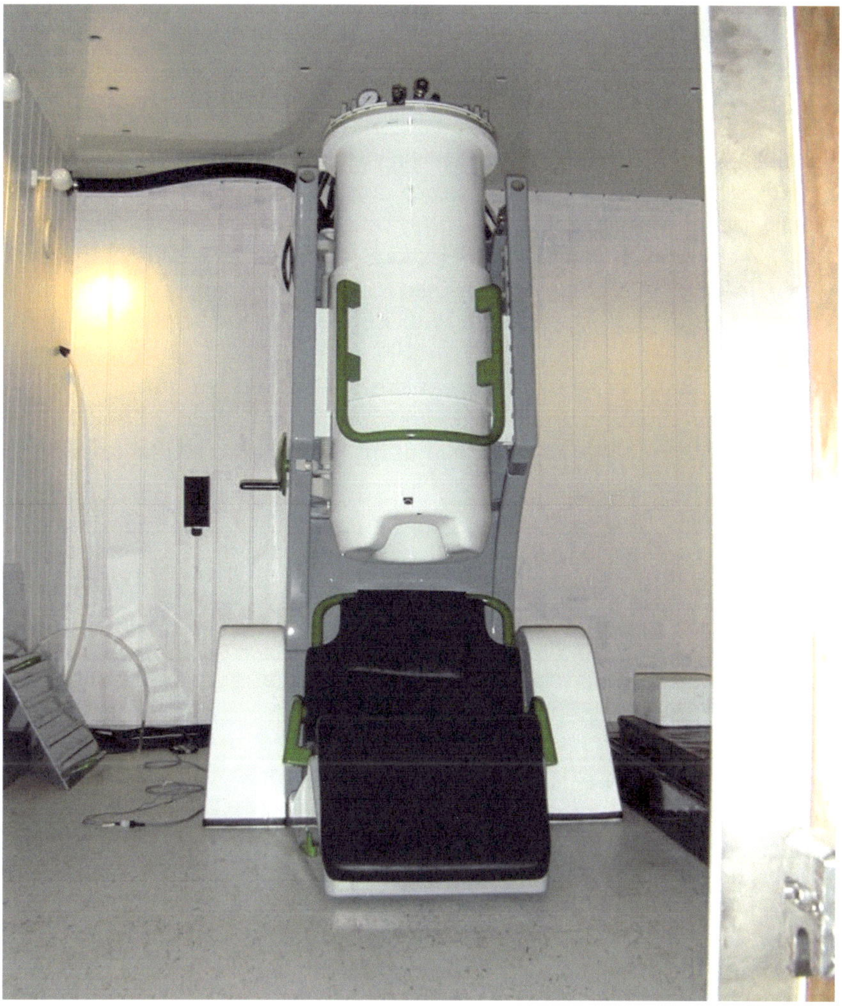

Fig. 1. The 122-channel-biomagnetometer

All MEG data were inspected carefully off-line for movement artifacts which were cut off from the data trace. The data were bandpass filtered between 0.03 and 130 Hz and sampled at 400 Hz. During off-line data analysis, we used a low-pass filter at 40 Hz and high-pass at 2-8 Hz to extract the spike component from the slower background activity.

When a clear dipole pattern was seen in the magnetic field distribution around the spike peak, the single equivalent current dipole (ECD) model was fitted in the patient's spherical head model to the recorded signals. We defined acceptable ECDs as those with a goodness-of-fit to the model of >80% and with ECD strength between 100 and 400 nAm (nano Ampere metre).

For the transformation of the ECD locations, the following coordinate system was used: x-axis perpendicular to the other two axes through the anterior commissure, y-axis passing

through the anterior and posterior commissure, and z-axis perpendicular to the y-axis through the anterior commissure at the middle plane of the brain.
Normal subjects of similar age who served as controls didn't show ECDs in their MEGs because normal controls did not have any spike activity on which to fit the data. The same sort of analyses was performed on the normal control data.

2.1 Results

Table 1 exhibits the clinical characteristics of each child. After the MEG signals were recorded, an ECD model was estimated at each time point, within the encompassing signal segment, using a single dipole model.
Two out of the 4 children shown ECD dipoles located at the right - temporal areas (**Figs.2,3,** child No 1,3), as active regions responsible for febrile seizures. These children were scheduled for future clinical examination with EEG due to the high number of events of febrile seizures (**Table 1**).
The children had a family history of febrile seizures. Their uncle (fathers' brother) had one event of febrile seizures and occurrence of epilepsy seizures during his life.
Figures 4, 5 exhibit the scalp MEG distribution for the children No.3,4 respectively. There are no ECD dipoles.

No of cases	Age	Sex	No of events of febrile seizures	Type of seizures	Duration of seizures	MEG
1	5 years	F	3	Generalized tonic - clonic Simple febrile seizures	1-2 min	ECD
2	4 years	F	1	Generalized tonic - clonic Simple febrile seizures	1-2 min	N
3	2.5 years	F	4	Generalized tonic - clonic Simple febrile seizures	1-2 min	ECD
4	15 months	F	1	Generalized tonic - clonic Simple febrile seizures	1-2 min	N

Table 1. The clinical characteristics of each child. F: Female; N: Normal, ECD: Equivalent Current Dipole

3. Conclusion

The most prevalent pathology following febrile seizures is a recurrence, which occurs in about one-third of the cases. The most reliable risk factors for the reappearance reported are the onset of first febrile seizures at less than 18 months of age and the family history of febrile seizures. Two other specific risk factors for reappearance are the peak temperature and the duration of the fever period prior to the seizure. The higher the peak temperature, the lower is the risk of recurrence and, the shorter the fever period before seizure, the higher

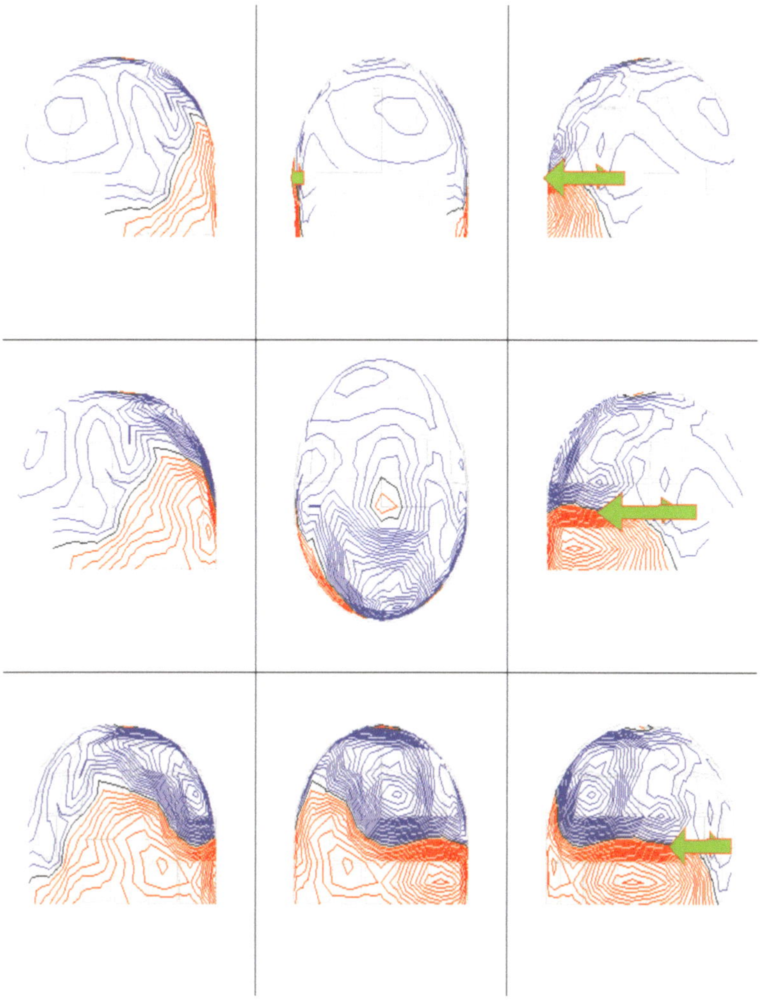

Fig. 2. The scalp MEG distribution and the ECD dipole indicated by the arrow in the child No.1 (Table 1). The coordinates are : x (left/right), y (anterior/posterior), and z (superior/inferior)

is the risk for recurrence. Furthermore fearing new seizures, the parents are faced with a concern of their child's chance of developing epilepsy or mental retardation (Østergaard, 2009; Berg et al., 1997).

There are only three reports in the literature investigating febrile seizures with MEG. Mayanagi et al. (1996) studied the clinical features of mesial temporal lobe epilepsy in 24 cases. A history of febrile convulsion, particularly in the form of status epilepticus, seemed to be a prognostic factor. For presurgical evaluation, EEG, MRI, MEG and single photon emission computed tomography (SPECT) were important tests.

Mohamed et al. (2007) referred to a previously healthy 10-year-old boy who developed generalized convulsive status epilepticus following a mild febrile illness. Ictal and interictal MEG demonstrated dipole sources projecting from the right mesial temporal region.

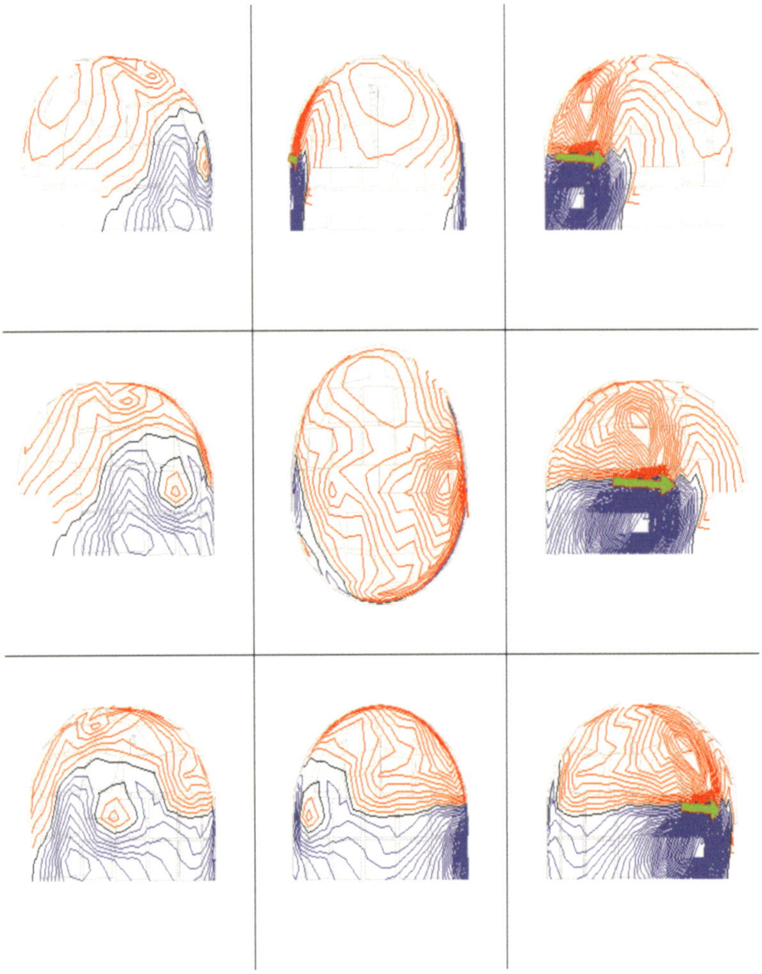

Fig. 3. The scalp MEG distribution and the ECD dipole indicated by the arrow in the child No.3 (Table 1). The coordinates are : x (left/right), y (anterior/posterior), and z (superior/inferior)

Diffusion-weighted imaging showed restricted diffusion involving the right hippocampus. Right anterior temporal lobectomy resulted in cessation of status epilepticus.

Anninos et al. (2010) studied 15 children within the age range of 2 - 7 years who experienced febrile seizures. Eight children showed ECDs located at the left-temporal, right-temporal, occipital, and frontal lobe, as active regions responsible for febrile seizures. They assumed that the interictal epileptiform discharges are a consequence of febrile seizures.

The most simple and widely used model that can explain a certain MEG surface map is the ECD, which assumes that the magnetic fields recorded at the surface can be accounted by a dipolar source. This model arises from the physiological observation that the main neuronal sources of MEG activity consist of palisades of cortical pyramidal cells, with elongated apical dendrites oriented perpendicularly to the cortical surface. The estimation of a dipole model is reasonable only if the magnetic field on the surface has focal characteristics(Sobel et al., 2000; RamachandranNair et al. 2007; Ramantani et al., 2006; Wilson et al., 2007;

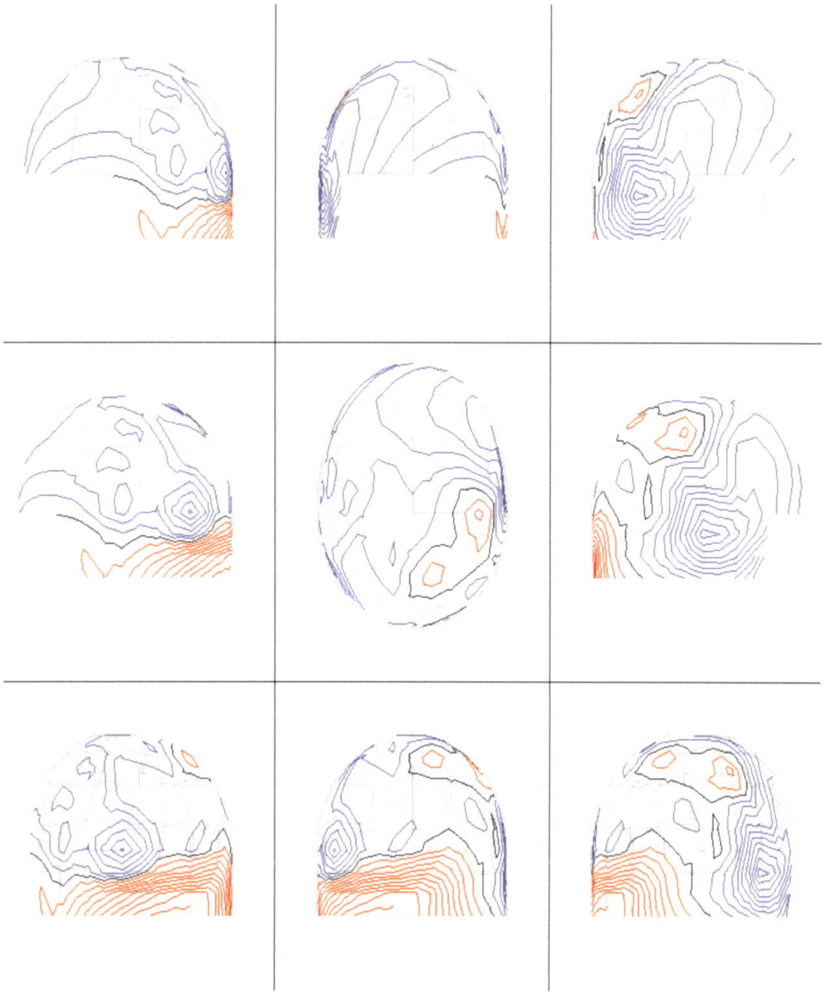

Fig. 4. The scalp MEG distribution in the child No2 (Table 1). The coordinates are : x (left/right), y (anterior/posterior), and z (superior/inferior)

Scheler et al. 2007; Papanicolaou et al., 2006; Wu et al., 2006;Chuang et al., 2006). This model allows characterization of the source of neuronal activity in the brain and is useful in focal epilepsies, in which small areas of brain tissue trigger the seizure and are important in obtaining a good spatiotemporal localization of the foci. However, MEG might be helpful in more complex epileptic patterns (generalized epilepsy).

We defined acceptable ECDs as those with a goodness of fit to the model of >80%. Standard ECD analysis defines the spatial extent of an epileptogenic zone when reliable ECD localizations are gathered to form a single cluster (Oishi et al., 2006; Iida et al.,2005). One single cluster of MEG spike sources can indicate the primary epileptogenic zone for complete resection and seizure control. Multiple clusters indicate complex and extensive epileptogenic zones and necessitate intracranial EEG monitoring. MEG is a technique for measuring the magnetic fields associated mainly with intracellular currents, while the EEG measures mainly extracellular field potentials. Intracellular currents are well modeled by the ECD model.

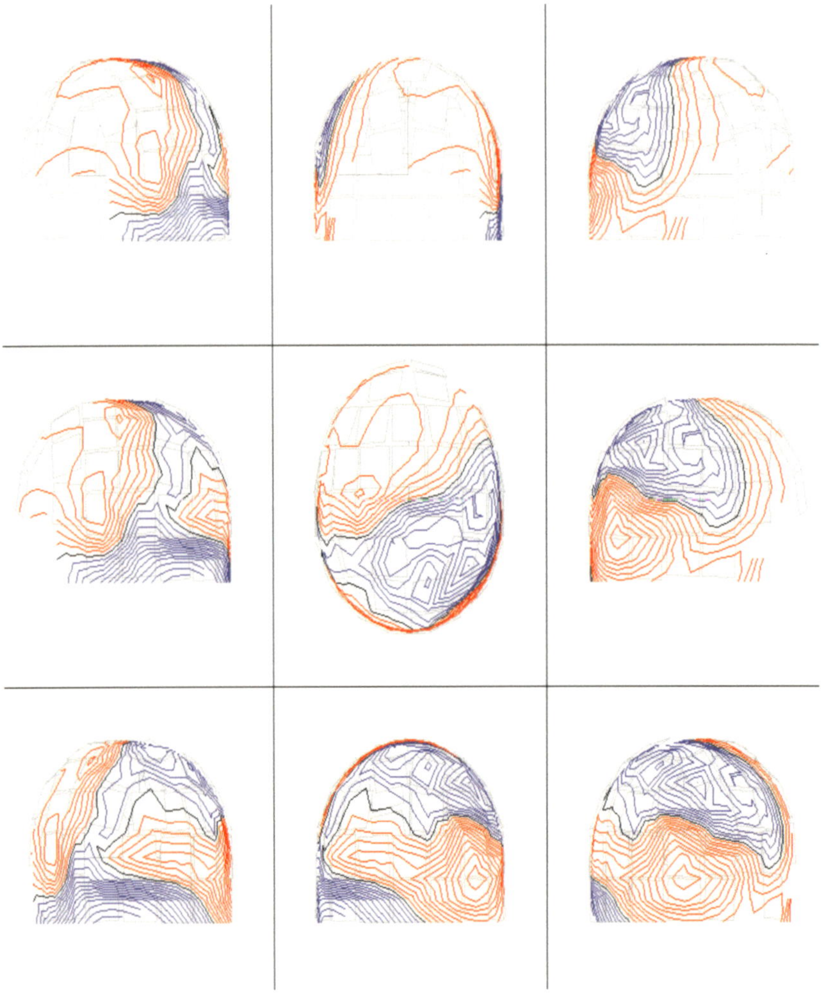

Fig. 5. The scalp MEG distribution in the child No.4 (Table 1). The coordinates are : x (left/right), y (anterior/posterior), and z (superior/inferior)

In our study, 2 out of 4 children were positive to ECDs, whereas the rest were negative. This fact depends on the activity of the patients' brain during the MEG measurements. If exhibits epileptic behavior, then we will observe ECDs, otherwise we would not. Neuroimaging studies are not necessary in children with simple febrile seizures. EEG's have been found to have limited value(Jones and Jacobsen, 2007). Abnormalities on EEG do not predict the occurrence of future seizures or the subsequent development of epilepsy. (Kuturec et al., 1997; Joshi et al., 2005). It is well known that EEG is an unhelpful diagnostic procedure and we use it only when we want to distinguish "febrile convulsions" from convulsions with fever (Panayiotopoulos, 2002; Püst, 2004; Chung et al., 2006).

Time domain analysis of neuromagnetic data give information about the underlying neuronal generators and especially is appropriate for transient behavior. The utility of the ECD algorithm depends on the goodness of fit between the structure of the sources in the model and the neuronal sources. Frequency domain localization of ECD sources is useful if the underlying neuronal generators are differentiated harmonic content and spatial distribution. The existence of such sources has been demonstrated by the determination of ECD components of activity with both a sharp spectral peak and localized source volume. Both frequency and time domain analysis may be applied to the same epoch of time. The coincident occurrence of spike activity localization in the time domain and slow activity localization in the frequency domain may be an interesting tool for localization of epileptic activity. The separation of a complex set of sources underlying spontaneous activity into distinct components is an initial step in determining the functional significance of spontaneous activity

Children with febrile seizures have a six-fold excess (3%) of subsequent afebrile seizures and epilepsy than controls. The risk is 2% after a simple and 5-10% after a complex febrile seizure. We tried to find a method that can supply us some prognostic indicators for possible epileptic behavior in children who experienced febrile seizures and have a family history of them. We assume that one of these prognostic indicators might be the existence of epileptiform discharges modeled by ECDs. Of course, further investigation is needed in order to assess the exact role of the ECDs and the occurrence of epilepsy in young children with a family history of febrile seizures.

4. Abbreviations

(ILAE) International League Against Epilepsy
(EEG) Electroencephalography
(CT) Computed tomography
(MRI) Magnetic resonance imaging
(SQUID) Superconductive Quantum Interference Device
(MEG) Magnetoencephalography
(fMRI) Functional magnetic resonance imaging
(SPECT) Single photon emission computed tomography
(ECD) Equivalent current dipole

5. References

American Academy of Pediatrics . Provisional committee on quality improvement: practice parameter: the neurodiagnostic evaluation of the child with a simple febrile seizure. Pediatrics. 1996; 97: 769–75

Anastasiasis P, Anninos PA, Diamantopoulos P, Sivridis E. Fetal magnetoencephalographic mapping in normal and preeclamptic pregnancies. J Obstet Gynaecol. 17(2), 1997, pp. 123-126.

Anninos P, Adamopoulos A, Kotini A, Tsagas N. Nonlinear analysis of brain activity in magnetic influenced Parkinson patients. Brain Topogr., 2000a, 13 (2) : 135-44.

Anninos P, Kotini A, Tsalkidis A, Dipla V, Chatzimichael A . MEG evaluation of febrile seizures in young children. J Child Neurol. 2010; 25:61-6

Anninos P.A., Anastasiadis P. & Kotini A. : Nonlinear analysis of biomagnetic signals recorded from the umbilical artery in normal and pre-eclamptic pregnancies. Eur J Obstet Gynecol Reprod Biol 85 (1999a), 159

Anninos P.A., Kotini A., Koutlaki N., Adamopoulos A., Galazios G. & Anastasiadis P. : Differential Diagnosis of Breast Lesions by use of Biomagnetic Activity and Non-Linear Analysis. Eur. J Gynaecol Oncol 21 (2000b) 591

Anninos PA, Adamopoulos A, Kotini A, Tsagas N. Nonlinear analysis of brain activity in magnetic influenced Parkinson patients. Brain Topography 2000c;13(2):135-144.

Anninos PA, and Raman S. Derivation of a mathematical equation for the EEG and the general solution within the brain and in space. Int. J. Theor. Phys. 12, 1975, pp. 1-9

Anninos PA, Anogianakis G, Lehnertz K,Pantev C, and Hoke M. Biomagnetic measurements using SQUID. Int. J.Neurosci. 37 :149-168(1987).

Anninos PA, Jacobson JI, Tsagas N, Adamopoulos A. Spatiotemporal stationarity of epileptic focal activity evaluated by analyzing magnetoencephalographic (MEG) data and the theoretical implications. Panminerva Med 1997;39:189-201.

Anninos PA, Kotini A, Adamopoulos A, Tsagas N. Magnetic stimulation can modulate seizures in epileptic patients. Brain Topography 2003;16(1):57-64

Anninos PA, Tsagas N, Jacobson, JI and Kotini A. The biological effects of magnetic stimulation in epileptic patients. Pannminerva Med. 41,1999b, pp.207-215

Anninos PA, Tsagas N, Sandyk R and Derpapas K. Magnetic stimulation in the treatment of partial seizures. Int. J. Neurosc. 60,1991, pp.141-171

Anninos, P.A. and Tsagas, N. Localization and cure of epileptic foci with the use of MEG measurements. Int. J. Neurosci., 1989a, 46: 235-242.

Anninos, P.A. Electromagnetic fields generated from neuronal activity TIT. Journal of Life Science 3, 1973, pp. 15

Anninos, P.A., Tsagas, N. and Adamopoulos, A. A brain model theory for epilepsy and the mechanism of treatment with experimental verification using SQUID measurements. In: R.M. Cotterill (Ed.), Models of Brain Function. New York Cambridge University Press, 1989b: 405-421.

Antoniou PE, Anninos PA, Piperidou H, Adamopoulos A, Kotini A, Koukourakis MI, Sivridis E. Non linear analysis of magnetoencephalographic signals as a tool for assessing malignant lesions of the brain: first results. Brain Topogr. 2004;17:117-23

Berg AT, Shinnar S, Darefsky AS, Holford TR, Shapiro ED, Salomon ME, Crain EF, Hauser AW . Predictors of recurrent febrile seizures. Arch Pediatr Adolesc Med. 1997; 151: 371–8

Braun C . Magnetoencephalography: a method for the study of brain function in neurosurgery. Z Med Phys. 2007;17:280-7

Chuang NA, Otsubo H, Pang EW, Chuang SH. Pediatric magnetoencephalography and magnetic source imaging. Neuroimaging Clin N Am. 16(1), 2006, pp.193-210.

Chung B, Wat LC, Wong V. Febrile seizures in southern Chinese children: incidence and recurrence. Pediatric Neurol. 34,2006, pp.121-126

Cohen D and Cuffin BD. EEG versus MEG localization accuracy:theory and experiment. Brain Topogr.4,95-103(1991).

Elger CE, Hoke M, Lehnertz K., et al. Mapping of MEG amplitude spectra: Its significance for the diagnosis of focal epilepsy. In: Maurer K, editor. Topographic brain mapping of EEG and evoked potentials. Berlin: Springer Verlag, 1989, 565-70.

Hamalainen M, Hari R, Ilmoniemi R, Knuutila J and Lounasmaa O. Magnetoencephalography-theory, instrumentation and applications to noninvasive studies of the working human brain. Rev. Mod. Phys 65: 1-93(1993).

Iida K, Otsubo H, Matsumoto Y, Ochi A, Oishi M, Holowka S, Pang E, Elliott I, Weiss SK, Chuang SH, Snead OC 3rd, Rutka JT . Characterizing magnetic spike sources by using magnetoencephalography-guided neuronavigation in epilepsy surgery in pediatric patients. J Neurosurg.2005; 102(Suppl 2):187-96

ILAE. Guidelines for epidemiologic studies on epilepsy.Epilepsia. 34(4):1993, pp. 592-596.

Jones T, Jacobsen SJ. Childhood Febrile Seizures: Overview and Implications. Int J Med Sci. 2007; 4(2): 110–114

Josephson BD. Possible effects in superconductivity tunneling. Phys. Lett.1, 1962, pp 252-256

Joshi C, Wawrykow T, Patrick J, Prasad A. Do clinical variables predict an abnormal EEG in patients with complex febrile seizures? Seizure. 2005;14:429–34

Kotini A, Anninos P, Adamopoulos A, Prassopoulos P. Low Frequency MEG Activity and MRI Evaluation in Parkinson's Disease. Brain Topogr 2005; 18:59-63

Kotini A, Anninos P, Tamiolakis D. MEG mapping in multiple sclerosis patients. Eura Medicophys 2007a; 43:345-8

Kotini A, Anastasiadis AN, .Koutlaki N, .Tamiolakis D, Anninos P, Anastasiadis P. Biomagnetism in Perinatal Medicine. Our experience in Greece. Clin Exp Obstet Gynaecol 2007b;34:42-6

Kotini A, Anninos P, Tamiolakis D, Prassopoulos P . Differentiation of MEG activity in multiple sclerosis patients with the use of nonlinear analysis. J Integr Neurosci. 2007c;6:233-40

Kotini A, Anninos P. Detection of non-linearity in schizophrenic patients using magnetoencephalography. Brain Topogr. 2002;15:107-13

Kotini A, Camposano S, Hara K, Salat D, Cole A, Stufflebeam S, Halgren E. Cortical thickness in a case of Congenital Unilateral Perisylvian Syndrome. Neurol Clin Neurophysiol 2004;4:1-4

Kotini A, Mavraki E, Anninos P, Piperidou H, Prassopoulos P . Meg evaluation of epileptic activity in the time and frequency domain. J Integr Neurosci. 2008;7:463-80

Kotini A, Mavraki E, Anninos P, Piperidou H, Prassopoulos P. Magnetoencephalographic Findings in Two Cases of Juvenile Myoclonus Epilepsy. Brain Topogr. 2010; 23:41-5

Kuturec M, Emoto SE, Sofijanov N, et al. Febrile seizures: is the EEG a useful predictor of recurrences? Clin.Pediatr.(Phila). 1997;36:31–6

Kylliäinen A, Braeutigam S, Hietanen JK, et al. Face and gaze processing in normally developing children: a magnetoencephalographic study. Eur J Neurosci. 2006 ;23:801-10

Lopes da Silva F and Van Rotterdam A. Biophysical aspects of EEG and magnetoencephalogram generation. In: Niedermeyer E, Lopes da Silva F (Eds). Electroencephalography. Baltimorc, Munich: Urban& Schwarzenberg ,29-41(1987).

Makela JP. Neurological application of MEG. Electroencephalogr. Clin. Neurophysiol. Supp. Review 47: 343-355(1996).

Mayanagi Y, Watanabe E, Kaneko Y. Mesial temporal lobe epilepsy: clinical features and seizure mechanism. Epilepsia. 1996; 37 (Suppl 3):57-60

Mohamed IS, Otsubo H, Imai K, Shroff M, Sharma R, Chuang SH, Donner E, Drake J, Snead OC 3rd .Surgical treatment for acute symptomatic refractory status epilepticus: a case report. J Child Neurol. 2007; 22:435-9

Oishi M, Kameyama S, Masuda H, Tohyama J, Kanazawa O, Sasagawa M, Otsubo H . Single and multiple clusters of magnetoencephalographic dipoles in neocortical epilepsy: significance in characterizing the epileptogenic zone. Epilepsia. 2006;47:355-64

Østergaard JR .Febrile seizures. Acta Paediatr. 2009; 98:771-3

Panayiotopoulos CP. A clinical guide to epileptic syndromes and their treatments 2002; 3:50-52

Papanicolaou AC, Pazo-Alvarez P, Castillo EM, et al. Functional neuroimaging with MEG: normative language profiles. Neuroimage. 33(1), 2006, pp.326-342.

Püst B. Febrile seizures: an update. Kinderkankenschwester 2004;23:328-31 (Review)

Ramachandran Nair R, Otsubo H, Shroff MM, et al. MEG predicts outcome following surgery for intractable epilepsy in children with normal or nonfocal MRI findings. Epilepsia. 48(1), 2007, pp.149-157.

Ramantani G, Boor R, Paetau R, et al. MEG versus EEG: influence of background activity on interictal spike detection. J Clin Neurophysiol. 23(6), 2006, pp.498-508.

Rose DF and Ducla-Soares R. Comparison of electroencephalography and magnetoencephalography. In: Sato S (Ed.),Magnetoencephalography. New York: Raven press,33-37(1990).

Rose DF, Smith PD and Sato S. Magnetoencephalography and epilepsy research. Science 238, 1987, pp. 329-335.

Scheler G, Fischer MJ, Genow A, et al. Spatial relationship of source localizations in patients with focal epilepsy: comparison of MEG and EEG with a three spherical shells and a boundary element volume conductor model. Hum Brain Mapp. 28(4), 2007, pp.315-322.

Shinnar S, Glauser TA . Febrile seizures. J Child Neurol. 2002;17: S44–S52

Sobel DF, Aung M, Otsubo H, Smith MC. Magnetoencephalography in Children with Landau-Kleffner Syndrome and Acquired Epileptic Aphasia. AJNR Am J Neuroradiol. 2000; 21:301-307

Tonoike M, Yamaguchi M, Kaetsu I, Kida H, Seo R, Koizuka I. Ipsilateral dominance of human olfactory activated centers estimated from event-related magnetic fields measured by 122-channel whole head neuromagnetometer using odorant stimuli synchronized with respirations. Ann NY Acad Sci 1998;855 : 579-590

Williamson SI and Kaufman L. Analysis of neuromagnetic signals. In : Gevins AS, Redmond A (Eds): Handbook of electroencephalography and Clinical Neurophysiology, Vol1.Methods and Analysis of Brain Electrical Signals. Elsevier, Amsterdam, 1987.

Wilson TW, Rojas DC, Reite ML, Teale PD, Rogers SJ. Children and adolescents with autism exhibit reduced MEG steady-state gamma responses. Biol Psychiatry. 62(3), 2007, pp.192-197.

Wu JY, Sutherling WW, Koh S, et al. Magnetic source imaging localizes epileptogenic zone in children with tuberous sclerosis complex. Neurology. 66(8), 2006, pp. 1270-1272.

8

Dense Array EEG & Epilepsy

Mark D. Holmes
Department of Neurology, Regional Epilepsy Center, University of Washington, Harborview Medical Center, Seattle USA

1. Introduction

Electroencephalographic (EEG) signals derive from the action of neuronal activity in the cerebral cortex, through the action of synchronously occurring post-synaptic potentials of neuronal masses (De Munck et al., 1992). Forming reciprocal combinations of interacting excitatory and inhibitory populations, these neuronal masses are believed to be the sources of the macroscopic EEG signal recorded on the scalp (Freeman, 1975; Wilson & Cowan, 1973; Lopes da Silva & van Leeuwen, 1978). In individuals with epilepsy, seizures emerge from ongoing cortical activity through incompletely understood mechanisms, but are likely related to a wide variety of biochemical, anatomic, physiologic, or genetic aberrations (Avanzini & Franceschetti, 2003; Bragin et al., 2002; D'Ambrosio et al., 2004; D'Ambrosio et al., 2005; Nemani & Binder, 2005; Noebels, 2003; Shah et al., 2004; Stables et al., 2002; White 2002).

For over 50 years the paroxysmal EEG signals ("spikes" or "sharp waves") recorded on the scalp, reflecting the abnormal behavior of cortical neuronal populations, have remained the most important laboratory findings in the clinical evaluation of patients with epilepsy (Niedermeyer, 1999). However, despite the indispensable role of the EEG, the standard assessment has significant limitations. Typically, 16-21 electrodes are placed over the upper portions of the cranium, and under these circumstances distances between individual electrodes are several cm, resulting in inadequate spatial resolution, and an even poorer assessment of cortical activity in basal brain regions. Research on the spatial frequency spectrum suggests that to maximize spatial information of the human EEG ("spatial Nyquist"), interelectrode distances on the cortical surface must be within 1.25 mm (Freeman et al, 2000), and on the scalp, less than 10 mm (Freeman, 2003). As a consequence, analysis of standard EEG recordings yields poor spatial resolution, often results in failure to detect significant pathology, and provides only limited insight into the extent of the involved cortical network and patterns of discharge propagation. It is anticipated that when detailed knowledge of the specific cortical regions activated during epileptiform discharges becomes readily available, that such information will prove to be critical in understanding the nature of an individual subject's seizures and in improving therapy (Spencer, 2002).

Major technological advances are becoming available and will likely change the role and utility of scalp-recorded EEG. One of these advances is the capability for rapid application of a dense array of electrodes, a technique that may also now be employed in the context of continuous longterm EEG video monitoring (LTM) (Thompson et al, 2008). Recording systems with up to 256 electrodes can provide coverage that includes face and neck, with the goal of "sampling" basal brain regions (e.g. inferior frontal and basal temporal areas), as well the convexity of the cerebrum. By increasing spatial sampling and decreasing the distance between electrodes, dense array EEG (dEEG) results in markedly improved spatial resolution from scalp EEG data (Lantz et al., 2003). Another important technological advance is in the development of physical models of head tissues that allow estimation of neural sources of the EEG (Michel et al., 2001). The combination of superior spatial resolution and sophisticated methods of source analysis, with results registered on realistic magnetic resonance imaging (MRI) models, results in more precise information on electrographic pathology that may be extracted from the scalp EEG (Phillips et al, 2002; Michel et al., 2004).

With this background in perspective, the purpose of this paper is to describe our research in dense array EEG as it applies to epilepsy. The review will include a discussion of the insight that this research has provided in understanding the nature of epileptic circuits, the potential role of dEEG in evaluating difficult seizures, and the direction of future technological developments.

2. Methodology

2.1 DEEG recordings

A 256-channel Geodesic Sensor Net (EGI, Inc, Eugene OR, USA) is applied to each person during the recordings, requiring 10-30 min for application and adjustment (Fig. 1). The net is constructed to include electrode coverage over the face and neck. For an average adult head, interelectrode distances are approximately 20-25 mm. The EEG-amplifier used in our research includes a bandpass of 0.1 to 400 Hz, sampling rate up to 1000 Hz, 16-bit analog-digital conversion, and noise levels engineered typically to 0.6 microvolts root-mean-square. Impedances are maintained at less than 50,000 ohms, consistent with the high input impedance amplifiers employed (Ferree et al., 2001). Continuous longterm EEG-video monitoring (LTM) with dEEG is also now feasible, and we have employed this technique to capture seizures in over 50 patients with medically refractory localization-related seizures, with continuous recordings up to 24-96 hours (Thompson et al., 2008). In our investigations on subjects with refractory generalized seizures, recordings are performed on an outpatient basis, with recording times of sufficient duration to record discharges (60-90 minutes) and with no reduction in subjects' antiseizure medications; these recordings include waking and, and in most cases, drowsy or sleep states.

The 256 channel dEEG is recorded with a common vertex reference, and re-referenced digitally to various montages for inspection, including the average reference. Because of the improved coverage of the inferior head surface, the average reference allows the potential at each index electrode to be examined with reference to an estimate of the zero potential of the head (Bertrand et al., 1985; Dien, 1998; Junghofer et al., 1999). The average-referenced EEG waveforms are examined with topographic waveform plots, a technique that allows inspection of geometric distribution of the potential fields. In addition, topographic maps are created with spherical spline interpolation (Perrin et al., 1987). Dynamic scalp topography of epileptiform discharges with animations can be created at variable time intervals (Tucker at al., 1994).

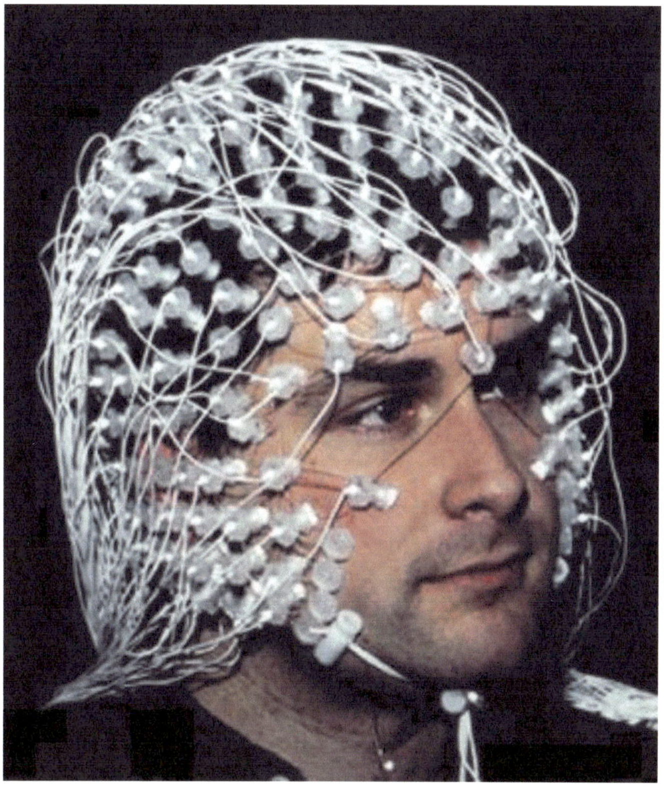

Fig. 1. This model is wearing the 256 channel dense array EEG net. Note the electrode coverage extending over the face and neck.

2.2 The "inverse problem"

The principal goal of our research efforts in dEEG is to noninvasively localize brain regions that are involved in the onset and distribution of epileptiform discharges. In other words, our efforts are aimed at solving the "inverse problem", which in this case is to determine the location of electrical signals originating from the cerebral cortex from recordings obtained on the closed surface of the head. Since there is no unique solution to the inverse problem, achieving viable answers begins with the construction of a brain and head model ("forward model"), based on biologically realistic assumptions, such as the geometry and the electrical properties of head tissues and assuming the cortical origin of scalp-recorded brain signals (Nunez & Srinivasan, 2006). In brief, the method of solving the inverse problem involves use of an appropriate forward model used in conjunction with an inverse algorithm for source analysis. It is important to emphasize that, regardless of the sophistication of the source analysis, the final results may be misleading if the scalp data lacks adequate spatial resolution, or if the researcher fails to recognize or account for non-cerebral artifacts (such as eye movements and muscle potentials) that often contaminate scalp EEG.

2.3 DEEG source analysis

As first step in this analysis, one technique of constructing the forward model is specification of an ellipsoidal head with four homogeneous shells: brain, cerebrospinal fluid

(CSF), skull, and scalp. Conductivity ratios that may be used include 1.0 (CSF), .3300 (brain), .0042 (skull), and .3300 (scalp); tissue thicknesses may be specified as 1.0 mm (CSF), 7.0 mm (skull), and 6.0 mm (scalp), with head radius set to 92.5 mm (Berg & Scherg, 1994). An improvement in the forward model may be accomplished by inclusion of a realistic model of head conductivity with finite difference computations (Salman et al., 2005). To provide solutions that are consistent with source analysis techniques regional sources are selected (with dipole moments in three orthogonal directions of space) that are most adequate to describe the discharge complex. Dipole locations are visualized in relation to a standard brain MRI model, with electrodes positioned in relation to skull landmarks in accordance with the international (10-20) EEG system (nasion, periaurcular points), and co-registered with the head conductivity model. The positions of the electrodes, with respect to the standard MRI model, are determined by fitting actual 256-channel locations used in the source localization software. These locations are the average cartesian coordinates of the digitized locations from five normal adult subjects.

Several independent methods have been employed in research in regard to the inverse algorithm component to identify electrographic sources, including linear inverse techniques (Pasqual-Marqui et al., 2002; Grave de Peralta Menendez et al., 2004) and equivalent dipole methods (Scherg & Ebersole, 1994; Scherg et al., 2002). Most of our research has utilized the linear inverse method of local autoregressive average (LAURA), which weights the solution distribution so that sources are continuous with nearby activity (Grave de Peralta Menendez et al., 2004). Because the vector fields of electrical sources fall off with the cube of distance (and the potential fields with the square of distance), the LAURA method constrains the solution with a weighting function that assumes the result will have a spatial smoothness with this physical property. The LAURA inverse solutions are implemented within the GeoSource software package used in our research (*http://www.egi.com*), using the head conductivity model and the probabilistic cortical gray matter locations from the Montreal Neurological Institute (MNI) probabilistic atlas (*www.bic.mni.mcgill.ca*) to constrain the location of 2400 source voxels on the standard MRI. Three orthogonal dipole moments (x,y,z) are defined and solved for each of the source voxels.

3. Studies of "localization-related" epilepsy

3.1 Comparison with intracranial EEG recordings

One method to test the validity of dEEG is with direct comparison with intracranial EEG recordings performed in the same patients (Holmes et al., 2008; Holmes et al., 2010a). In order to accomplish this, seizures must be captured using dEEG LTM. We have studied 10 consecutive patients with medically refractory localization-related epilepsy, all surgical candidates, who underwent noninvasive evaluation with dEEG LTM studies prior to intracranial EEG recordings. At least twelve months of postoperative clinical outcome for each patient is available.

Standard methods in these 10 subjects, which included, as appropriate in each case, high resolution MRI examinations, standard scalp EEG LTM, single photon emission tomography (SPECT) imaging, positron emission tomography (PET) imaging, neuropsychological testing, and detailed neurological examination, failed to provide adequate ictal localization. For this reason, all individuals required invasive EEG studies to define ictal onsets. Patients with skull defects or previous brain surgery were not offered dEEG studies, since these would affect source analysis methods. The subjects included 7 males and 3 females, with age range 12-49 years

Prior to intracranial monitoring, the subjects were hospitalized and underwent continuous video-EEG recording long enough to capture one or more habitual seizure, using the 256 channel EEG system, with the exception of one subject, who was studied with 128 channels. The hospital stay was generally shorter (24-96 hours), compared to standard LTM.

The first steps in evaluating the data include screening for artifacts, and removing or digitally interpolating channels degraded by artifact or poor contact (Perrin et al., 1987); from zero to 10 channels were interpolated in the typical 256 dEEG LTM recording in this series. The next phase of analysis typically includes the following: 1) Before actual EEG review, the video recordings are analyzed to determine ictal semiology and time of onset of clinical seizures. 2) The initial electrographic analysis consists of review of the continuous EEG data. Montages using the traditional clinical 10-20 electrode array (30 mm/sec) are first inspected for the purposes of orienting to the head topography and to obtain a general estimate when the ictal onset most likely occurs. 3) EEG characteristics that signify the onset of the seizure are then isolated. This part of the evaluation is complex and subjective because there are often multiple clues to the onset of the seizure, as with any clinical EEG evaluation. Such clues may take place across a considerable amount of time, ranging from milliseconds to seconds, to even minutes. It is not possible simply to select one sample for source localization and consistent findings across multiple seizures increase confidence in the results. The clinical neurophysiologist's interpretation is required to separate the electrographic signs of seizure onset from other EEG features, many of which may be pathological but not indicative of the seizure. For example, in some patients recurring spikes are observed prior to the fully developed seizure; often these early spikes are important for localizing the potential onset of the seizure. In other patients, the EEG may appear relatively "quiescent" prior to the onset of the seizure and more subtle clues are sought, such as slow oscillations (0.5-7 Hz), or focal rhythmic or arrhythmic slowing proximal to the fully developed seizure. 4) Review of the topographic EEG display (topographic waveform plot) of all 256 channels further aids in spatially isolating distinct epileptiform patterns that occur prior to and during the onset of the seizure. With an accurate average reference formed from 256 surface potential channels (approximating the zero sum of all cortical dipoles), the topographic waveform plot illustrates the phase reversals and thus approximate neural sources of epileptiform events. In many cases, ictal patterns emerge when all 256 channels are displayed that are not obvious using only subsampled, standard 10-20 chart views (Fig. 2). 5) Topographic mapping examinations of the electrical potentials at the surfaces of the brain are often aided by two-dimensional Laplacian (the spatial second derivative) computations, using the potentials with spherical splines, in order to estimate radial scalp current density (Tucker et al., 1994).

The invasive EEG recordings obtained in all 10 cases were necessitated by the fact that the initial standard noninvasive evaluation failed to reveal adequate information upon which surgical therapy could be planned. The indications, type of electrodes (subdural grid or strip electrodes), location of electrode placement, and duration of recordings were based on standard clinical criteria. The neurosurgeon was aware of the dense array recordings prior to placement of subdural arrays. However, interpretations of the invasive recordings were made without reference to the dense array predictions of seizure onset, and brain resections were based solely on the analysis of ictal onsets obtained from the invasive EEG recordings.

Of the nine subjects who underwent surgery, eight underwent resections, while one underwent multiple subpial transections (MST), since her seizures originated, in part, within hand motor cortex (Morrell et al., 1989). One subject, who had bitemporal epilepsy, was judged not to be a candidate for resective surgery.

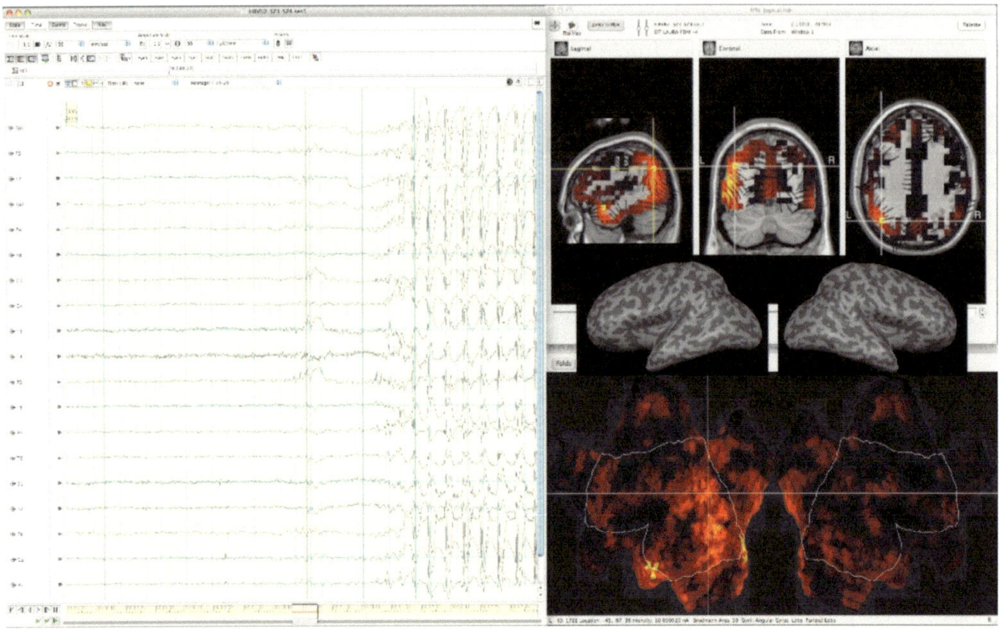

Fig. 2. This figure demonstrates the seizure onset of one subject. The standard EEG (left side) shows that the seizure is heralded by poorly localized discharges over left posterior quadrant. Source analysis of one dEEG-recorded seizure suggests that the onset is localized to left parietal cortex (top right). The "flatmap" of flattened cortical surface of standard MRI used in source analysis denotes regions of maximal intensity with crosshairs (bottom right). See also Fig. 3.

We found ictal localization, estimated from dense array EEG studies, convergent (within approximately 3 cm) in 8 of 10 patients with the intracranial data (Fig. 3). In the two cases where we found divergence of ictal localization, lateralization was the same using both modalities. In two subjects, we found more than one ictal focus with intracranial studies; one of the two foci for each of these two cases was found with dense array recordings. In all instances, the recording times for intracranial LTM (range 7-20 days) exceeded that of dense array LTM. More seizures were recorded during invasive studies compared to dense array recordings, as a result of the longer recording time for intracranial recordings, in nine of the 10 patients.

All patients in the series have been followed at least twelve months after surgery (range 12-40 months). Recorded outcomes are based on both an approximate percentage of seizure reduction and the corresponding Engel classification of postsurgical outcome (Engel et al., 1993). The nine patients who underwent resections or MST were either seizure-free (two patients) or had a clinically significant improvement in seizure frequency or severity at the time of most recent postoperative clinic visit (Engel class 1, 2, or 3). Nonspecific gliosis proved to be the most commonly observed pathological finding.

A detailed study of one case report in this series is illustrative (Holmes et al., 2008). A 13 y/o girl presented with medically refractory, daily complex partial seizures since age 5. Her attacks, each lasting 30-60 sec, consist of the onset of confusion with orofacial and upper extremity automatisms. Standard EEG studies disclosed left occipital and left parietal spikes. Ictal onsets from standard LTM were found to be of probable left posterior quadrant onset, but were poorly localized. MRI was normal. DEEG LTM studies captured one of her typical seizures and disclosed that the seizure originated from left posterior inferior occipital lobe. Within one sec, ictal propagation to right posterior temporal-occipital cortex, and then back to left parietal cortex was found. The patient subsequently underwent invasive LTM, with intracranial subdural grid electrodes placed over left posterior quadrant, and subdural strip electrodes placed bilaterally over posterior quadrants and basal temporal regions. Both ictal onsets and propagation patterns recorded from the invasive EEG studies corresponded closely to that found on the dEEG studies. Surgery was carried out, based on the results of the invasive studies, and the patient has been seizure-free 35 months after resection.

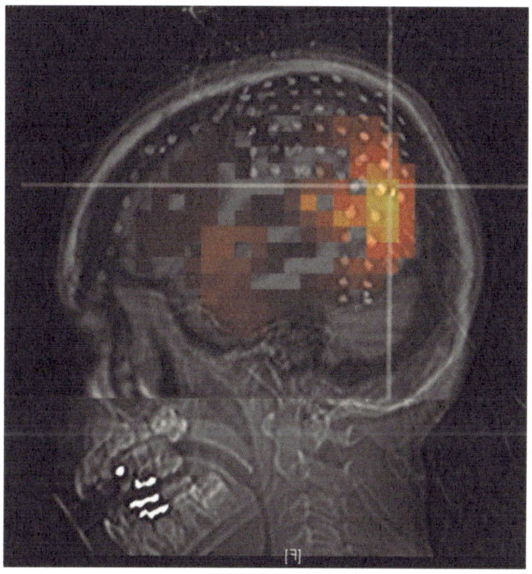

Fig. 3. Source analysis of onset of seizure of subject shown in Fig. 2, co-registered on standard MRI model suggests origin in left parietal cortex (yellow color, with maximal intensity at crosshairs). The figure is also co-registered with subsequent computed tomography showing intracranial electrode placement. Invasive studies revealed left parietal cortical origin of the subject's seizures.

3.2 Analysis of interictal spikes in localization-related epilepsy

Interictal dense array EEG studies may be conducted on a short-term, outpatient basis (Phillips et al., 2002; Holmes et al., 2005; Michel et al., 2004) to capture interictal epileptiform discharges. In a study (Holmes et al., 2005) of eight subjects, all surgical candidates, spikes were detected with Reveal software (http://www.eeg-persyst.com), and confirmed by visual analysis. For each patient spikes were clustered into populations and each spike population was subjected to source analysis at 10 msec intervals along the time course of the spike, utilizing the linear inverse method of LAURA. Although standard visual analysis suggested that all spike populations in all patients were confined to one temporal lobe region, more complex spatiotemporal patterns of spike propagation were often observed in the dense array EEG data. In some cases, sources indeed remained confined to one temporal lobe throughout the duration of the spike. In other instances, however, propagation spread rapidly from basal temporal to lateral temporal lobe, to orbitofrontal cortex, and finally to the opposite temporal lobe. These findings may give credence to the concept that temporal lobe epilepsy may be a bilateral corticolimbic network disturbance in some patients (Spencer, 2002; Ebersole, 1997). A recent study that compared simultaneously dEEG with intracranial subdural recordings in subjects with temporal lobe epilepsy offers confirmatory evidence that dEEG, when used in conjunction with realistic source analysis and head model, accurately localizes intertictal discharges to medial temporal structures (Yamazaki et al., 2010). This same study also shows that 47% of all intracranial-recorded spikes are detected by dEEG, with the average detectable dEEG spike approximately 1 μV in amplitude. Furthermore, the findings in this comparative study suggests that dEEG provides more precise information regarding deep spike foci than either conventional EEG or magnetoencephalography. Future research is necessary to answer the question as to whether or not spike propagation patterns encapsulate the cortical network involved during clinical seizures.

4. Studies of "generalized" seizures

4.1 Absence seizures

The conventional classification of epileptic seizures is based on the International League Against Epilepsy dichotomy that epileptic seizures are either "partial" (localization-related) or "generalized" (Commission on Classification and Terminology of the International League Against Epilepsy, 1989). This scheme implies that partial seizures have discrete focal origins, while generalized seizures are assumed to occur without lateralizing or localizing features that include bilateral, global cortical activation at ictal onset (Panayiotopoulos, 2002). Experimental evidence that implicates thalamic and thalmocortical mechanisms in the pathophysiology of generalized seizures has been offered as an explanation for the apparently "generalized" nature of these seizures (Gloor, 1978; McCormick, 2002; Slaght et al., 2002).

The absence seizure is often considered the prototypic idiopathic generalized seizure. Although the concept of generalized seizures persists in clinical practice, traditional EEG visual analysis emphasized a frontal preponderance of the spike-wave complexes in absence (Niedermeyer, 1999) and early studies in source analysis suggested that, although bilateral at onset, the ictal patterns in absence localized to frontal cortex (Rodin et al., 1994). Research using dense array EEG provides further evidence that the traditional concept of "generalized" epilepsy may not be accurate. Recent studies of absence in five patients using 256 channel dEEG recordings showed that both at onset and during propagation, the discharges in absence are associated with activation of only discrete regions of mainly medial frontal and orbital frontal cortex (Holmes et al., 2004). Detailed studies of the ictal discharges in absence, the onsets of which develop rapidly, suggest that the waveforms may best be described as "wave-spike", rather than "spike-wave". Though individual variability between subjects may exist, typically the intial slow wave follows oscillations localized to medial frontal regions, then exhibits anterior propagation and abrupt transition over the frontal pole as a positive spike displaces the diffuse anterior negative slow wave, with the discharge then sweeping posteriorly along the orbital frontal cortex.

Separately, Tucker et al (Tucker et al., 2007) analyzed the same data collected for the Holmes et al., 2004 study, using the LAURA inverse, and an improved high resolution finite difference head conductivity model, that showed a "flatmap" display of the cortical surface using GeoSource software. Overall, the results were convergent with the earlier report. For each seizure in each patient the slow wave of the wave-spike cycle engaged networks of mainly medial frontal, and occasionally temporal, cortical networks. Invariably, this was followed by primary current source distribution in ventromedial frontal cortex during the abrupt wave-spike transition. Although differences were found between individual patients, particularly during in the slow wave and the oscillatory EEG changes in the second or so prior to ictal onset, each seizure rapidly progressed to a stereotyped pattern with major spike discharges localized to midline frontal networks.

4.2 Studies in juvenile myoclonic epilepsy

We also evaluated epileptiform discharges in 10 patients with the idiopathic generalized epilepsy syndrome of juvenile myoclonic epilepsy (JME) (Holmes et al, 2010b). In this syndrome, seizures begin typically in adolescence, do not remit, and may be characterized by absence, myoclonic, or generalized tonic-clonic attacks. The neurological examination and magnetic resonance imaging studies are normal, and discharges (based on standard EEG) is classically shown to exhibit generalized 4-6 Hz spike or multiple spike-slow wave complexes. In this study, each subject underwent 1-2 hours of outpatient recording using a 256 channel dEEG system and epileptiform discharges were captured in all cases. Analysis of epileptiform patterns disclosed that in many cases the results were, not surprisingly, similar to absence, with activation of mesial frontal and orbital frontal regions found in all cases (Figs 4, 5). Involvement of other midline regions (anterior or posterior cingulum) was observed in 4/10 subjects. Importantly, in 6/10 (60%) of the patients, the epileptiform circuit included mesial temporal lobe. The common denominator in all cases of JME is engagement of orbitofrontal and medial frontal cortical regions. Independent research findings from other investigators who have examined JME and absence epilepsy with other modalities, including MRI volumetric analysis (Tae et al., 2008), diffuse tensor imaging (Deppe et al., 2006), magnetic resonance spectroscopy (Lin et al., 2009), and functional MRI (Bai et al, 2010) have all implicated focal cortical involvement in "generalized epilepsies", particularly discrete regions of frontal and temporal lobe

Epileptic seizures may involve only specific cortical networks. Analysis of ictal patterns in both generalized and localization-related seizures with dense array EEG leads to an interpretation that all seizures, including those classified as "generalized", involve only specific cortical networks. The standard classification of epileptic seizures is a reflection of the inadequacy of conventional EEG analysis, where spatial resolution is at best limited. Furthermore, consideration of the regions of cortical involvement at the onset and during propagation may also lead to the hypothesis that epileptic seizures may be considered as fundamentally corticothalamic or corticolimbic in nature. Discharges in absence seizures and in JME invariably involve discrete regions of orbital and medial frontal cortex, and by inference that is based on mammalian research, the thalamic reticular nucleus (TRN), with sparing of limbic circuits (Futatsugi & Riviello, 1998; Steriade, 2003). Absence may be the prototype of the corticothalamic ("generalized") seizure in which corticothalmic mechanisms interact with TRN networks and therefore influence thalamocortical projections and widespread cortical regions (Zikopoulos & Barbas, 2006). In contrast, the temporal lobe seizure may be the prototype of the corticolimbic ("localization-related" or "partial" seizure. However, some frontal lobe seizures may also show spread to ventomedial frontal cortex, in a manner similar to absence, and thus may also be considered as "corticothalamic" seizures. On the other hand, some extratemporal seizures show propagation to temporal lobe structures. Seizures classically considered to be localization-related may therefore exhibit patterns consistent with primary involvement of either corticothalamic or corticolimbic circuits. The detailed study of the specific networks involved in the major types of epileptic seizures may have broader implications as well. Close examination of how consciousness breaks down in epileptic seizures most certainly offers clues to the underlying mechanisms that bind consciousness within the large-scale networks of the cerebral cortex (Tucker & Holmes, 2011).

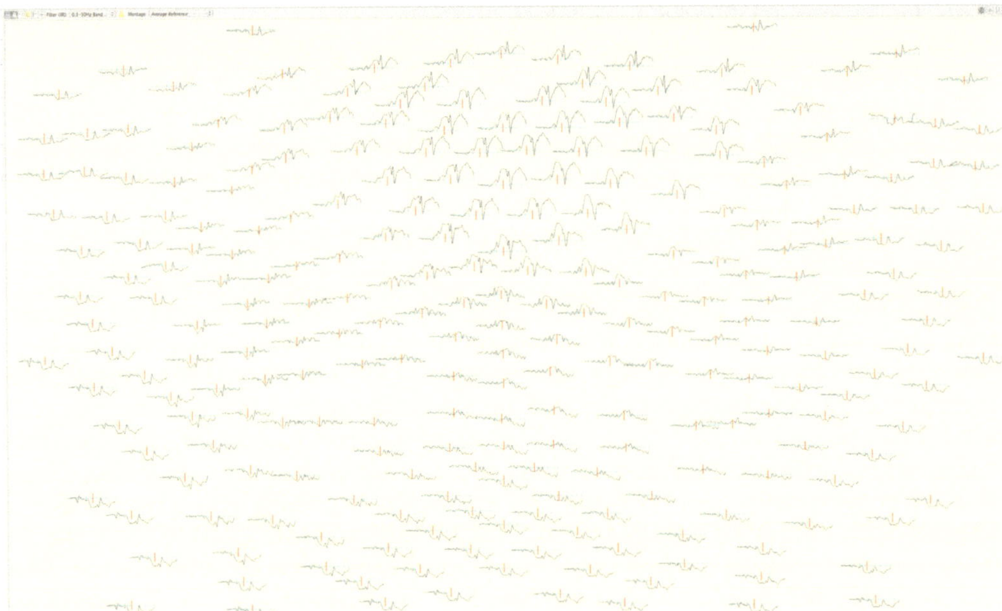

Fig. 4. Topographic display of onset of epileptiform discharges in subject with juvenile myoclonic epilepsy. Note that the discharges are not "generalized", but rather are maximal in amplitude in anterior-midline regions, and slightly lateralized to the left side. See also Fig. 5.

5. The potential role of dense array EEG in the presurgical evaluation

In addition to suggesting new insights into anatomical mechanisms of epilepsy, dEEG may be useful in assisting in localizing the site of seizure onset. Ideally, this determination should be made noninvasively, but in, practice, at least 30-50% of surgical candidates will require some form of intracranial EEG evaluation, including the majority of individuals with difficult extratemporal epilepsy (Holmes, 2006). DEEG may hold the promise to assist in ictal localization, when standard EEG methods fail, and may reduce the need for invasive studies. However, the present evidence is preliminary, as presented earlier in this chapter, and further research and validation studies are needed to establish the precise role of this technique in the presurgical evaluation; such research is necessary since complete concordance of dEEG and intracranial EEG findings is not yet available. At the very least, however, it is likely that dEEG will eventually assist in guiding the placement of invasive electrodes in some cases. As a corollary, the method may also eventually assist in planning the intracranial placement of novel treatment devices (Motamedi & Lesser, 2006). Unique methods of analyzing interictal segments of dEEG may also prove useful in localizing the epileptogenic zone. A recent study that analyzed one-minute randon, interictal segments of seizure and spike-free dEEG found that the intracranially proven epileptogenic zone corresponded closely to regions of focal increases in scalp dEEG 20-50 Hz synchronization and simultaneous decreases in coupling of theta and gamma frequencies (Fig. 6) (Ramon et al., 2008)

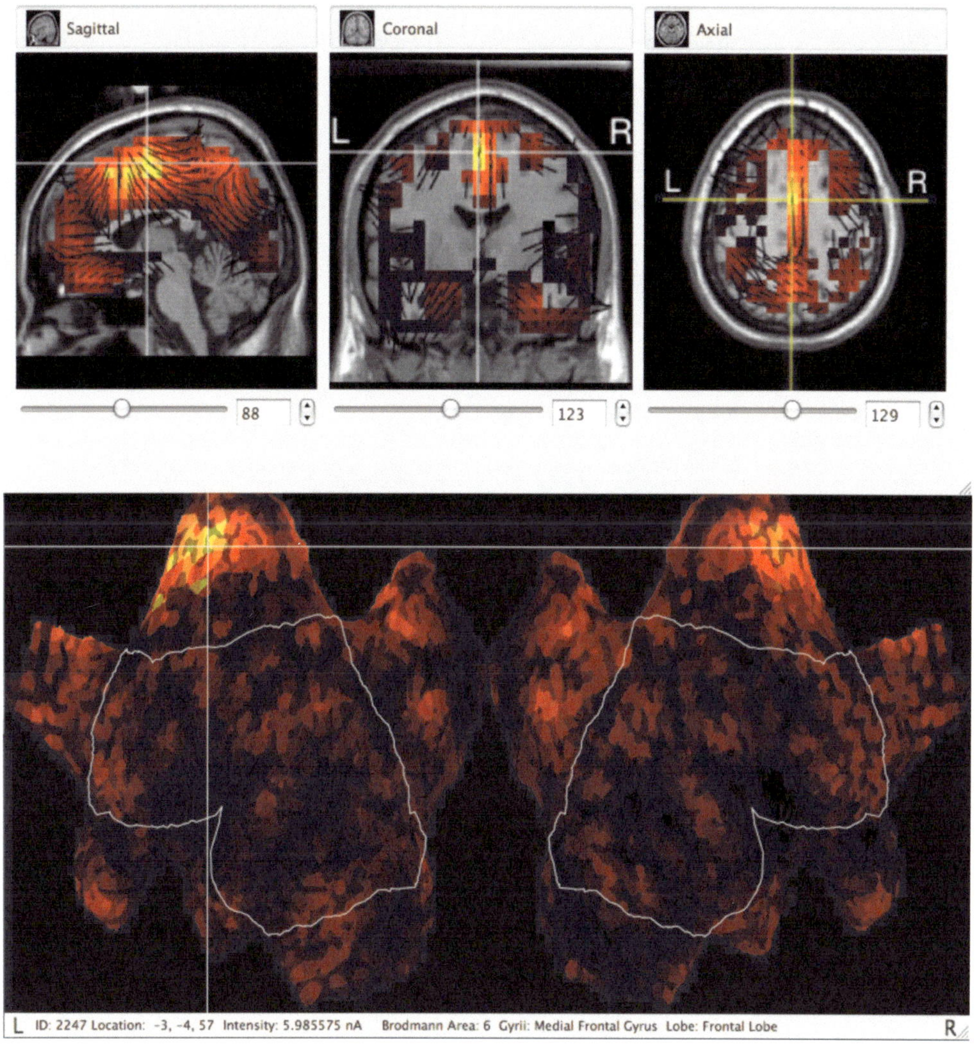

Fig. 5. Source analysis of onset of discharges in Fig. 4 (top) suggest localization of onset in medial frontal cortex. The flatmap (bottom) shows the flattened cortical surface of the standard MRI model used in source analysis, with regions of maximal intensity denoted by crosshairs.

In addition to the role that the method may play in assisting in defining the epileptogenic in the presurgical evaluation, dEEG may also prove useful in lateralizing, and even localizing, essential language regions and motor function. A recent study in surgical candidates that exmained covert naming revealed that focal increases in power of 3-7 Hz and 20-50 Hz frequencies on dEEG lateralized to the same language-dominant side as predicted by the Wada test (Ramon et al., 2009a). These patterns are not apparent on standard EEG, again emphasizing the importance of improved spatial resolution provided by dEEG. Another study that examined motor mapping of thumb and little finger using subject-specific head models and simultaneous dEEG and fMRI demonstrated convergence between the two modalities (Luu & Tucker, 2010).

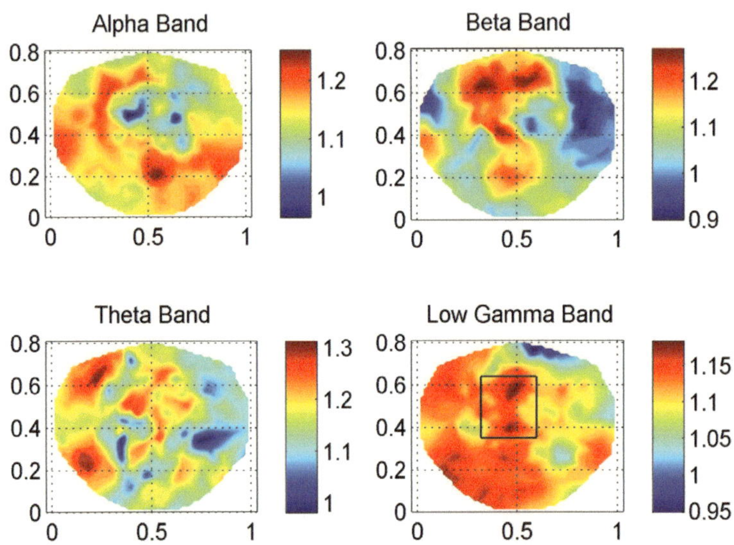

Fig. 6. Random segment of interictal dEEG free of visually apparent epileptiform discharges discloses focal increases in low gamma power (30-50 Hz) that corresponds to intracranially proven epileptogenic zone (in box, left medial frontal region) (Ramon et al, 2008).

6. Future research

Technological development in dense array EEG is anticipated in several areas with the aims of improving methodology and reliability. Firstly, the current forward model used in source analysis calculations, which utilizes a standard MRI or ellipsoidal multi-shell model, may be replaced by the individual patient's own MRI. Research is currently underway to feasibly incorporate patient-specific MRIs into source analysis algorithms. Secondly, more than 256 electrodes may eventually be recorded simultaneously from the scalp. Given that the spatial Nyquist of the human scalp EEG necessitates intersensor distances less than 3-5 mm (Freeman et al, 2003), as many as 1500 electrodes, or more, may be required to reduce interelectrode distances to achieve the ideal dimension. Furthermore, recent studies also suggest that when optimal scalp EEG spatial resolution is obtained, examination of spatial frequency patterns even make possible the extraction of details of the cortical surface anatomy, including gyral and sulcul patterns (Ramon et al., 2009b). Other future developments are likely to include the incorporation of advances in the quantitative evaluation of the onset and propagation of ictal EEG patterns, including analysis of direct current (ultraslow) frequencies (Vanhatalo et al., 2003; Miller et al., 2007), high frequency EEG (Worrell et al., 2004), and coherence and spatial pattern analysis (Freeman et al., 2006). Finally, the utility of dense array EEG in source localization of cortical activity can be evaluated, and improved, through joint recordings with whole-head magnetoencephalography (Liu et al., 2002). Future research will establish the clinical utility and role of each of these newer methods in extending the information from scalp EEG recordings.

7. Disclosure statement

The author has received no financial support, consulting fees, or research funding for the work described in this manuscript. He has no conflict of interest, financial or otherwise, in regard to the research described in this report

8. References

Avanzini G & Franceschetti S. (2003). Cellular biology of epileptogenesis. *Lancet Neurology* 2(1):33-42.

Bai X, Vestal M, Berman R, Negishi M, Spann M, Vega C, Desalvo M, Novotny E, Constable R & Blumenthal H. (2010). Dynamic time course of typical absence seizures: EEG, behavior, and functional magnetic imaging. *J Neurosci* 30(17):5884-5893.

Berg P & Scherg M. (1994). A fast method for forward computation of multiple-shellspherical head models. *Electroencephalogr Clin Neurophysiol* 90:58-64.

Bertrand O, Perrin F & Pernier J. (1985). A theoretical justification of the average-reference in topographic evoked potential studies. *Electroencephalogr Clin Neurophysiol* 62:678-695.

Bragin A, Mody I, Wilson C & Engel J Jr. (2002). Local generation of fast ripples iin epileptic brain. *J Neurosci* 22:2012-2021.

Commission on Classification and Terminology of the International League Against Against Epilepsy. (1989). Proposal for revised classification of epilepsies and epileptic syndromes. *Epilepsia* 30:389-99.

D'Ambrosio R, Fairbanks J, Fender J, Born D, Doyle D & Miller J. (2004). Post-traumatic epilepsy following fluid percussion injury in the rat. *Brain* 127:304-314.

D'Ambrosio R, Fender J, Fairbanks J, Simon E, Born D, Doyle D & Miller J. (2005). Progression from fronto-parietal to mesial-temporal epilepsy after fluid percussion injury in the rat. *Brain* 128(Pt 1):174-188.

De Munck J, Vijn P & Lopes da Silva F. (1992). A random dipole model for spontaneous brain activity. *IEEE Biomed Eng* 39:791-804.

Deppe M, Kellinghaus C, Duning T, Moddell G, Mohammadi S, Deppe K, Schiffbauer H, Kugel H, Keller S, Ringelstein E & Knecht S. (2008). Nerve fiber impairment of anterior thalamic circuitry in juvenile myoclonic epilepsy. *Neurology* 71;1981-1986

Dien J. (1998). Issues in the application of the average reference: review, critiques, and recommendations. *Behav Res Method Instrum Comput* 30:34-43.

Ebersole J. (1997). Defining epileptogenic foci: past, present, and future. *J Clin Neurophysiol* 14(6):470-483.

Engel J Jr, Van Ness P, Rasmussen T & Ojemann L. Outcome with respect to epileptic seizures. (1993) In: *Surgical Treatment of the Epilepsies,* Engel J Jr (ed), pp 609-621. Raven Press, New York.

Ferree T, Luu P, Russell G & Tucker D. (2001) Scalp electrode impedance, infection risk, and EEG data quality. *Clin Neurophysiology* 112: 536-544.

Freeman W. (1975). *Mass Action in the Nervous System*. Academic Press, New York.

Freeman W, Rogers L, Holmes M & Silbergeld D. (2000). Spatial spectral analysis of human electrocorticograms including the alpha and gamma Bands. *J Neurosci Methods* 15; 95(2):1111-1121.

Freeman W, Holmes M, Burke B & Vanhatalo S. (2003). Spatial spectra of scalp EEG and EMG from awake humans. *Clin Neurophysiol* 114:1053-1069.

Freeman W, Holmes M, West G & Vanhatalo S. (2006). Fine-grain spatiotemporal infrastructure of phase in human intracranial EEG. *Clin Neurophysiol* 117:1228-1243.

Grave de Peralta Menendez R, Murray M, Michel C, Martuzzi R & Gonzalez Andino S. (2004). Electrical neuroimaging based on biophysical constraints. *Neuroimage* 21:527-539.

Futatsugi Y & Riviello J. (1998). Mechanisns of generalized absence epilepsy. *Brain & Development* 20:75-79.

Gloor P. (1978). Generalized epilepsy with bilateral synchronous spike and wave discharges: new findings concerning its physiological mechanisms. *Electroencephalogr Clin Neurophysiol* Suppl 34:245-249.

Holmes M, Brown M & Tucker D. (2004). Are "generalized" seizures truly generalizes? Evidence of localized mesial frontal and frontopolar discharges in absence. *Epilepsia* 45(12):1568-1579.

Holmes M, Brown M & Tucker D. (2005). Dense array EEG and source analysis reveal spatiotemporal dynamics of epileptiform discharges. *Epilepsia* 46 (Suppl 8):136 (abstract).

Holmes M. (2006). Neurophysiological Studies. In: *Epilepsy Surgery: Principles & Controversies*, Miller J, Silbergeld D (eds). pp 247-269. Francis & Taylor, New York.

Holmes M, Brown M, Tucker D, Saneto R, Miller K, Wig G & Ojemann J. (2008). Localization of extratemporal seizure with noninvasive dense array EEG. *Pediatric Neurosurgery* 44(6):474-479.

Holmes M, Tucker D, Quiring J, Hakimian S, Miller J & Ojemann J.(2010a). Comparing dense array EEG and intracranial EEG for source localization of seizures. *Neurosurgery* 66 (2):354-362.

Holmes M, Brown M & Tucker D. (2010b) Evidence that juvenile myoclonic epilepsy is disorder of frontothalamic corticothalamic networks. *Neuroimage* 49(1):80-93.

Junghofer M, Elbert T, Tucker D & Braun C. (1999). The polar average reference effect:a bias in estimating the head surface integral in EEG recording. *Clin Neurophysiol* 110:1149-1155.

Lantz G, Grave de Peralta R, Spinelli L, Seeck M & Michel C. (2003). Epileptic source localization with high density EEG: how many electrodes are needed? *Clin Neurophysiol* 114:63-69

Lin K, Carrette H Jr, Lin J, Peruchi M, Filho G, Guaranha M, Guilhoto L, Sakamoto A & Yacubian E. (2009). Mahnetic resonance spectroscopy reveals an epileptic network in juvenile myoclonic epilepsy. *Epilepsia* 50(5):1191-2000

Liu A, Dale A & Belliveau J. (2002). Monte Carlo simulation studies of EEG and MEG localization accuracy. *Hum Brain Mapp* 16:47-62.

Lopes da Silva F, Storm van Leeuwen W (1978). The cortical alpha rhythm in dog: The depth and surface profile of phase. In: *Architectonics of Cerebral Cortex.* Brazier M, Petsche H (eds). Raven Press, New York.

Luu P & Tucker D. (2010). Simultaneous EEG-fMRI recordings of activity from primary motor cortex in asingle subject. *Human Brain Mapping Conference*, June 5-10, Barcelona, Spain (abstract).

McCormick D. (2002). Cortical and subcortical generators of normal and abnormal rhymthmicity. *Int Rev Neurobiol* 49:99-114.

Michel C, Thut G, Morand S, Khateb A, Pegna A, Grave de Peralta R, Gonzales S, Seeck M & Landis T. (2001). Electric source imaging of human brain function. *Brain Res Rev* 36:108-118.

Michel C, Murray M, Lantz G, Gonzales S, Spinelli L & Grave de Peralta R. (2004). EEG source imaging. *Clin Neurophysiol* 115(10):2194-2222.

Miller J, Kim W, Holmes M & Vanhatalo S. (2007). Ictal localization by source analysis analysis of infraslow activity in DC-coupled scalp EEG recordings. *Neuroimage* 35 (2):583-597.

Morrell F, Whisler W, Bleck T. (1989) Multiple subpial transaction: a new approach to the surgical treatment of focal epilepsy. *J Neurosurg* 70:231-239.

Motamedi G & Lesser R. (2006). Prospects for developing electrical stimulation of the cortex for treatment of intractable seizures. In: *Epilepsy Surgery: Principles & Controversies*, Miller J, Silbergeld D (eds). pp 810-819, Francis & Taylor, New York.

Nemani V & Binder D. (2005). Emerging role of gap junctions in epilepsy. Histol Histopathol 20(1):253-259.

Niedermeyer E. (1999). Abnormal EEG patterns: epileptic and paroxysmal. In: *Electroencephalography: Basic Principles, Clinical Applications, and Related Fields* (4th edition). Niedermeyer E, Lopes da Silva F (eds). pp 235-260, Williams & Wilkins, Baltimore.

Noebels J. (2003). The biology of epilepsy genes. *Annu Rev Neurosci* 26:599-625.

Nunez P, Srinivasan R. (2006). *Electric Fields of the Brain: Neurophysics of EEG* (2nd edition). Oxford University Press, New York.

Pasqual-Marqui R, Essen M, Kochi K & Lehmann D. (2002). Functional imaging with low-resolution brain electromagnetic tomography (LORETA): a review. *Method Find Exp Clin Pharmacol* 24 Suppl C:91-95.

Panayiotopoulos C. (2002). Idiopathic generalized epilepsies. In: *A Clinical Guide to Epileptic Syndromes and their Treatment*, Panayiotopoulos C. pp 114-160, Bladen Medical Publishing, Oxfordshire, UK.

Perrin F, Pernier J, Bertrand O, Giard M & Echallier J (1987). Mapping of scalp potentials by surface spline interpolation. *Electroencephalogr Clin Neurophysiol* 66:75-81.

Phillips C, Rugg M & Friston K. (2002). Anatomically informed basis functions for EEG source localization: Combining functional and anatomical constraints *Neuroimage* 16:678-695.

Ramon C, Holmes M, Freeman W, McElroy R & Rezvanian E. (2008). Comparative analysis of temporal dynamics of EEG and phase synchronization of EEG to localize epileptic sites from high density scalp EEG interictal recordings. *30th Conf Proc IEEE Eng Med Biol Soc* 4538-4550.

Ramon C, Holmes M, Freeman W, Gratkowski M, Eriksen J & Haueisen J. (2009a), Power spectral density changes and language lateralization during covert object naming tasks measured with high-density EEG recordings. *Epilepsy Behav* 14:54-59.

Ramon C, Freeman W, Holmes M, Ishimaru A, Hauseien J, Schimpf P & Rezvanian E (2009b). Similarities between simulated spatial spectra of scalp EEG, MEG, and structural MRI. *Brain Topogr* 22:191-196.

Rodin E, Rodin M & Thompson J. (1994). Source analysis of generalized spike-wave wave complexes. *Brain Topogr*7:113-119.

Salman A, Turovets S, Malony A, Eriksen J & Tucker D. (2005). Computational modeling of human head conductivity. Paper presented at *Computational Science-ICCS 5th International Conference*. Atlanta, GA, USA (abstract).

Scherg M & Ebersole J. (1994). Brain source imaging of focal and multifocal epileptiform EEG activity. *Clin Neurophysiol* 24:51-60.

Scherg M, Ille N, Bornfleth H & Berg P. (2002). Advanced tools for digital EEG review: virtual source montages, whole-head mapping, correlation, and phase ananlysis. *J Clin Neurophysiol* 19:91-112.

Shah M, Anderson A, Leung V, Lin X, & Johnston D. (2004). Seizure-induced plasticity of *h* channels in entorhinal cortical layer III pyramidal neurons. *Neuron* 44(3):495-508.

Slaght S, Leresche N, Deniau J, Crunelli V & Charpier S. (2002). Activity of thalamic reticular neurons during spontaneous genetically determined spike and wave discharges. *J Neurosci* 22:2323-2334.

Spencer S. (2002). Neural networks in human epilepsy: evidence of and implications for treatment. *Epilepsia* 43(3):219-227.

Stables J, Bertram E, White H, Coulter D, Dichter M, Jacobs M, Loscher W, Lowenstein D, Moshe S, Noebels J & Davis M (2002). Models for epilepsy and epileptogenesis: Report from the NIH workshop, Bethesda, Maryland. *Epilepsia* 43(11): 1410-1420.

Steriade M (2003). *Neuronal Substrates of Sleep and Epilepsy*. New York: Cambridge University Press.

Tae W, Kim S, Joo E, Han S, Kim I, Kim S, Lee J-M & Hong S. (2008). Cortical thickness abnormality in juvenile myoclonic epilepsy. *J Neurol* 255(4):561-566.

Thompson P, Rae J, Weber L, Pearson C, Goldshtein Z & Holmes M. (2008). Long- term seizure monitoring using a 256 contact dense array system. *Am J END Tech* 48:93-106.

Tucker D, Liotti M, Potts G, Russell G & Posner M. (1994). Spatiotemporal analysis of brain electrical fields. *Hum Brain Mapp* 1:134-152.

Tucker D, Brown M, Luu P & Holmes M. (2007). Discharges in ventromedial frontal cortex during absence spells. *Epilepsy Behav* 11 (4):546-557.

Tucker D & Holmes M. (2011). Fractures and bindings of consciousness: studying how seizures impair awareness may yield clues to the way that cconscious experience is organized within large-scale cerebral networks. *American Scientist* January-February: 32-39.

Vanhatalo S, Holmes M, Tallgren P, Voipio J, Kaila K & Miller J. (2003). Very slow EEG responses lateralizes temporal lobe seizures: a noninvasive DC-EEG study. *Neurology* 60(7):1098-1103.

White H. (2002). Animal models of epileptogenesis. *Neurology* 59(9) Suppl 5: S7-S14.

Wilson H & Cowan J. (1973). A mathematical theory of the functional dynamics of cortical and thalamic nervous tissue. *Kybernetik* 13:55-80.

Worrell G., Parish L, Cranstoun S, Jonas R, Baltuch G & Litt B. (2004). High- frequency oscillations and seizure generation in neocortical epilepsy. *Brain* 127(Pt7), 1496-1506.

Yamazaki M, Tucker D, Fujimoto A, Yamazoe T, Okanishi Tohru T, Yokota T, Enoki H & Yamamoto T. (2010). Comparison of dense array EEG with simultaneous intracranial ECoG for interictal spike detection and localization. *American Epilespy Society Annual Meeting*, San Antonio Tx, Dec 4-7 (abstract).

Zikopoulos B & Barbas H. (2006). Prefrontal projections to the thalamic reticular nucleus from a unique circuit for attentional mechanisms. *J Neurosci* 26 (28):7348-7361.

Part 5

Psychosocial Aspect of Epilepsy

9

Positive Psychosocial Variables and Outcome Variables in Persons with Epilepsy

J. Pais-Ribeiro[1] and R. F. Meneses[2]
[1]*FPCE-Universidade do Porto*
[2]*FCHS-Universidade Fernando Pessoa*
Portugal

1. Introduction

Epilepsy is a chronic disease and the world's most common serious neurological disorder (International League Against Epilepsy [ILAE], 2003a; Jacoby, 2002). Epilepsy is the name for a group of functional disorders of the brain, characterised by repetitive seizures, caused by abnormal, excessive electric discharges of the nerve cells or neurones in the brain (ILAE, 2003b). Between 5% (ILAE, 2003b) and 11% of the population experience at least one seizure at some point (Hauser & Hesdorffer, 1990), but not everybody who experiences an epileptic seizure will develop epilepsy. A diagnosis of epilepsy requires that the patient has had a minimum of two unprovoked seizures (ILAE, 2003b).

Nowadays, the new generation of antiepileptic drugs and treatment adherence (i.e., proper use of pharmacological agents and compliance to life style orientations) guarantee that the majority of patients do not have seizures and can maintain a normal life, with a low cognitive and aesthetic impact of the disease. Nevertheless, epilepsy therapy may be prolonged and a cure not always attainable.

The prognosis for seizure control is very good, and with appropriate therapy approximately 75% of patients with epilepsy become seizure free (ILAE, 2003a). Epilepsy is, nonetheless, a chronic disease, i.e., a disorder that persists for an extended period and affects a person's ability to function normally. Seizure control (caused by pharmacological treatment or surgery, for instance) does not necessarily mean absence of epilepsy.

The impact of epilepsy may be greater than that of some other chronic conditions, partly because of the unpredictability of seizures, and partly because of the associated stigma. In fact, research indicates that seizure disorders are often associated with a variety of psychological and social problems, as well as malaise (Collings, 1990, 1995; Jacoby et al., 1996) and social and political isolation. Thus, as any other chronic illness, epilepsy has the potential to induce profound changes in a person's life, resulting in negative effects on quality of life (QOL) and wellbeing (de Ridder et al., 2008).

In this context, improvement of the psychosocial health of people with epilepsy is a relevant issue for researchers and clinicians, making it important to understand psychosocial dimensions associated with the disease that facilitate epilepsy patients' adjustment. Psychosocial health depends on adjustment to epilepsy. It is a process that has a start and an end point: it can be assessed by the results, or as an end point, and can be viewed by its positive side (positive adjustment) and not as an adjustment disorder.

2. Adjustment to chronic disease

What does it mean to adjust to a chronic disease? The literature suggests three main conclusions: (a) a chronic disease requires adjustment across multiple life domains, (b) adjustment unfolds over time, and (c) there is marked heterogeneity across individuals in how they adjust to chronic disease.

Adjustment is a process that begins at the presentation of symptoms and continues throughout the course of the illness and responds to changes in illness status (Sharp & Curran, 2006). It can be defined as a response to a change in the environment that allows an organism to become more suitably adapted to that change (Sharpe & Curran, 2006). It refers to the healthy rebalancing by patients to their new circumstances (de Ridder et al., 2008). However, for about 30% of patients, the adjustment phase is prolonged and sometimes unsuccessful (de Ridder et al., 2008). The above definition implies that adjustment occurs over time, and often refers to a desirable state or endpoint. de Ridder et al. (2008) and Stanton et al. (2007) report key elements of successful adjustment to a chronic illness: (a) the successful performance of adaptive tasks (e.g., adjustment to disability, maintained emotional balance, and preservation of healthy relationships); (b) the absence of psychological disorders; (c) the presence of low negative affect and high positive affect; (d) adequate functional (e.g., work) status; (e) and the satisfaction and wellbeing in various life domains.

Several models have been proposed on how patients could achieve these outcomes, namely (de Ridder et al., 2008): the model of cognitive adaptation, which emphasises illness acceptance and perceptions of control over illness; the personality model that emphasises the role of personality factors in adjustment; and the stress and coping model that emphasises strategies used by patients to deal with adaptive tasks imposed by disease. All the models presuppose relationships between different kinds of psychosocial and behavioural variables.

In other words, the adjustment process includes contextual, disease, and personal characteristics, more stable (like personality) or more elusive (more easily influenced by training or education, like stigma perception, coping, positive psychological state, adherence to treatment, social support, psychosomatic symptoms, spiritual beliefs, and life events), and their conjoint impact on outcome variables (health status perception, health related quality of life - HRQOL -, and subjective happiness).

In this context, the objective of the present study is to discuss the role of psychosocial variables in adjustment to everyday life in persons with epilepsy.

3. Adjustment challenges

When adjustment is unsuccessful, mental health problems/personality disorders may become (more) evident or more intense. Inversely, these situations can make adjustment more difficult. One should, nevertheless, bear in mind that what can be seen as a personality trait may, in fact, be an attempt to compensate deficits, namely, cognitive deficits (Devinsky & Najjar, 1999; Hermann & Whitman, 1984; Perrine & Kiolbasa, 1999). It is also worth stressing that the concept of epileptic personality has become, a long time ago, obsolete, since only a part of patients is at risk of developing characteristic personality traits (that present themselves in a highly variable degree) (Blumer, 1991, 1999). However, some epileptic patients present "strange" personalities that do not fulfill the criteria for specific psychiatric disorders (Perrine & Kiolbasa, 1999).

In this context, timing may be a crucial element. In fact, research data suggest that epilepsy onset in adolescence influences the development of adult personality traits: patients with epilepsy onset during adolescence had higher neuroticism compared with normative data and other patients; high neuroticism, particularly when accompanied by lower extraversion, predisposed to poor adjustment to chronic epilepsy as reflected by impaired mood and difficulties with family functioning (Wilson et al., 2009).

But even when psychological and psychosomatic symptoms are absent, and the patient is successfully adjusting to living with epilepsy, there are no guaranties that significant others will not have difficulty adjusting to the situation. In fact, epilepsy has a significant impact on both the physical and psychological functioning of family members and other informal carers (Lee et al., 2002). Behrouzian and Neamatpour (2010), for example, report that the prevalence of symptoms of depression and anxiety was increased in mothers of epilepsy patients.

3.1 Psychological/psychiatric symptoms

Research suggests that personality traits or psychiatric presentation of patients with epilepsy have special features, resulting in a higher prevalence of psychiatric diagnoses, such as depression and psychosis, when compared with the general population (Locke et al., 2010). Vuilleumier and Jallon (1998) report that the overall prevalence of psychiatric disturbances in epileptic patients can be estimated between 20 and 30 per cent, with psychotic disorders, depression, and suicide as the three most common among interictal disturbances. An epidemiological study with 36,984 subjects, aiming to explore numerous aspects of mental health in persons with epilepsy in the community, compared with those without epilepsy, found an increased prevalence of mental health disorders, including a higher prevalence of suicidal ideation, when compared with the general population (Tellez-Zenteno et al., 2007). However, data about psychiatric disorders associated with epilepsy are heterogeneous with great variability and discordance in results encountered in epidemiologic studies.

Psychiatric disturbances correlate positively with the multiplicity of seizures but often inversely with their frequency. The overall risk might be the highest during the first years after diagnosis of epilepsy, as well as in patients with temporal lobe foci, previous depression, or psychosis. In a study with 2152 persons with epilepsy in Norway, Naess, et al. (2007) found that seizure frequency, medication side effects, and co-morbidity are strongly related to self-reported psychological distress. In another study, comparing people with intellectual disability and epilepsy with people with intellectual disability and no epilepsy, Arshad et al. (2011) found that rates of mental health problems, including those in the schizophrenia spectrum, personality and anxiety disorders, were significantly lower among patients with epilepsy.

Depressive disorders are the most common type of psychiatric co-morbidity in patients with epilepsy: they have various clinical presentations, some typical of the different types of mood disorders in non-epileptic patients, others constituting rather frequent atypical presentations that can easily go unrecognized (Kanner & Balabanov, 2002). The prevalence of anxiety symptoms is also higher in patients with epilepsy than in the general population or with other chronic medical disorders (Beyenburg et al., 2005).

Studying anxiety and depression in persons with epilepsy, Meneses et al. (2008), Pais-Ribeiro et al. (2007), and Trueman and Duthie (1998) found that patients reported having both anxiety and depression levels characterised as mild, moderate and severe, although comparisons with other groups of persons with other chronic diseases, or no disease, showed lower levels of anxiety and depression.

3.2 Psychosomatic symptoms

Unsuccessful adjustment may also be accompanied by psychosomatic symptoms. "The psychosomatic symptom (PS) remains without an aetiological explanation, albeit the innumerous studies from diverse areas of biological and psychological knowledge" (Salim, 2007, p. 234). Consequently, Salim presents a review of the psychoanalytic theory of the PS and other lines of thought central to his aim: "to present the hypothesis that the etiology of the PS has a relationship with traumatic recurrence and autistic withdrawal", both of which are "instinctive biological responses to soothe and prolong life" (2007, p. 234). He finishes his article stressing the need to develop more studies involving psychoanalysts, psychiatrists and neuroscientists" (Salim, 2007, p. 238).

In this context, Nagane et al. (2009) investigated individual variation in the levels of growth hormone in healthy students (21-22 years) and had them rate their psychosomatic symptoms, with a self-assessment questionnaire (five items pertaining to physical symptoms - drowsiness, poor appetite, heaviness in the head, dizziness, whole-body fatigue - and five to mental symptoms - lack of motivation, easily irritated, feelings of melancholy, desire to rest, anxiety), twice a day. They concluded that "psychosomatic symptoms may be associated with circadian dysfunction, as inferred from blunted rhythmicity in growth hormone secretion".

In a more recent study, Åslund et al. (2010) asked students between 13-18 years old how often they suffered from: headache, stomach ache, feelings of nervousness, feelings of irritation, and sleep problems, as a mean to assess their psychosomatic symptoms. Based on the answers, 6.4% of the boys and 20.4% of the girls were classified as having many psychosomatic symptoms; girls reported more psychosomatic symptoms; individuals within the group with low neighbourhood social capital had approximately double the odds of having many psychosomatic symptoms compared with those with high neighbourhood social capital, while individuals within the group with low general social trust had a more than a three times increased odds of having many psychosomatic symptoms compared with the group with high general social trust; parental unemployment and low subjective SES were also related to psychosomatic symptoms.

Consequently, it is surprising to verify that, although psychosomatic symptoms have been studied for so long, there are fewer articles than could be expected on the psychosomatic symptoms of individuals with epilepsy, suggesting that the scientific community hasn't been very interested in analyzing them.

3.3 Stigma perception

Dell (1986) defined stigma as a distinctive feature in an individual and the devaluation society places on that difference. Stigmatisation is most effective if the stigmatised person holds the same belief as the society, as it often occurs in people with epilepsy. Despite the important actual clinical and therapeutic progress, people with epilepsy continue to suffer from discrimination (ILAE, 2003d). In fact, epilepsy is often surrounded by prejudice and myth, which can be overcome only with enormous difficulties (Austin et al., 2004).

These difficulties can be even greater in some developmental periods. For instance, in adolescents with epilepsy, stigma is a complex concept to investigate because it involves personal attitudes and beliefs, elements of secrecy and disclosure management, and influences from the social environment (Austin et al., 2004). It is widely expected that reducing stigma should help adolescents (and older patients) with epilepsy experience an improved QOL (Austin et al., 2002).

In fact, DiIorio et al. (2003) found that participants reporting higher levels of perceived stigma also reported lower levels of self-efficacy to manage epilepsy, more negative outcome expectancies related to treatment and seizures, lower levels of medication management, medication adherence, and patient satisfaction, greater management of information related to seizures. They also found that other demographic and disease variables, like income, age at first seizure, seizures during the past year, lower self-efficacy, negative outcome expectancies for seizures, and satisfaction explained important variance in perceived stigma. Stigma was also associated with interactions of seizure worry and employment status, self-efficacy and social support, and quality care and age at seizure onset (Smith et al., 2009) and predicted depressive symptoms at baseline, 3 months, and 6 months (Reisinger & DiIorio, 2009), as well as QOL at a later time (Whatley et al., 2010).

As a result, stigma-reducing interventions focused on individuals with epilepsy probably reduce epilepsy's health burden and decrease the emotional impact of epilepsy (Birbeck, 2006).

Research found that there are cross-cultural significant differences in stigma perception between patients from European countries (Baker et al., 1999). Baker (2002) report that the factors that best predict epilepsy stigma are seizure frequency, knowledge of epilepsy, duration of epilepsy, and seizure type.

All that has been said so far underscores the importance of knowing the (psychosocial) variables associated to successful adjustment. In fact, variables like hope, optimism, and spirituality are among the positive variables useful to consider when organizing programs to help patients adjust to a life with disease.

4. Adjustment and psychosocial variables

4.1 Hope

Hope is defined as the perceived capability to derive Pathways to desired goals, and motivate oneself via Agency thinking to use those pathways (Snyder, 2002). The hope construct includes agency thoughts that "tape the perceived capacity to initiate (causal capacity) and sustain (agentic capacity and action-control beliefs) movement toward desired goals" (Little et al., 2006, p. 72).

Rustøen et al. (2005) found that hope scores differed significantly between hospitalized heart failure patients and the general population (for 7 of the 12 items and global score), being that patients reported higher (better) hope. Hope was associated with patients' level of satisfaction and number of associated comorbid diseases, and was predicted by self-assessment of health and satisfaction with life.

In another study, patients with end stage renal disease identified hope as central to the process of advance care planning: it helped them determine future goals of care and provided insight into the benefits of advance care planning and their willingness to engage in end of life discussions (Davison & Simpson, 2006).

Additionally, research suggests that people with higher levels of hope cope with disease more effectively (Chi, 2007; Elliott et al., 1991; Snyder, 2002). Nonetheless, research on patients' hope (namely, epileptic patients) is not easy to find (cf. Lohne, 2001).

4.2 Optimism

Optimism is a global generalized tendency to believe that one will usually experience good versus bad outcomes in life (Scheier & Carver, 1985, 1992). Research asserts that optimism and pessimism strongly influence physical health and help people cope with chronic diseases (Aspinwall et al., 2001; Ebert et al., 2002; Scheier & Carver, 1992).

In a sample of general medical outpatients, a pessimistic explanatory style (Optimism-Pessimism scale of the Minnesota Multiphasic Personality Inventory) was significantly associated with a self-report of poorer physical and mental functioning (SF-36) 30 years later; scores on all 8 health domains were significantly poorer in the pessimistic group than in both the optimistic and the mixed group (Maruta et al., 2002). Moreover, it is believed that optimism can serve as a protective factor when facing difficulties in life such as illness (Fournier et al., 2002; Giltay et al., 2004, 2006).

The same happens with epilepsy: Pais-Ribeiro et al. (2007) found that optimism is the variable that best contributes to mental health status perception and QOL in persons with epilepsy. It was found that: (a) optimism/pessimism are strong predictors of QOL; (b) optimism/pessimism do not predict objective health (assessed by the objective physical disability rating scale); (c) optimism does not have a stronger effect on objective health or QOL for one diagnostic group relative to the other (right temporal lobe epilepsy, left temporal lobe epilepsy, psychogenic non-epileptic seizures) (Kent, 2008); (d) explanatory style (i.e., optimistic explanations for negative events are attributed to external causes that temporarily affect specific domains of one's life) are not good predictors of seizure load in individuals with temporal lobe epilepsy (Donnelly, 2010); and (e) in adults with intractable epileptic seizures and psychogenic nonepileptic seizures, both optimism and pessimism are good predictors of seizure group, and attributional style is an index of personality and cognitive response to stress (Griffith, 2008). Nevertheless, optimism seems an under-recognised variable in the context of epilepsy research.

4.3 Self-efficacy

Self-efficacy or "efficacy expectation is the conviction that one can successfully execute the behaviour required to produce the outcomes" (Bandura, 1977, p. 193), predicting "with considerable accuracy the level of performance" (Bandura & Adams, 1977, pp. 303-304). I.e., "given appropriate skills and adequate incentives... efficacy expectations are a major determinant of people's choice of activities, how much effort they will expend, and of how long they will sustain effort in dealing with stressful situations" (Bandura, 1977, p. 194).

Being so, this variable has been occupying a central place on Health Psychology (Ribeiro, n.d.). In epilepsy research, the development of an instrument to measure self-efficacy in persons with epilepsy, based on Bandura's self-efficacy theory (Dilorio et al., 1992), would suggest this context presents no exception. Furthermore, considering the concept's definition, one would expect studies on self-efficacy to increase in the context of the Positive Psychology movement. But this does not seem to be the case.

Be as it may, research has showed that self-efficacy (in epilepsy) correlates or predicts social support, self-management, lifestyle management, depressive symptoms, and QOL (Amir et al., 1999; Begley et al., 2010; Dilorio et al., 1992; Lee et al., 2010; Robinson et al., 2008). Additionally, self-management, depressive symptoms, and seizure severity predict self-reported epilepsy self-efficacy, as do patient satisfaction and stigma, while social support and regimen-specific support do not (DiIorio et al., 2006).

Moreover, improvements in (seizure) self-efficacy of individuals with epilepsy can be obtained with interventions like WebEase, an Internet-based self-management program (DiIorio et al., 2009), and even with an educational intervention without a psychological component (Frizzell et al., 2011).

4.4 Social support

Social support can be defined as the existence or availability of individuals in whom we can trust, that show us they care about us, value us, and like us (Sarason et al., 1983). Nevertheless, there is no consensus on its definition, since there are numerous ways to characterize/classify the social domain (Berkman, 1984; Bruhn & Philips, 1984; Cassel, 1976; Cobb, 1976; Cohen, 1988; Kaplan et al., 1977; Taylor, 1990), and several types/dimensions of social support (Cohen & McKay, 1984; Cramer et al., 1997; Dunst & Trivette, 1990; Singer & Lord, 1984; Weiss, 1974). Researchers tend, however, to agree on the multidimensionality of social support and that its different aspects have diverse effects on individuals or groups (e.g., Ridder & Schreurs, 1996).

Even though the process is not clear (Pais-Ribeiro, 1999), the strong relation between social support and numerous health/disease indicators is very robust (Broadhead et al., 1983; Ell et al., 1992; Hanson et al., 1989; Kessler et al., 1985; Ornelas, 1996; Rutter & Quine, 1996; Schwarzer & Leppin, 1989, 1991; Thomason et al., 1996; Wethingston & Kessler, 1986).

In epilepsy patients, social support is related to/predicts: self-rated health status, life satisfaction (Elliott et al., 2011), depressive symptoms (Lee et al., 2010; Reisinger & DiIorio, 2009; Robinson et al., 2008), self-management (Begley et al., 2010), and QOL (Amir et al., 1999; Choi-Kwon et al., 2003; Whatley et al., 2010). Social support is also a mediator between disease severity and mastery (Amir et al., 1999).

Consequently, it is not surprising that researchers defend that clinicians should encourage epilepsy patients to improve their social support (e.g., Elliott et al., 2011), developing programs that improve it (e.g., DiIorio et al., 2009).

4.5 Spiritual beliefs

Spirituality, namely spiritual beliefs, has been increasingly considered when caring for and studying chronic patients (cf. Meneses, 2006). Among all the theoretical contradictions (Hill & Pargament, 2003; Miller & Thoresen, 2003), one thing is certain - spirituality and religiosity are not interchangeable: spirituality implies "a polyhedron-like relation with the transcendent that can be experienced through religiosity and its expressions (doctrinal, celebrative and/or moral-behavioural) or through occurrences associated with art, philosophy, nature, etc." (Valiente-Barroso & García-García, 2010, p. 226).

Similarly, Koenig et al. (2001, as cited in Moreira-Almeida & Koenig, 2006, p. 844) argue that religion "is an organized system of beliefs, practices, rituals, and symbols designed to facilitate closeness to the sacred or transcendent (God, higher power, or ultimate truth/reality)", while spirituality "is the personal quest for understanding answers to ultimate questions about life, about meaning, and about relationship with the sacred or transcendent, which may (or may not) lead to or arise from the development of religious rituals and the formation of community".

Gardner (2001, as cited in Valiente-Barroso & García-García, 2010, p. 226) refers to a "spiritual intelligence", an ability included in the "existential intelligence", i.e., "the ability to place oneself in relation with the cosmos, and in relation with existential traces of the human condition, like the meaning of life, the meaning of death, interpersonal love or the artistic experience". In this context, Emmons et al. (1998, as cited in Valiente-Barroso & García-García, 2010, p. 227) present a list of abilities of the spiritual intelligence: transcendence, ability to reach enlightened consciousness states (mystic experience regarding the sacred), ability to give significance to the activities and events with a sense of sacred, ability to reuse spiritual resources to solve life problems, and ability to behave in a virtuous manner".

In the past decades spirituality has caught the attention of organizations like the World Health Organization and various spirituality indicators have been analyzed in diverse populations, namely those outside the healthcare system (e.g., Panzini et al., 2011). In university students, for instance, it was found that: (a) reports were very heterogeneous; (b) those with religion reported higher Connectedness to a spiritual being or force, Spiritual strength and Faith; (c) those without health problems reported higher Inner peace/serenity/harmony; (d) longer duration of health problems was related to higher Awe, Wholeness & integration, Spiritual strength, Inner peace/serenity/harmony, and Hope & optimism, stressing the need for longitudinal studies to clarify the role Inner peace/serenity/harmony has throughout the course of disease; (e) spirituality was related to QOL (Meneses et al., 2010a, 2010b). Nurses' spiritual well-being was found to be globally positive, with most nurses referring it was important to offer patients spiritual assistance, even though most had no training (undergraduate, graduate or other Nursing courses) to give spiritual assistance (Pedrão & Beresin, 2010).

In fact, spirituality seems to play an important role in the QOL, health, disease (progression) and even cure (p.e., Chattopadhyay, 2007; Gallagher et al., 2002; Koenig, 2000, 2004; Mueller et al., 2001; Pais-Ribeiro et al., 2004; Post et al., 2000; Rippentrop, 2005; Seawaerd, 2000; Tate & Forchheimer, 2002), and religious needs assessments, as well as spiritually focused therapy may positively impact illness adjustment (Lavery & O'Hea, 2010). There have been, nevertheless, plenty of contradictory data, whose meaning remains uncertain (cf. Powell et al., 2003; Rippentrop, 2005). Some even question if spirituality can, or should, be scientifically studied (Miller & Thoresen, 2003).

When searching for research reports on epilepsy patients' spiritual beliefs, one essentially finds studies on complementary/traditional/alternative healing methods (e.g., traditional spiritual healing), not always regarding epilepsy, even though many go beyond epilepsy patients (Azaizeh et al., 2010; Coleman et al., 2002; Ismail et al., 2005; Shaikh & Hatcher, 2005; Winkler et al., 2010).

Valiente-Barroso and García-García (2010), reviewing some of the phenomena regarding altered consciousness states associated with spirituality, in order to clarify its neurological basis, focused on some forms of epilepsy related to religious spirituality and on mystic states due to hallucinogens. They argued that "regarding the interictal spiritual phenomenology, one should consider not only the underlying neurological mechanisms, but also the influence of psychosocial factors in order to gain a deeper understanding of this phenomenon" (Valiente-Barroso & García-García, 2010, p. 230).

Giovagnoli et al. (2009) explored the role of spirituality (defining it as the complex of personal transcendence, connectedness, purpose, and values) in determining QOL in chronic neurological disorders (epilepsy, brain tumors, ischemic or immune-mediate brain damage), comparing patients with healthy controls. Patients reported worse QOL, with no difference between the patient subgroups. Mood, Cognition, Inner Energy, schooling, and subjective health status correlated with QOL, but only Mood and Inner Energy predicted QOL.

In another study, QOL indicators of focal epilepsy patients were significantly predicted by spiritual (namely, Awe and Transcendence), mood, and cognition factors, highlighting the contribution of spirituality to QOL in epilepsy (Giovagnoli et al., 2006).

4.6 Coping

A recurrent construct seems to be coping, since it is through it that several variables "operate". For instance, life events (e.g., a chronic diagnosis) may have a smaller impact on an individual (e.g., on his/her QOL) if s/he is able to use adequate coping resources/strategies. Additionally, conceptualizing religious coping multidimensionally, one might find a negative relationship between negative religious coping and illness adjustment (Lavery & O'Hea, 2010).

Having seizures and/or taking care of someone with seizures can be a challenge for an individual personal coping style, i.e., "person's typical response when dealing with stressful life-events or smaller problems in daily life" (Westerhuis et al., 2011, p. 37). In fact, research has shown that partial epilepsy patients used mainly palliative reaction patterns, active confronting, and avoidance; the prevalence of their coping styles differed from the coping styles of the reference Dutch population; and a passive coping style predicted QOL (Westerhuis et al., 2011).

According to the Turkish version of the Ways of Coping Inventory, and to a two dimensional coping styles - problem-focused efficient ways of coping (self-confidence, optimism, seeking social support) and emotion-focused inefficient ways of coping (submissiveness, helplessness), adolescents with epilepsy had lower self-confidence and overall lower problem-focused ways of coping than controls; lower self-esteem and emotion-focused coping and higher self-esteem and problem-focused ways of coping were associated; those with higher total problem behaviors also had lower problem-focused ways of coping (Çengel-Kültür et al., 2009).

Piazzini et al. (2007) also found differences in coping responses, but between other samples: drug-resistant patients seemed to adopt the "denial" and the "exclusion" strategies more, while seizure-free subjects used the "control" strategy more; and "control" was associated with better social adaptation.

Furthermore, patients with refractory epilepsy tend to present themselves in a clinical encounter with a neurologist as resourceful and in control of their condition, but analyzing subtle linguistic and interactional features it becomes clear that some find their disorder quite difficult to cope with (Monzoni & Reuber, 2009).

The same can be said of epilepsy patients' families, since a child's illness is a critical event that places additional stress and burden on families (McCubbin & Patterson, 1983, as cited in Modi, 2009). Parents of children with new-onset epilepsy reported the highest levels of stress regarding finances, disciplining their child with epilepsy, concerns about education, and their marital relationships, but no significant differences were found between patients' parents and controls (without epilepsy) on parenting stress (Modi, 2009). In another sample, mothers' coping profiles were not correlated with the adolescents' and there were no significant differences between the coping profiles of mothers of the epilepsy and the control group (Çengel-Kültür et al., 2009).

Be as it may, given that parental coping may have a negative effect on the child's adjustment to disease, and that stress is a frequent precipitant of seizures, it is essential to identify ways to facilitate parents' and patients' positive coping skills (Arida et al., 2009; Duffy, 2011).

Exercise can be a powerful strategy among stress reduction therapies for the treatment of seizures (Arida et al., 2009). Moreover, the Coping Openly and Personally with Epilepsy (COPE), an intervention based on cognitive-behavioral techniques and focused on epilepsy education, primary and secondary coping skills, was considered, by caregivers and youth with epilepsy, as highly satisfying, and promising in terms of feasibility and accuracy (Wagner et al., 2011).

4.7 Treatment adherence

The first problem one faces when considering treatment adherence is concept definition. In fact, compliance may be defined as to "obey, submit, defer or accede to instructions" (Donovan & Blake, 1992, as cited in Eatock & Baker, 2007, p. 117); adherence as "what is expected of the patient as opposed to compliance being told what to do" (Barofsky, 1978, as cited in Eatock & Baker, 2007, p. 118), involving more co-operation and agreement; and concordance as advocating "a decision-making process where patients can feel more comfortable with their treatment" (Marinker & Shaw 2003, as cited in Eatock & Baker, 2007, p. 118).

Non-adherence to medication encompasses taking too few doses, too large a dose, too many tablets, or at the wrong time, accidentally (through forgetfulness, misunderstanding, or uncertainty about clinician's recommendations) or intentionally (due to expectations of treatment, side-effects, and lifestyle choice), which has implications for intervention (Eatock & Baker, 2007).

To make matters worse, the three concepts can encompass not only medication but also lifestyle changes that have been recommended to promote health. In effect, a larger proportion of adults with epilepsy reported higher self-efficacy for medication management behaviors than for healthful lifestyle behaviors (Kobau & DiIorio, 2003).

A second problem has to do with assessment, since the constructs in question have been measured in different ways, each of which with important limitations (Eatock & Baker, 2007). This heterogeneity may be one of the causes of divergence in research results, namely those concerning factors associated with better/worse adherence, but it is certainly not the only one.

Briesacher et al. (2008), for instance, found modest variation in the adherence to newly started drug therapies in privately insured adults. They also found that adherence improved across seven different diseases, except seizure disorders, with increasing age and that add-on therapy and a history of trying other drugs for the condition before starting the new therapy improved adherence in association with seizure disorders, but not all the other conditions.

Others have found that co-morbid chronic disease, self-driving, seizure after a missed dose, and self-efficacy are significantly associated with medication compliance (Chen et al., 2010). Non-compliance with the pharmacological treatment was also associated with: lack of money to buy the medicine, patient's failure to acknowledge the disease, poor response to treatment, belief that the treatment was useless, and factors associated with the relationship between physician and patient (Enríquez-Cáceres & Soto-Santillana, 2006). Moreover, treatment adherence was negatively associated with the presence of adverse effects and correlated with better QOL (Martins et al., 2009). Additionally, certain medications convey differential risks of poor adherence in patients with epilepsy (Zeber et al., 2010).

Since medication adherence is critical to prevent/minimize seizures and their impact on patients'/families' QOL, researchers have been trying to identify factors (e.g., psychological characteristics, drug regime, family support, impact on everyday life, relationship with the clinician) that predict (non-)adherence and interventions that promote adherence (Eatock & Baker, 2007).

Even though the aim of WebEase, a multicomponent, interactive, Internet-based self-management program, is "to encourage people with epilepsy to take their medications as prescribed, practice strategies to reduce stress and adopt strategies to facilitate adequate sleep" (DiIorio et al., 2009, p. 186), for most measures, but not all, there were no statistically significant gains. In epilepsy self-management and one measure of adherence there were, nonetheless, improvements.

Some other interventions (e.g., intensive reminders and "implementation intention") have potential to improve adherence to antiepileptic mediations, but additional evidence on their efficacy is needed (Al-Aqeel & Al-Sabhan, 2011). "What is increasingly clear… is that total adherence is an unrealistic goal" (Eatock & Baker, 2007, p. 129).

5. Adjustment and outcome variables

5.1 Health status perception

Ross (2010), as other authors before her, presents health as a complex construct, with several dimensions, arguing that "perception influences health status and how people responded to policy interventions and other solutions" and that self-reported health status and objective health status are "outcomes of the socio-economic and behavioral situation of the individual" (Ross, 2010, p. 10). In addition, she refers that "it is expected that these two measures, objective and subjective, will reinforce each other to create a single health status perception for an individual.… Unfortunately, there is evidence that this is not always the case, which leads to the gap between perception and reality" (Ross, 2010, pp. 4-5). Nevertheless, "the perception of health status by the individual is a more significant indicator than clinical indicators. Researchers use this indicator to understand the value the individual assigns to health" (Bordoni et al., 2006, p. 68).

In practice, subjective health status is measured by an individual's self-reported health status, and objective health status is defined by visible health metrics (i.e., health characteristics that provide sensory feedback to individuals - fever, rash, increased waist measurement, etc.) and technical health metrics (which tend not to provide overt feedback/to be asymptomatic) (Ross, 2010, p. 5).

To make matters worse, self-reported health status is "the result of a complex aggregation process, involving information and weights known only to the individual, consciously and sub-consciously" (Ross, 2010, p. 4). Consequently, "measuring health status is a complex process that requires the use of indicators that evaluate health both in terms of disease and of the impact the health-disease- care process has on the quality of life" (Bordoni et al., 2006, p. 68).

Li et al. (2007) present part of the Phase VI of the Demonstration Project (DP) on Epilepsy, part of the Global Campaign Epilepsy Out of the Shadows-WHO-ILAE-IBE in Brazil, with a mean follow-up of 26 months (1-38). They report a model of epilepsy treatment at primary health level with which people with epilepsy can be treated with important reductions in seizure frequency and other improvements: the opinions of patients, relatives, and physicians regarding the overall health status at the end of the DP were similar and indicate considerable improvements.

In adults with epilepsy receiving antiepileptic drugs for treatment, Perucca et al. (2009) tried to identify patterns of association of adverse effects and their relationships with subjective health status at baseline and over a prospective 4-month follow-up. The self-report health assessments include the Adverse Event Profile, the Quality of Life in Epilepsy Inventory-89, and the Beck Depression Inventory. Their results agree with clinical and research data: patients taking antiepileptic drugs usually report more than one adverse effect, revealing the important burden of toxicity associated with antiepileptic drugs; in patients with refractory epilepsy, adverse effects and mood disorders may be more important than seizure frequency in determining subjective health status.

Pais-Ribeiro et al. (2007) results showed that epilepsy patients' optimism was the best predictor of mental health status perception and QOL, whereas cognitive functioning perception was the best predictor of physical health status. In the same study, seizure control was a significant predictor of physical health status perception but not of mental health status perception or QOL.

I.e., there are some psychosocial variables that are associated with health in persons with a chronic disease: those variables are buffers reducing the impact of disease on health. This perspective assumes a positive health perspective. Seligman (2008) explains that positive health describes a state beyond the mere absence of disease and is definable and measurable as it is defined by the World Health Organization (a state of complete positive physical, mental, and social well-being and not merely the absence of disease or infirmity (WHO, 1948)).

Positive health acts as a buffer against chronic diseases. Positive health in general populations and in people with chronic diseases predicts longevity, quality adjusted life years and/or disability adjusted life years that individuals go on to live, less costs for health and illness among individuals in positive health, positive progression of disease and how well an individual responds to the challenges of disease, high status on the subjective, social and work functional variables.

5.2 (Health-related) Quality of life

QOL is recognised as a vague and ethereal entity, something that many people talk about, but which nobody knows very clearly what to do about (Pais-Ribeiro, 2004). However, QOL becomes an important primary end-point in clinical intervention (Bucher et al., 1999).

We can find many definitions. Farquhar (1995) proposes an organization of QOL definitions as: global definitions, component definitions (research-specific and non-research-specific), focused definitions (explicit or implicit), combination definitions and lay definitions.

ILAE (2003c) propose the following QOL definition: an individual's emotional response to his or her life circumstances, the gap between these circumstances and their expectations, and their ability to meet their personal needs. When considered in the health/disease field, QOL is sometimes named HRQOL and tends to include items, or domains, specific for the focused disease.

Pais-Ribeiro (2004) remembers that there is a wide disagreement about the meaning of the term "quality of life" and how to measure it. Different researchers or professionals prefer definitions and measures influenced by the preoccupations of their respective disciplines. The same happens with the diseases and clinical settings.

QOL measures tend to incorporate five broad domains: physical, occupational, psychological, social, and somatic (ILAE, 2003c).

Research suggest that there are no differences between QOL of persons with epilepsy and persons without epilepsy (Liou et al., 2005; Montanaro et al., 2004; Raty et al., 2003).
Neuropsychological variables seem to be related with QOL, with some QOL dimensions more intimately related with cognitive performance than others (Devinsky et al., 1995; Giovagnoli & Avanzini, 2000; Meneses et al., 2009; Perrine et al., 1995).
The most consistent pattern that has emerged from these inquiries is that QOL in epilepsy is a function of the interaction of factors, including clinical variables (e.g., seizure frequency, severity, illness duration, treatment side effects, and psychiatric co-morbidity), and social variables (e.g., divorce, unemployment, social stigma, family caregiver characteristics, and social support) (Ohaeri et al., 2009; Pais-Ribeiro et al., 1998).
Kendrick and Trimble (1994) report and suggest different QOL measures in epilepsy, namely: (a) The Washington Psychosocial Seizure Inventory and the Social Effects Scale; (b) The Epilepsy Surgery Inventory and the Quality of Life in Epilepsy with 31 items (QOLIE-31); (c) The Liverpool QOL Battery.
To improve the QOL of people with epilepsy it is important to educate, not only the people with epilepsy but also the media and the general public, as well as the professionals (ILAE, 2003d).
Other positive outcomes, like subjective well-being and happiness are, in some way, similar to QOL for many experts, if not conceptually, at least in terms of assessment indicators. In a study with 2152 persons with epilepsy in Norway, Naess et al. (2007) found that seizure frequency, medication side effects, and co-morbidity are strongly related to well-being and life satisfaction.

6. Conclusion

Living with epilepsy (as a patient or as a patient's significant other) is challenging. The complex biopsychosocial characteristics of the condition and its treatment require adjustment. The adjustment process includes contextual, disease, and personal characteristics, and their conjoint impact on outcome variables (e.g., health status perception, HRQOL).
Scientific research and clinical practice have been showing that a number of psychosocial variables are associated with better adjustment. Unsuccessful adjustment may be accompanied (e.g., as cause or consequence) by mental health problems, personality disorders, psychological, psychiatric and/or psychosomatic symptoms, and stigma (perception).
Consequently, it is important to understand psychosocial dimensions associated with the disease that facilitate patients' adjustment and be aware of interventions that have a positive impact on adjustment. For example, several psychosocial variables and interventions are highly correlated with treatment adherence, very important for adjustment and an unquestionable concern for health care professionals. Nevertheless, research on epileptic patients' psychosocial variables, mainly positive psychosocial variables, is not always easy to find (cf., for instance, the number of articles indexed in the Pubmed database and retrievable using "epilepsy" and most of the variables mentioned in this study).
With the present study, whose aim was to discuss the role of psychosocial variables in adjustment to everyday life in persons with epilepsy, the authors hope to contribute to an area of expertise that is central to the development of comprehensive interventions aimed at epilepsy patients and their significant others, without forgetting healthcare professionals and the society as a whole.

7. References

Al-Aqeel, S., & Al-Sabhan, J. (2011). Strategies for improving adherence to antiepileptic drug treatment in patients with epilepsy. *The Cochrane database of systematic reviews [electronic resource]*, Vol.19, No.1:CD008312.

Amir, M., Roziner, I., Knoll, A., & Neufeld, M. Y. (1999). Self-efficacy and social support as mediators in the relation between disease severity and quality of life in patients with epilepsy. *Epilepsia*, Vol.40, No.2, pp.216-224.

Arida, R. M., Scorza, F. A., Terra, V. C., Scorza, C. A., de Almeida, A. C., & Cavalheiro, E. A. (2009). Physical exercise in epilepsy: What kind of stressor is it? *Epilepsy & Behavior*, Vol.16, No.3, pp.381-387.

Arshad, S., Winterhalder, R., Underwood, L., Kelesidi, K., Chaplin, E., Kravariti, E., Anagnostopoulos, D., Bouras, N., McCarthy, J., & Tsakanikos, E. (2011). Epilepsy and intellectual disability: does epilepsy increase the likelihood of co-morbid psychopathology? *Research in Developmental Disabilities*, Vol.32, No.1, pp.353-357.

Åslund, C., Starrin, B., & Nilsson, K. W. (2010). Social capital in relation to depression, musculoskeletal pain, and psychosomatic symptoms: a cross-sectional study of a large population-based cohort of Swedish adolescents. *BMC Public Health*, Vol.10, pp.715.

Aspinwall, L., Richter, L., & Hoffman III, R. (2001). Understanding how optimism works: an examination of optimists' adaptive moderation of belief and behaviour. In: Edward C. Chang (Edt.) *Optimism and Pessimism: Implications for Theory, Research, and Practice* (pp.217-238). Washington: American Psychological Association.

Austin, J., MacLeod, J., Dunn, D., Shen, J., & ,Perkins, S. (2004). Measuring stigma in children with epilepsy and their parents: instrument development and testing. *Epilepsy & Behavior*, Vol.5, pp.472–482.

Austin, J., Shafer,P., & Deering,J. (2002). Epilepsy familiarity, knowledge, and perceptions of stigma: report from a survey of adolescents in the general population. *Epilepsy & Behavior, 3*, pp.368–375.

Azaizeh, H., Saad, B., Cooper, E., & Said, O. (2010). Traditional Arabic and Islamic Medicine, a Re-emerging Health Aid. *Evidence-based complementary and alternative medicine : eCAM*, Vol.7, No.4, pp.419–424.

Baker, G. (2002). People with epilepsy: what do they know and understand, and how does this contribute to their perceived level of stigma? *Epilepsy & Behavior*, Vol.3, pp.S26–S32.

Baker, G., Brooks, J., Buck, D., & Jacoby, A. (1999). The Stigma of Epilepsy: A European Perspective. *Epilepsia*, Vol.41, No.1, pp.98-104.

Bandura, A. (1977). Self-efficacy: Toward a unifying theory of behavioral change. *Psychological Review*, Vol. 84, No.2, 191-215.

Bandura, A., & Adams, N. E. (1977). Analysis of self-efficacy theory of behavioral change. *Cognitive Therapy and Research*, Vol.1, No.4, pp.287-310.

Begley, C. E., Shegog, R., Iyagba, B., Chen, V., Talluri, K., Dubinsky, S., Newmark, M., Ojukwu, N., & Friedman, D. (2010). Socioeconomic status and self-management in epilepsy: comparison of diverse clinical populations in Houston, Texas. *Epilepsy & Behavior.*, Vol.19, No.3, pp.232-238.

Behrouzian, F., & Neamatpour, S. (2010). Parental knowledge and mental health in parents of children with epilepsy. *Pakistan Journal of Medical Sciences,* Vol.26, No.1, pp. 191-194.

Berkman, L. F. (1984). Assessing the physical health effects of social networks and social support. *Annual Review of Public Health,* Vol. 5, pp.413-432.

Beyenburg, S., Mitchell, A., Schmidt, D., Elger, C., & Reuber, M. (2005). Anxiety in patients with epilepsy: Systematic review and suggestions for clinical management. *Epilepsy & Behavior,* Vol.7, pp.161–171.

Birbeck, G. (2006). Interventions to reduce epilepsy-associated stigma. *Psychology, Health & Medicine,* Vol.6, No.3, pp.364-366.

Blumer, D. (1991). Personality in epilepsy. *Seminars in Neurology,* Vol.11 , No.2, pp.155-166.

Blumer, D. (1999). Evidence supporting the temporal lobe epilepsy personality syndrome. *Neurology,* Vol. 53 , No. Suppl. 2, pp.S9-S12.

Bordoni, N., Cadile, M. C., Sotelo, R., & Squassi, A. (2006). Teachers' perception of oral health status. Design and validation of an evaluation instrument. *Acta odontológica latinoamericana : AOL.,* Vol.19, No.2, pp.67-74.

Briesacher, B. A., Andrade, S. E., Fouayzi, H., & Chan, K. A. (2008). Comparison of drug adherence rates among patients with seven different medical conditions. *Pharmacotherapy,* Vol.28, No.4, pp.437–443.

Broadhead, W., Kaplan, B., James, S., Wagner, E., Schoenbach, V., Grimson, R., Heyden, S., Tibblin, G., & Gehlbach, S. (1983). The epidemiologic evidence for a relationship between social support and health. *American Journal of Epidemiology,* Vol.117, No.5, pp.521-537.

Bruhn, J. G., & Philips, B. U. (1984). Measuring social suport: a synthesis of current approaches. *Journal of Behavioral Medicine,*Vol. 7, No.2, pp.151-169.

Bucher, H., Guyatt, G., Cook, D., Holbrook, A., & McLister, F. (1999). Users' guides to the medical literature: XIX. Applying clinical trial results: A. How to use an article measuring the effect of an intervention on surrogate end points. *The Journal of the American Medical Association,* Vol.25, 271–278.

Cassel, J. (1976). The contribution of the social environment to host resistance. *American Journal of Epidemiology,* Vol.104, No.2, pp.107-123.

Çengel-Kültür, S. E., Ulay, H. T., & Erdağ, G. (2009). Ways of coping with epilepsy and related factors in adolescence. *The Turkish Journal of Pediatrics,* Vol. 51, pp.238-247.

Chang, E., & Sanna, L.(2001).Optimism, Pessimism, and Positive and Negative Affectivity in Middle-Aged Adults: A Test of a Cognitive-Affective Model of Psychological Adjustment. *Psychology and Aging,* Vol.16, No.3, pp.524-531.

Chattopadhyay, S. (2007). Religion, spirituality, health and medicine: Why should Indian physicians care? *Journal of Postgraduate Medicine,* Vol.53, pp.262-266.

Chen, H. F., Tsai, Y. F., Lin, Y. P., Shih, M. S., & Chen, J. C. (2010). The relationships among medicine symptom distress, self-efficacy, patient-provider relationship, and medication compliance in patients with epilepsy. *Epilepsy & Behavior,* Vol.19, No.1, pp.43-49.

Chi, G. (2007). The role of hope in patients with cancer. *Oncology Nursing Forum,* Vol.34, No.2, pp.415-424.

Choi-Kwon, S., Chung, C., Kim, H., Lee, S., Yoon, S., Kho, H., Oh, J., Lee, S. (2003). Factors affecting the quality of life in patients with epilepsy in Seoul, South Korea. *Acta neurologica Scandinavica.,* Vol.108, No.6, pp.428-434.

Cobb, S. (1976). Social support as a moderator of life stress. *Psychosomatic Medicine,* Vol.38, No.5, pp.300-314.

Cohen, S. (1988). Psychosocial models of the role of social support in the etiology of psysical disease. *Health Psychology,* Vol.7, No.3, 269-297.

Cohen, S., & McKay, G. (1984). Social suport, stress, and the buffering hypotesis; a theoretical analysis. In A. Baum, S. Taylor, & J. Singer (Eds.), *Handbook of psychology and health* (Vol. IV, pp. 253--268). New Jersey: Laurence Erlbaum Associates.

Coleman, R., Loppy, L., & Walraven, G. (2002). The treatment gap and primary health care for people with epilepsy in rural Gambia. *Bulletin of the World Health Organization,* Vol.80, No.5, pp.378-383.

Cramer, D., Henderson, S., & Scott, R. (1997). Mental health and desired social support: a four-wave panel study. *Journal of Social and Personal Relationships,* Vol.14, No.6, pp.761-775.

Davison, S. N., & Simpson, C. (2006). Hope and advance care planning in patients with end stage renal disease: qualitative interview study. *British medical journal,* Vol.333, pp.886.

de Ridder, D., Geenen, R., Kuijer, R., & van Middendorp, H. (2008). Psychological adjustment to chronic disease. *The Lancet,* Vol. *372,* pp.246–255.

Dell, J.L. (1986). Social dimensions of epilepsy: stigma and response. In: S.Whitman, & B.P.Hermann (eds.) *Psychopathology in epilepsy* (pp .185-210). New York: Oxford University Press.

Devinsky, O., & Najjar, S. (1999). Evidence against the existence of a temporal lobe epilepsy personality syndrome. *Neurology,* Vol.53 , No.Suppl. 2, pp. S13-S25.

Devinsky, O., Vickrey, B.G., Cramer, J., Perrine, K., Hermann, B., Meador, K., et al. (1995). Development of the Quality of Life in Epilepsy Inventory. *Epilepsia,* Vol.36, No.11, pp.1089–1104.

DiIorio, C., Escoffery, C., McCarty, F., Yeager, K. A., Henry, T. R., Koganti, A., Reisinger, E. L., & Wexler, B. (2009).Evaluation of WebEase: an epilepsy self-management Web site. *Health Education Research,* Vol.24, No.2, pp.185–197.

DiIorio, C., Shafer, P. O., Letz, R., Henry, T. R., Schomer, D. L., Yeager, K., & Project EASE Study Group. (2006). Behavioral, social, and affective factors associated with self-efficacy for self-management among people with epilepsy. *Epilepsy & Behavior,* Vol. 9, No.1, pp.158-163.

DiIorio, C., Shafer, P., Letz,R., Henry, T., Schomer, D., Yeager,K., and the Project EASE Study Group (2003). The association of stigma with self-management and perceptions of health care among adults with epilepsy. *Epilepsy & Behavior,* Vol.4, pp. 259–267.

Dilorio, C., Faherty, B., & Manteuffel, B. (1992). The development and testing of an instrument to measure self-efficacy in individuals with epilepsy. *The Journal of neuroscience nursing : journal of the American Association of Neuroscience Nurses,* Vol.24, No.1, pp.9-13.

Donnelly, K. M. (2010). Optimism as a potential moderator of the effects of emotional distress on seizure control in adults with temporal lobe epilepsy. Part of the requirements for the degree of Master of Arts in Psychology, Graduate School of the University of Cincinnati. Available from http://etd.ohiolink.edu/send-pdf.cgi/Donnelly%20Kiely%20M.pdf?ucin1265990186

Duffy, L. V. (2011). Parental coping and childhood epilepsy: the need for future research. *The Journal of neuroscience nursing : journal of the American Association of Neuroscience Nurses*, Vol.43, No.1, pp.29-35.

Dunst, C., & Trivette, C. (1990). Assessment of social support in early intervention programs. In S. Meisels, & J. Shonkoff (Eds.), *Handbook of early childhood intervention* (pp. 326-349). New York: Cambridge University Press.

Eatock, J., & Baker, G. A. (2007). Managing patient adherence and quality of life in epilepsy. *Neuropsychiatric Disease and Treatment,* Vol.3, No.1, pp.117-131.

Ebert,S.,Tucker, D., & Roth, D.(2002).Psychological resistance factors as predictors of general health status and physical symptom reporting. *Psychology, Health & Medicine,* Vol. 7, No.3, pp.363-375.

Ell, K., Nishimoto, R., Mediansky, L., Mantell, J., & Hamovitch, M. (1992). Social relations, social support and survival among patients with cancer. *Journal of Psychosomatic Research,* Vol.36, No.6, pp.531-541.

Elliott, J. O., Charyton, C., Sprangers, P., Lu, B., & Moore, J. L. (2011). The impact of marriage and social support on persons with active epilepsy. *Epilepsy & Behavior* [Epub ahead of print]

Elliott, T., Witty, T., Herrick, S., & Hoffman, J. (1991). Negotiating reality after physical loss: Hope, depression, and disability. *Journal of Personality and Social Psychology,* Vol. 73, pp.1257-1267.

Enríquez-Cáceres, M., & Soto-Santillana, M. (2006). [Non-compliance with pharmacological treatment in patients with epilepsy]. *Revista de neurologia.,* Vol.42, No.11, pp.647-654.

Farquhar, M. (1995). Definitions of quality of life: a taxonomy. *Journal of Advancing Nursing,* Vol.22, pp.502–508.

Foster, D., & Vilendrer, S. (2009). Two treatments, one disease: childhood malaria management in Tanga, Tanzania *Malaria Journal*, Vol.8, pp.240.

Fournier, M., de Ridder, D., & Bensing,J. (2002). How optimism contributes to the adaptation of chronic illness. A prospective study into the enduring effects of optimism on adaptation moderated by the controllability of chronic illness. *Personality and Individual Differences*, Vol.33, No.7, pp.1163-1183.

Frizzell, C. K., Connolly, A. M., Beavis, E., Lawson, J. A., & Bye, A. M. (2011). Personalised epilepsy education intervention for adolescents and impact on knowledge acquisition and psychosocial function. *Journal of paediatrics and child health,* [Epub ahead of print]

Gallagher, E. B., Wadsworth, A. L., Stratton, T. D. (2002). Commentary. Religion, spirituality and mental health. *The Journal of Nervous and Mental Disease,* Vol.190, pp.697-704.

Giltay, E., Geleijnse, J., Zitman, F., Hoekstra, T., & Schouten, E. (2004). Dispositional Optimism and All-Cause and Cardiovascular Mortality in a Prospective Cohort of

Elderly Dutch Men and Women. *Archives of General Psychiatry,* Vol.61, pp.1126-1135.

Giltay, E., Kamphuis, M., Kalmijn, S., Zitman,F., & Kromhout, D.(2006). Dispositional Optimism and the Risk of Cardiovascular Death: The Zutphen Elderly Study. *Archives of Internal Medicine,* Vol.166, pp.431-436.

Giovagnoli, A. R., Martins da Silva, A., Federico, A., & Cornelio, F. (2009). On the personal facets of quality of life in chronic neurological disorders. *Behavioural neurology,*Vol.21, No.3, pp.155-163.

Giovagnoli, A. R., Meneses, R. F., & Silva, A. M. (2006). The contribution of spirituality to quality of life in focal epilepsy. *Epilepsy & Behavior,* Vol.9, pp.133-139.

Giovagnoli, A.R., Avanzini, G. (2000). Quality of life and memory performance in patients with temporal lobe epilepsy. *Acta Neurologica Scandinavica,* Vol.101, pp.295–300.

Griffith, N. M. (2008). Attributional style and depressive symptoms in adult patients with intractable seizure disorders: optimism and pessimism as predictors of seizure group. Part of the requirements for the degree of Ph. D. in Psychology dissertation submitted to Division of Research and Advanced Studies of the University of Cincinnati. Available from http://etd.ohiolink.edu/send-pdf.cgi/Griffith%20Nathan%20M.pdf?ucin1211900492

Hanson, B., Isacsson, S., Janzon, L., & Lindell, S. (1989). Social network and social support influence mortality in elderly mem. *American Journal of Epidemiology,* Vol.130, No.1, pp.100-111.

Hermann, B. P., & Whitman, S. (1984). Behavioral and personality correlates of epilepsy: A review, methodological critique, and conceptual model. *Psychological Bulletin,* Vol.95, No.3, pp.451-497.

Hill, P. C., & Pargament, K. I. (2003). Advances in the conceptualization and measurement of religion and spirituality: Implications for physical and mental health research. *American Psychologist,* Vol.58, No.1, pp.64-74.

ILAE (2003a). Epidemiology. *Epilepsia,* Vol.44, No.Suppl. 6, pp.17–18.

ILAE (2003b). Introduction: Definition of Epilepsy. *Epilepsia,* Vol.44, No.Suppl. 6, pp.15–16.

ILAE (2003c). Quality of Life: General Considerations. *Epilepsia,* Vol.44, No.Suppl. 6, pp.57–58.

ILAE (2003d). Introduction: The History and Stigma of Epilepsy. *Epilepsia,* Vol. 44, No.Suppl. 6, pp.12-14.

Ismail, H., Wright, J., Rhodes, P., & Small, N. (2005). Religious beliefs about causes and treatment of epilepsy. *The British journal of general practice : the journal of the Royal College of General Practitioners,* Vol.55, No.510, pp.26-31.

Kanner, A.M., & Balabanov, A. (2002). Depression and epilepsy: how closely related are they? *Neurology,* Vol.58, No.8 Suppl 5, pp.S27-S39.

Kaplan, B., Cassel, J., Gore, S. (1977). Social support and health. *Medical Care,* Vol.15, No.5, pp.47-58.

Kendrick, A.M., & Trimble, M.R.(1994). Repertory grid in the assessment of quality of life in patients with epilepsy: the quality of life assessment schedule. In: M.R.Trimble & W.E. Dodson (eds.). *Epilepsy and quality of life* (pp.151-163). New York: Raven Press.

Kent, G. P. (2008). Optimism, pessimism, and health: Implications for individuals with seizure disorders. Part of the requirements for the degree of Doctor of Philosophy in Psychology, Division of Research and Advanced Studies of the University of Cincinnati. Available from http://etd.ohiolink.edu/view.cgi?acc_num=ucin1227243421

Kessler, R., Price, R., & Wortman, C. (1985). Social factors in psychopathology: stress, social support, and coping process. *Annual Review of Psychology,* Vol. 36, pp.531-572.

Khine, H., Weiss, D., Graber, N., Hoffman, R. S., Esteban-Cruciani, N., & Avner, J. R. (2009). A cluster of children with seizures caused by camphor poisoning. *Pediatrics,* Vol.123, No.5, pp.1269-1272.

Kobau, R., & DiIorio, C. (2003). Epilepsy self-management: a comparison of self-efficacy and outcome expectancy for medication adherence and lifestyle behaviors among people with epilepsy. *Epilepsy & Behavior,* Vol.4, No.3, pp.217-225.

Koenig, H. G. (2000). Religion, spirituality, and Medicine: Application to clinical practice. *The journal of the American Medical Association*, Vol.284, No.13, pp.1708.

Koenig, H. G. (2004). Religion, spirituality, and Medicine: Research findings and implications for clinical practice. *Southern Medical Journal,* Vol.97, No.12, pp.1194-1200.

Lavery, M. E., & O'Hea, E. L. (2010). Religious/spiritual coping and adjustment in individuals with cancer: Unanswered questions, important trends, and future directions. *Mental Health, Religion & Culture,* Vol.13, No.1, pp.55-65.

Lee, M., Lee, T., Ng ph, k , Hung, A, Au.,A , Wongvc,N. (2002)Psychosocial Well-Being of carers of people with epilepsy in Hong Kong. *Epilepsy & Behavior,* Vol.*3*, pp.147-157.

Lee, S. A., Lee, S. M., & No, Y. J. (2010). Factors contributing to depression in patients with epilepsy. *Epilepsia,* Vol.51, No.7, pp.1305-1308.

Li, L. M., Fernandes, P. T., Noronha, A. L. A., Marques, L. H. N., Borges, M. A., Borges, K., Cendes, F., Guerreiro, C. A. M., Zanetta, D. M. T., de Boer, H. M., Espíndola, J., Miranda, C. T., Prilipko, L., & Sander, J. W. (2007). Demonstration project on epilepsy in Brazil: Outcome assessment. *Arquivos de neuro-psiquiatria,* Vol.65, No.Supl 1, pp.58-62.

Liou, H.H., Chen, R.C., Chen, C.C., Chiu, M.J., Chang, Y.Y., Wang, J.D.(2005). Health related quality of life in adult patients with epilepsy compared with a general reference population in Taiwan. Epilepsy Research, Vol.64, pp.151–159.

Little, T., Snyder, C., & Wehmeyer, M. (2006). The agentic self: on the nature and origins of personal agency across life span. In: D. Mroczek & T.Little (Edts.). *Handbook of personality development* (pp.61-79). New Jersey: Lawrence Erlbaum Associates, Publishers.

Locke,D.. Fakhoury, T., Berry, D., Locke, T., & Schmitt,F. (2010). Objective evaluation of personality and psychopathology in temporal lobe versus extratemporal lobe epilepsy. *Epilepsy & Behavior,* Vol.17, 172–177.

Lohne, V. (2001). Hope in patients with spinal cord injury: A literature review related to nursing. *Journal of Neuroscience Nursing*, Vol.33, No.6, pp.317-325.

Martins, H. H., Alonso, N. B., Guilhoto, L. M. F. F., Guaranha, M. S. B., Yacubian, E. M. T. (2009). Adherence to treatment in patients with juvenile myoclonic epilepsy:

Correlation with quality of life and adverse effects of medication. *Journal of Epilepsy and Clinical Neurophysiology,* Vol.15, No.4, pp.192-196.

Maruta, T., Colligan, R. C., Malinchoc, M., & Offord, K. O. (2002). Optimism-pessimism assessed in the 1960s and self-reported health status 30 years later. *Mayo Clinic proceedings,*Vol.77, pp.748-753.

Meneses, R. F. (2006). Espiritualidade na óptica da Psicologia da Saúde. In I. Leal (Coord.), *Perspectivas em Psicologia da Saúde* (pp. 203-230). Coimbra: Quarteto.

Meneses, R. F., Miyazaki, C., & Pais-Ribeiro, J. (2010a). Correlatos da espiritualidade, religião e crenças pessoais de estudantes universitários portugueses. *Psicologia, Saúde & Doenças,* Vol.11, No.S1, pp. 44.

Meneses, R. F., Miyazaki, C., & Pais-Ribeiro, J. (2010b). Estudantes universitários: Perfil sócio-demográfico, de espiritualidade, religiosidade e crenças pessoais associado a pior qualidade de vida. *Psicologia, Saúde & Doenças,* Vol.11, No.S1, pp.74-75.

Meneses, R., Pais-Ribeiro, J., Martins da Silva, A., & Giovagnoli, A R. (2008). Portuguese Hospital Anxiety and Depression Scale (HADS): Usefulness in Focal Epilepsy. *The Internet Journal of Mental Health,* Vol.5, No.2,pp.1-29.

Meneses, R.F., Pais-Ribeiro, J., Martins da Silva, A., & Giovagnoli, A.R. (2009). Neuropsychological predictors of quality of life in focal epilepsy. *Seizure,* Vol.18, pp.313-319.

Miller, W. R., & Thoresen, C. E. (2003). Spirituality, religion, and health: An emerging research field. *American Psychologist,* Vol.58, No.1, pp.24-35.

Modi, A. C. (2009). The impact of a new pediatric epilepsy diagnosis on parents: Parenting stress and activity patterns. *Epilepsy & Behavior,* Vol.14, No.1, pp.237-242.

Montanaro, M., Battistella, P.A., Boniver, C., & Galeone, D. (2004). Quality of life in young Italian patients with epilepsy. *Neurological Sciences,25,* pp.264-273.

Monzoni, C., & Reuber, M. (2009). Conversational displays of coping resources in clinical encounters between patients with epilepsy and neurologists: A pilot study. *Epilepsy & Behavior,* Vol.16, No.4, pp.652-659.

Moreira-Almeida, A., & Koenig, H. G. (2006). Retaining the meaning of the words religiousness and spirituality: A commentary on the WHOQOL SRPB group's "A cross-cultural study of spirituality, religion, and personal beliefs as components of quality of life". *Social Science & Medicine,* Vol.63, No.4, 843-845.

Mueller, P. S., Plevak, D. J., & Rummans, T. A. (2001). Religious involvement, spirituality, and medicine: Implications for clinical practice. *Mayo Clinic Proceedings,* Vol.76, pp.1125-1135.

Naess, S., Eriksen, J., & Tambs, K. (2007). Psychological well-being of people with epilepsy in Norway. *Epilepsy & Behavior,* Vol.11, pp.310-315.

Nagane, M., Yoshimura, K., Watanabe, S.-I., & Nomura, M. (2009). A possible connection between psychosomatic symptoms and daily rhythmicity in growth hormone secretion in healthy Japanese students. *Journal of Circadian Rhythms,* Vol.7, pp.10.

Ohaeri, J.U., Awadalla, A.W., Farah, A.A. (2009) . Quality of life in people with epilepsy and their family caregivers. An Arab experience using the short version of the World Health Organization quality of life instrument. *Saudi Medical Journal,* Vol.30, No.10, pp.1328-1235.

Ornelas, J. (1996). Suporte social e doença mental. *Análise Psicológica,* Vol.14, No.2-3, pp.263-268.

Pais-Ribeiro, J. (2004). Quality of life is a primary end-point in clinical settings. *Clinical Nutrition,* Vol.23, pp.121–130.

Pais-Ribeiro, J. L. (1999). Escala de Satisfação com o Suporte Social (ESSS). *Análise Psicológica,* Vol.XVII, No.3, pp.547-558.

Pais-Ribeiro, J., Martins da Silva, A., Meneses, R., & Falco, C. (2007). Relationship between optimism, disease variables, and health perception and quality of life in individuals with epilepsy. *Epilepsy & Behavior,* Vol.11, pp.33–38.

Pais-Ribeiro, J., Martins da Silva, A., Meneses, R., & Falco, C. (2004). O *coping* no ajustamento à epilepsia. In J. L. P. Ribeiro, & I. Leal (Eds.), *5º Congresso Nacional de Psicologia da Saúde- Actas* (pp. 437-444). Lisboa: Instituto Superior de Psicologia Aplicada.

Pais-Ribeiro, J., Silva, I., Ferreira,T., Martins, A., Meneses, R. & Baltar, M. (2007). Validation study of a Portuguese version of the hospital anxiety and depression scale. *Psychology, Health and Medicine,* Vol.12, No.2, pp.225-237.

Pais-Ribeiro, J.L., Mendonça, D., Martins da Silva, A. (1998). Impact of epilepsy on QOL in a Portuguese population: exploratory study. *Acta Neurologica Scandinavica,* Vol.97 , No.5, pp.287-294.

Panzini, R. G., Maganha, C., Rocha, N. S., Bandeira, D. R., & Fleck, M. P. (2011).Validação brasileira do Instrumento de Qualidade de Vida/espiritualidade, religião e crenças pessoais. *Revista de saúde pública,* Vol. 45, No.1, pp.153-165.

Pedrão, R. B., & Beresin, R. (2010). Nursing and spirituality. *Einstein,* Vol.8(1 Pt 1), pp. 86-91.

Perrine, K., & Kiolbasa, T. (1999). Cognitive deficits in epilepsy and contribution to psychopathology. *Neurology,* Vol.53 , No..Suppl. 2, pp. S39-S48.

Perrine, K., Hermann, B.P., Meador, K.J., Vickrey, B.G,, Cramer, J.A., Hays, R.D., et al. (1995). The relationship of neuropsychological functioning to quality of life in epilepsy. Archives of Neurology, Vol.52, pp.997–1003.

Perucca, P., Carter, J., Vahle, V., & Gilliam, F. G. (2009). Adverse antiepileptic drug effects: Toward a clinically and neurobiologically relevant taxonomy. *Neurology,* Vol.72, pp.1223–1229.

Piazzini, A., Ramaglia, G., Turner, K., Chifari, R., Kiky, E. E., Canger, R., & Canevini, M. P. (2007). Coping strategies in epilepsy: 50 drug-resistant and 50 seizure-free patients. *Seizure,* Vol. 16, No.3, pp.211-217.

Post, S. G., Puchalski, C. M., & Larson, D. B. (2000). Physicians and patient spirituality: professional boundaries, competency, and ethics. *Annals of Internal Medicine,* Vol.132, No.7, pp.578-583.

Powell, L. H., Shahabi, L., & Thoresen, C. E. (2003). Religion and spirituality: Linkages to physical health. *American Psychologist,* Vol.58, No.1, pp.36-52.

Raty, L.K.A., Larsson, B.M.W., & Soderfeldt, B.A. (2003). Health-related quality of life in youth: a comparison between adolescents and young adults with uncomplicated epilepsy and healthy controls. Journal of Adolescent Health, Vol.33, pp.252–258.

Reisinger, E. L., & DiIorio, C. (2009). Individual, seizure-related, and psychosocial predictors of depressive symptoms among people with epilepsy over six months. *Epilepsy & Behavior,* Vol. 15, No.2, pp.196-201.

Ribeiro, J. L. P. (1995). Adaptação de uma escala de avaliação da auto-eficácia geral. In: L. Almeida e I. Ribeiro (Edts.). *Avaliação Psicológica: formas e contextos.* (pp.163-176). Braga: APPORT.

Ridder, D., & Schreurs, K. (1996). Coping, social support and chronic disease: a research agenda. *Psychology, Health & Medicine,* Vol.1, pp.71-82.

Rippentrop, A. E. (2005). A review of the role of religion and spirituality in chronic pain populations. *Rehabilitation Psychology,* Vol. 50, No.3, pp.278-284.

Robinson, E., DiIorio, C., DePadilla, L., McCarty, F., Yeager, K., Henry, T., Schomer, D., & Shafer, P. (2008). Psychosocial predictors of lifestyle management in adults with epilepsy. *Epilepsy & Behavior,* Vol.13, No.3, pp.523-528.

Ross, K. (2010). Assessing differences in perceptions and actual health status: A national cross-sectional analysis. A Dissertation submitted in partial fulfillment of the requirements for the degree Doctor of Philosophy, Department of Agricultural Economics, College of Agriculture, Kansas State University, Manhattan, Kansas. Available from http://krex.k-state.edu/dspace/bitstream/2097/6652/1/KaraRoss2010.pdf

Rustøen, T., Howie, J., Eidsmo, I., & Moum, T. (2005). Hope in patients hospitalized with heart failure. *American Journal of Critical Care,* Vol.14, pp.417-425.

Rutter, D., & Quine, L. (1996). Social psychological mediators of the relationship between demographic factors and health outcomes: a theoretical model and some preliminary data. *Psychology and Health,* Vol.11, pp.5-22.

Salim, S. A. (2007). A etiologia do sintoma psicossomático: Sua relação com a reincidência traumática e o retraimento autista [Etiology of psychosomatic symptoms: its relationship with traumatic recurrence and autistic withdrawal]. *Revista de Psiquiatria do Rio Grande do Sul,* Vol.29, No.2, pp.233-238.

Sarason, I. G., Levine, H. M., Basham, R. B., & Sarason, B. R. (1983). Assessing social support: the social support questionnaire. *Journal of Personality and Social Psychology,* Vol.44, No.1, pp.127-139.

Scheier, M. F, & Carver, C. S. (1992). Effects of optimism on psychological and physical well-being: theoretical overview and empirical update. *Cognitive Therapy and Research,* Vol.16, No.2, pp.201-228.

Scheier, M. F., & Carver, C. S. (1985). Optimism, coping, and health: assessment and implications of generalized outcome expectancies. *Health Psychology,* Vol. 4, pp.219-247.

Schwarzer, R., & Leppin, A. (1989). Social support and health: A meta-analysis. *Psychology and Health,* Vol.3, No.1, pp.1-15.

Schwarzer, R., & Leppin, A. (1991). Social support and health: A theoretical and empirical overview. *Journal of Social and Personal Relationships,* Vol.8, pp.99-127.

Seawaerd, B. L. (2000). Stress and human spirituality 2000: at the cross roads of physics and metaphysics. *Applied Psychophysiology and Biofeedback,* Vol.25, pp.241-246.

Seligman, M. (2008). Positive Health. *Applied psychology: an international review,* Vol.57, pp.3–18.

Shaikh, B. T., & Hatcher, J. (2005). Complementary and Alternative Medicine in Pakistan: Prospects and Limitations. *Evidence-based complementary and alternative medicine : eCAM,*Vol.2, No. 2, pp.139-142.

Sharpe, L., & Curran, L. (2006). Understanding the process of adjustment to illness. *Social Science & Medicine* Vol. 62, pp.1153–1166.

Singer, J. E., & Lord, D. (1984). The role of social support in coping with chronic or life-threatening illness. In A. Baum, S. Taylor, & J. Singer (Eds.), *Handbook of psychology and health* (Vol. IV, pp. 269-278). New Jersey: Laurence Erlbaum Associates.

Smith, G., Ferguson, P. L., Saunders, L. L., Wagner, J. L., Wannamaker, B. B., & Selassie, A. W. (2009). Psychosocial factors associated with stigma in adults with epilepsy. *Epilepsy & Behavior,* Vol. 16 No.3, pp.484-490.

Snyder, C.R. (2002). Hope theory: rainbows in the mind. *Psychological Inquiry,* Vol.13 No.4, pp.249–275.

Stanton, A., Revenson, T., and Tennen, H. (2007). Health Psychology: Psychological Adjustment to Chronic Disease. *Annual Review of Psychol.ogy,* Vol.*58,* pp.565–592.

Tate, D. G., & Forchheimer, M. (2002). Quality of life, life satisfaction, and spirituality. *American Journal of Physical Medicine & Rehabilitation,* Vol.81, pp.400-410.

Taylor, S. E. (1990). Health psychology: the science and the field. *American Psychologist, 45,* 40-50.

Tellez-Zenteno, J.F., Patten, S.B., Jetté, N., Williams, J., & Wiebe, S. (2007). Psychiatric comorbidity in epilepsy: a population-based analysis. *Epilepsia,* Vol.48 No.12, pp.2336-2344.

Thomason, B., Jones, G., McClure, J., & Brantley, P. (1996). Psychosocial co-factors in HIV illness: an empirical-Based model. *Psychology and Health, 11,* pp.385-393.

Trueman, P., & Duthie, T. (1998). Use of the Hospital Anxiety and Depression Scale (HADS) in a Large, General Population Study of Epilepsy. *Quality of life newsletter,* Vol.19, pp.9-10.

Valiente-Barroso, C., & García-García, E. (2010). Aspectos neurológicos relativos a estados alterados de conciencia asociados a la espiritualidad [Article in Spanish; Neurological aspects related to altered consciousness states associated with spirituality]. *Revista de Neurologia,* Vol. 51 No.4, pp.226-236.

Vuilleumier P, & Jallon P. (1998). Epilepsie et troubles psychiatriques: données épidémiologique. *Revue Neurologique,* Vol.154 No.4, pp.305-317.

Wagner, J. L., Smith, G., Ferguson, P., van Bakergem, K., & Hrisko, S. (2011). Feasibility of a pediatric cognitive-behavioral self-management intervention: Coping Openly and Personally with Epilepsy (COPE). *Seizure* [Epub ahead of print]

Weiss, R. (1974). The provisions of social relations. In Z. Rubin (Ed.), *Doing unto others.* Englewood Cliffs, New Jersey: Prentice-Hall.

Westerhuis, W., Zijlmans, M., Fischer, K., van Andel, J., & Leijten, F. S. (2011). Coping style and quality of life in patients with epilepsy: a cross-sectional study. *Journal of Neurology,* Vol.258 No.1, pp.37-43.

Wethingston, E., & Kessler, R. C. (1986). Perceived support, received support, and adjustment to stressfull life evets. *Journal of Health and Social behavior,* Vol.27, pp.78-89.

Whatley, A. D., DiIorio, C. K., & Yeager, K. (2010).Examining the relationships of depressive symptoms, stigma, social support and regimen-specific support on quality of life in adult patients with epilepsy.Health education research, Vol.25 No.4, pp.575-584.

WHO. (1948). Officials Records of the World Health Organization, no.2, p. 100. United Nations, World Health Organization. Geneve, Interim Comission.

Wilson, S. J., Wrench, J. M., McIntosh, A. M., Bladin, P. F., & Berkovic, S. F. (2009). Personality development in the context of intractable epilepsy. *Archives of Neurology,* 66 No.1, pp.68-72.

Winkler, A. S., Mayer, M., Ombay, M., Mathias, B., Schmutzhard, E., & Jilek-Aall, L. (2010). Attitudes towards african traditional medicine and christian spiritual healing regarding treatment of epilepsy in a rural community of northern Tanzania. *African journal of traditional, complementary, and alternative medicines,* Vol. 7 No.2, pp.162-170.

Zeber, J. E., Copeland, L. A., & Pugh, M. J. V. (2010). Variation in antiepileptic drug adherence among older patients with new-onset epilepsy. *The Annals of Pharmacotherapy,* Vol.44, No. 12, pp.1896-1904.